THE PHYSICIAN'S PRACTICE

Educational Communications
P.O. Box 87
Pomona, New York 10970
—
(914) 354-7446

THE PHYSICIAN'S PRACTICE

Edited by

JOHN M. EISENBERG, M.D., M.B.A.

Chief, Section of General Medicine
Solomon Katz Assistant Professor of General Medicine
Department of Medicine
University of Pennsylvania School of Medicine
Philadelphia, Pennsylvania

SANKEY V. WILLIAMS, M.D.

Assistant Professor of Medicine
Section of General Medicine
Department of Medicine
University of Pennsylvania School of Medicine
Associate Director, National Health Care Management Center
University of Pennsylvania
Philadelphia, Pennsylvania

with

ELLEN S. SMITH, M.B.A.

Coordinating Editor
Administrator
Robert Wood Johnson Foundation Clinical Scholars Program
and Primary Care Residency Program
University of Pennsylvania School of Medicine
Philadelphia, Pennsylvania

A WILEY MEDICAL PUBLICATION
JOHN WILEY & SONS
New York • Chichester • Brisbane • Toronto

Library of Congress Cataloging in Publication Data
Main entry under title:

The Physician's practice.

(A Wiley medical publication)
Includes index.
1. Medicine—Practice.   2. Medical offices—Manage-
ment.   3. Medicine—Practice—United States.   I.
Eisenberg, John M.   II. Williams, Sankey V.   III.
Smith, Ellen S. [DNLM: 1. Practice management,
Medical.   W80 P578]
R728.P53   610'.68   80-13691
ISBN 0-471-05469-0

Printed in the United States of America

10 9 8 7 6 5 4 3 2 1

We dedicate this book to *Samuel P. Martin, III, M.D.,* our mentor and advisor during and after our years as Robert Wood Johnson Foundation Clinical Scholars, a program that he has directed at the University of Pennsylvania since its inception in 1974.

Contributors

Kathryn J. Bowman, R.N., M.S.N., Family Nurse Clinician, Medical Group Practice; Section of General Medicine, Department of Medicine; Adjunct Instructor, Graduate Division, School of Nursing, University of Pennsylvania, Philadelphia, Pennsylvania

Frank Caliri, III, M.B.A., C.L.U., San Gabriel, California

Joan Bonner Conway, D.S.W., A.C.S.W., Director, Department of Social Work, Hospital of the University of Pennsylvania; Lecturer, School of Social Work, University of Pennsylvania, Philadelphia, Pennsylvania

Joan L. Davies, Sc.M., Research Specialist, Clinical Epidemiology Unit, Section of General Medicine, Department of Medicine, University of Pennsylvania School of Medicine, Philadelphia, Pennsylvania

John M. Eisenberg, M.D., M.B.A., Chief, Section of General Medicine, Solomon Katz Assistant Professor of General Medicine, Department of Medicine, University of Pennsylvania School of Medicine, Philadelphia, Pennsylvania

Judith Frank Hirschwald, M.S.W., A.C.S.W., Director, Social Service Department, Magee Memorial Rehabilitation Center; Patient Systems Coordinator, Regional Spinal Cord Injury Center of Delaware Valley; Lecturer, School of Social Work, University of Pennsylvania, Philadelphia, Pennsylvania

Lawrence G. Hrebiniak, Ph.D., Associate Professor of Management, The Wharton School, University of Pennsylvania, Philadelphia, Pennsylvania

Vasilios J. Kalogredis, J.D., C.P.B.C., Medical Practice Management Consultant, Management Consulting for Professionals, Inc., Bala Cynwyd, Pennsylvania

Denis J. Lucey, III, M.D., Consultant, Oberfest Associates, Philadelphia, Pennsylvania

Veronica C. Oestreicher, M.P.H., Health Policy Analyst, Health Standards and Quality Bureau, Health Care Financing Administration, Department of Health and Human Services, Washington, D.C.

Arnold J. Rosoff, J.D., Associate Professor of Legal Studies and Health Care Systems, The Wharton School, University of Pennsylvania, Philadelphia, Pennsylvania

Ellen S. Smith, M.B.A., Administrator, Robert Wood Johnson Foundation Clinical Scholars Program and Primary Care Residency Program, University of Pennsylvania School of Medicine, Philadelphia, Pennsylvania

Helen L. Smits, M.D., Director, Health Standards and Quality Bureau, Health Care Financing Administration, Department of Health and Human Services, Washington, D.C.

William C. Steinmann, M.D., Formerly, Robert Wood Johnson Foundation Clinical Scholar; Fellow, Milbank Memorial Fund Clinical Epidemiology Program; Assistant Professor, Section of General Medicine, Department of Medicine, University of Pennsylvania School of Medicine, Philadelphia, Pennsylvania

Paul D. Stolley, M.D., Professor of Medicine; Director, Clinical Epidemiology Unit, Section of General Medicine, Department of Medicine, University of Pennsylvania School of Medicine, Philadelphia, Pennsylvania

Michael T. Walsh, J.D., M.B.A., Associate Director, Advanced Underwriting, Penn Mutual Life Insurance Company, Philadelphia, Pennsylvania

Ross Arkell Webber, Ph.D., Professor of Management, The Wharton School, University of Pennsylvania, Philadelphia, Pennsylvania

Sankey V. Williams, M.D., Assistant Professor of Medicine, Section of General Medicine, Department of Medicine, University of Pennsylvania School of Medicine; Associate Director, National Health Care Management Center, University of Pennsylvania, Philadelphia, Pennsylvania

Robert A. Zelten, Ph.D., Associate Professor of Insurance, The Wharton School, University of Pennsylvania, Philadelphia, Pennsylvania

Andrea Zubick, R.N., M.S.N., Formerly, Family Nurse Clinician, Medical Group Practice, Section of General Medicine, Department of Medicine; Adjunct Instructor, Graduate Division, School of Nursing, University of Pennsylvania, Philadelphia, Pennsylvania

Preface

When physicians complete their clinical training, they generally are well prepared to deal with the clinical problems that are encountered in medical practice. By contrast, they are seldom prepared to make decisions about the practice itself. This book is designed for the practicing physician and for the physician preparing to enter practice. It will provide an introduction to the organizational, financial, and legal aspects of practicing medicine. We expect that other health care professionals, such as nurses, physician's assistants, and social workers, also will find the book useful.

It is important for all physicians to understand the practical aspects of medical practice, but it is especially important for physicians in primary care. Since the primary care physician is so often called upon to integrate the clinical and nonclinical aspects of patient care, it is the primary care physician who most needs information about the workings of the health care system. Patients expect this from their primary care physician. The physician is often the leader of a team of other professionals and may supervise a busy office staff, so it is important that the principles of leadership and management be understood. Since the successful practice depends on successful business techniques, the physician must be familiar with the organizational and financial aspects of the practice. As more physicians join group practices and as group practices grow more complex, these skills are becoming more important. The increasing prominence of regulation in medical practice demands that the physician be familiar with the legislative and administrative rules that affect the practice.

In 1976, the Department of Medicine and the Department of Pediatrics at the University of Pennsylvania established a seminar series in the practice of medicine for residents in primary care internal medicine and pediatrics and for students in the Family Nurse Clinician Program of the School of Nursing. This seminar series has become a central component of primary care residency training at the University of Pennsylvania. The course is taught by faculty from the School of Medicine, the Wharton School, the Law School, and the Faculty of Arts and Sciences at the University of Pennsylvania and by professionals who advise practicing physicians about the problems of running a practice. As an outgrowth of the seminar series, this book provides other physicians and physicians in training with an opportunity to learn how to deal with similar problems.

Most of the chapters offer practical information about managing an office practice. In the first chapter, we review the available practice opportunities from solo practice to health maintenance organizations. In the next five chapters, Kalogredis presents an extensive discussion of how to develop an efficient and effective office practice. Walsh and Caliri review the principles of personal finance, and Zelten explains the details of health insurance. Rosoff explains aspects of health care law that affect medical practice. Lucey and Smith describe the process of health planning, while Oestreicher and Smits describe the process of peer review and quality assurance, especially as it is coordinated by professional standards review organizations. Both chapters explain how the physician can cope with the regulation of health care.

Because of the importance of professionals other than physicians, Bowman and Zubick describe the roles of the nurse practitioner and physician's assistant, while Conway and Hirschwald explain the role of social workers. The chapters by Webber and Hrebiniak provide an introduction to the principles of management, which physicians will find useful in making changes in their organizations, dealing with employees and other professionals, and planning for the future. The chapters by Steinmann and by Stolley and Davies will enable the physician to better understand the literature of medicine and to answer clinical questions about his or her own practice.

Much of the material contained in this book can be learned by experience as the new physician struggles with the problems of establishing a practice. Most practicing physicians will, no doubt, recognize information that they have learned in this way as they read our book. Our intention in collecting this material has been to make it easier for new physicians to create effective practices and to help established physicians fill in any gaps in their knowledge created by the haphazard approach that they have been forced to use in the past.

John M. Eisenberg, M.D., M.B.A.
Sankey V. Williams, M.D.

Acknowledgments

In developing this book, we are indebted to the people who have supported primary care residency training in medicine and pediatrics at the University of Pennsylvania, especially those who helped establish the residency's seminar series on primary care in practice, which served as the outline for this book.

Edward Stemmler, M.D., Dean of the School of Medicine, has stimulated and encouraged primary care residency training. Arnold S. Relman, M.D., and Laurence E. Earley, M.D., the chairmen of our Department of Medicine, have provided guidance and continuing support since we first began to plan a primary care residency in 1975. Laurence Beck, M.D., Associate Chairman of the Department of Medicine, has provided wise advice, innovative ideas, and skilled teaching. Jean Cortner, M.D., chairman of the Department of Pediatrics, has supervised the development of the residency in primary care pediatrics, and we are indebted to our colleagues in pediatrics, David Cornfeld, M.D., William Schwartz, M.D., and George Peckham, M.D., for their role in the development of the seminar series that prompted us to develop this book. We depended on the advice of our residents when developing the seminar series, and we thank them for their sympathetic yet challenging support. It was Annie Lea Shuster of the Robert Wood Johnson Foundation who first suggested that we develop a book based on the course and Leif Beck, J.D., who helped us formulate the book's outline. We also thank John de Carville of John Wiley & Sons for his guidance and patience. Without the cooperation and participation of faculty from the Leonard Davis Institute of Health Economics and the National Health Care Management Center (DHHS Grant HS 02577), this book would not have been possible. We also thank our colleagues in the School of Nursing of the University of Pennsylvania who participated in the seminar series. Finally, we thank Nancie Lucera and Sandra Pascale, who typed the manuscript.

The Residency Program in General Medicine and General Pediatrics, from which the seminar series on primary-care practice developed, has been supported by the Robert Wood Johnson Foundation and the Bureau of Health Professions, Public Health Service, Department of Health and Human Services (DHHS Grant 2 D28 PE 13157).

John M. Eisenberg, M.D., M.B.A.
Sankey V. Williams, M.D.

Contents

1
Modes of Practice

John M. Eisenberg
Sankey V. Williams

When preparing to enter medical practice, the physician is confronted with a diverse array of medical practice modes. Should he or she enter a group practice or practice in a solo arrangement? Should he or she join a prepaid plan or a fee-for-service practice? What are the advantages and disadvantages of the alternative forms of ownership of the practice—sole proprietorship, association, partnership, incorporation, and institutional practice? In this chapter the various modes of practice are reviewed, including their organization, their implications for salary, benefits, and taxes, their practice characteristics, and the liability assumed by physicians.

Several principles are applicable to all types of practice—group or solo, prepaid or fee-for-service, and regardless of the ownership of the practice. First, the new physician who is entering practice or the experienced physician who is considering a change in style of practice should proceed with caution. Since the practice may be a lifelong commitment, careful and deliberate consideration should be given to the advantages and disadvantages of each alternative. Second, the physician should seek professional assistance. Although friends and medical acquaintances may be well intentioned, they may be misinformed, biased by their own peculiar experience, or influenced by personal considerations. A professional consultant experienced in assisting physicians may seem expensive when financial constraints exist, but the investment in one's future practice is well spent. Generally speaking, the consultant will be a lawyer, an accountant, or a person trained in a school of health care administration. Third, if the physician remains unsure of his preference for styles of practice, a trial practice of one or two years may be helpful. When starting, joining, or reorganizing a practice, gradual transitions can be made from one practice to another and may be preferable to leaping into an inflexible practice arrangement prematurely.

GROUP OR SOLO PRACTICE?

The first decision is whether the physician wants to practice in a group or in a solo practice. Although many would define a group practice as any arrangement where two or more physicians practice together, the American Medical Association (AMA) has adopted a more rigorous definition:

> Medical group practice is the provision of health care services by a group of at least three licensed physicians engaged in a formally organized and legally recognized entity; sharing equipment, facilities, common records, and personnel involved in both patient care and business management (1).

According to the AMA criteria, a 1975 survey showed that there were 8,483 medical groups in the United States and its possessions, with a total of 66,842 physicians. In 1969, 18% of nonfederal physicians were members of group practices; by 1975, 24% were members. The average size of these groups was 7.9 physicians. Eight percent of the group practices offered prepayment plans (a financial arrangement discussed later in this chapter). The prepaid group practices employed 13,534 doctors in 1975 (2). According to another survey, the AMA's Tenth Periodic Survey of Physicians in 1975, 50.4% of American physicians practice in solo arrangements (3). Therefore, approximately half of American physicians are in solo practice, and 25% practice in formal groups of three or more.

Group practice first became popular in the Midwest, and large group practices are still concentrated in the Midwest. Various arrangements exist for the distribution of income among the physicians. In 30.2% of group practices, income is distributed equally among all physicians, whereas 9.0% distribute income according to each physician's productivity in generating revenue. Another 20.1% pay physicians according to a straight salary, and 33.3% use a formula that considers some combination of salary, equal distribution, and productivity. For example, half the income may be distributed equally among all physicians and the other half according to productivity (4).

The principal advantage of group practice is the opportunity to share with other physicians—to share schedules, clinical responsibility, expenses, space, and knowledge. The principal disadvantage is the obvious loss of independence. In addition, the administrative burden of a group practice is usually greater than that of a solo practice. Conversely, solo practice offers the physician ultimate independence but presents problems in obtaining coverage for absences, potential inefficiency in the use of resources, and the risk of professional isolation.

Beck and Kalogredis have reviewed the advantages and disadvantages of group practice and have pointed out the advantages of coverage on nights and days off, weekends, and vacations (5) (see also Chap. 2). However, the practice usually continues or accelerates its growth as the additional physicians establish their practices and the burden of coverage multiplies. Other advantages of group practice include the simple appeal of bigness, peer communication and review, and the opportunity to select physicians with specific skills for the practice.

In establishing any group practice, physicians need to develop an understanding and appreciation of how they will work together, including patient responsibilities. A group may operate as a true team practice in which patients are shared or, alternatively, as a federation of independent practices with little or no responsibility for other members' patients (6).

PRACTICE OWNERSHIP AND ORGANIZATION

There are four principal types of ownership and organization of medical practice. First, in sole proprietorship, one physician owns the practice. This physician may practice in a solo arrangement or may employ other physicians, but in either case this physician is the only owner of the practice. Second, two or more physicians may retain sole ownership of their practices but practice together in a group, sharing resources. This arrangement is called an association and is sometimes known as office sharing. Third, physicians may join together in a partnership. Last, they may form a professional corporation. These forms of practice and other less common forms will be discussed in detail.

Sole Proprietorship

In a sole proprietorship, one physician owns the practice in an unincorporated form and employs other physicians to work in the practice. If the decision is made to practice in a group, the physician may employ other physicians as well as nurses, aides, clerks, and additional office staff. The employer physician has exclusive right and title to all capital and is solely responsible for the financial obligations of the practice. Therefore, the employees, including the employee physicians, have limited financial liability and carry professional (malpractice) liability only for themselves and those whom they directly supervise. However, the employer may allow the other physicians to participate in practice management and decision-making.

The physician who is considering entering such a practice as an employee should establish a clear policy about his or her future ability to join the practice as a partner and should assure the right of first refusal to purchase the practice in case the employer dies, retires, or decides to sell the practice (7). In addition, the contract between the employer physician and the employee physician should clearly spell out the compensation arrangement and amount, the term of the job and the method of termination, the rights of the employee, clinical responsibilities, especially regarding night and weekend coverage, insurance to be purchased by the employer (medical, life, and disability), vacation, fringe benefits, and the plan for expense sharing. The employer-employee arrangement offers the new physician a chance to try out the practice without investing capital or taking a financial risk. However, the physician's future income and professional flexibility may be limited by a rigid employer-employee arrangement.

Associations

When two or more physicians choose to retain ownership of their own practices but do not want to practice independently, they may enter a formal association. Although there is no legal connection between their practices, the physicians may agree to share space, staff, and call schedules. Economy may thus be gained by practicing on a larger scale, and convenience may be gained by sharing some clinical responsibilities. Income is not shared, however, and both physicians retain much of their independence, depending on the degree of sharing. Associations are usually temporary arrangements and are often established by physicians who are considering a partnership or corporation together but desire a "trial marriage" at first.

Partnership

Two or more physicians who choose to practice together may form a partnership, which legally defines them as "co-owners of an unincorporated business for profits" (8,9). Generally speaking, a partnership involves two or three physicians of the same specialty who are partners, but the partnership may be multispecialty and may employ other physicians who will be employees rather than partners.

In most states, all members of a partnership must be physicians. In general, a partnership is established by a written agreement, but physicians practicing together in an association may be considered legally to be in partnership unless they make their independence clear to creditors and patients. Because of the legal principle of estoppel, which implies that one is liable for leading another person to rely on a misconception to his detriment, these partnerships are called "partnerships by estoppel." Many of the legal aspects of partnerships are based on the Uniform Partnership Act, which has been adopted by many states (8).

There are several important issues that should be agreed upon in the written partnership agreement. The obligation of each partner to contribute to the capital (both financial and physical) of the practice should be clarified. It is also important to clarify the way in which a new partner may buy into the practice, including the method of assigning value to practice capital (10). This point will be important in calculating the value of one partner's share in the event of death, retirement, or dissolution of the partnership. In addition to agreements regarding contribution to the capital and the value of the practice, the partnership agreement should stipulate the process of decision-making in the practice, each partner's duties, the definition of full-time partnership and agreement about restraints on practice outside the partnership, the way in which practice expenses will be paid and what expenses the partnership will pay, how accounts receivable will be handled, methods for termination of the partnership, and how depreciation and tax credits will be allocated.

Most important, the partnership agreement should stipulate the way in which income will be distributed. The Center for Research in Ambulatory Health Care Administration suggests several alternatives (8).

1. *Equal distribution.* In 7 of 21 partnerships that were surveyed, income is distributed equally. All these groups distribute laboratory, radiology, and clinical income equally among all partners. In an equal-distribution compensation plan, fringe benefits generally are more liberal than in other forms of income distribution. A group will often offer a monthly salary to each partner and divide the remaining funds equally on a periodic basis.

2. *Guaranteed minimum.* Other practices guarantee each member a minimum income but base the total income for each partner on such factors as productivity. Newcomers to partnerships are often offered minimum incomes, even if more senior physicians are not, and sometimes the founder of the practice is

guaranteed a minimum income. Guarantees to different physicians in the partnership need not be equal.

3. *Productivity.* The physicians' income may be determined by the amount of net income (after expenses) that each one generates for the partnership. Other groups divide income in proportion to relative receipts or charges generated. One observer has suggested that about 40–60% of net earnings for physician compensation can be effectively distributed on the basis of productivity. Less than 40% seems to be inadequate reward for hard workers, whereas more than 60% tends to create strong independent competition within the group (11).

4. *Combination of equality and productivity.* This alternative provides a base salary that is common to all members of the partnership and a bonus based on the physician's productivity. For example, the physicians could distribute the first half of the partnership's income equally and divide the second half according to the physician's contribution to group revenue. This arrangement is different from income based on productivity with a guaranteed minimum.

5. *Point system.* If the group wishes to base compensation on factors other than productivity, it may use a point system, in which a physician is awarded points for particular characteristics and income is divided according to the number of points each physician has accumulated. For example, points may be awarded for seniority, number of referrals to other partners, publications or research, teaching, community service, continuing education, administrative activity, or specialty (especially in multidisciplinary groups where one specialty generates more revenues than another and the group wants to equalize income). Conversely, points may be deducted if a physician's operation is especially costly to the practice, such as in staff assistance.

Note that compensation may be in direct income or in other forms, such as retirement-plan contributions or fringe benefits. However, because the partnership does not pay its own tax, as professional corporations do, all net income is considered to be the personal income of the partners whether it is distributed or not. Each partner pays a personal income tax based on his or her proportionate share of the partnership's taxable income.

For pension benefits, the partner or sole proprietor may establish a Keogh plan. This form of contribution to retirement benefits is a legitimate business expense but has certain limitations, according to the Employee Retirement Income Security Act of 1974 (ERISA). This act, also known as the Pension Reform Act, raised the Keogh contribution limits to 15% of net income or $7,500, whichever is less (12). The partners are taxed as self-employed co-owners of a for-profit business. The partnership need only file an informational return with the Internal Revenue Service (9). Retirement plans are discussed in greater detail in Chapter 7.

The principal advantages of a partnership are those of group practice—cross coverage, economies of scale, and professional stimulation. In addition, the formal compensation arrangement eliminates some of the financial risk of solo practice or an association of sole proprietors, especially in the early years of a physician's professional life.

In exchange for these advantages of partnership, there are several disadvantages. The partners must accept a loss of some independence in practice and risk personality or philosophical conflicts with their partners. Second, anytime the composition of the partnership changes, the partnership must be dissolved and reestablished with the new group of partners. Therefore, in the event of any partner's departure, be it through death, retirement, or expulsion, the partnership must be dissolved and reestablished with a new partnership agreement. Similarly, whenever a new partner is added, a new partnership agreement must be made. The most important disadvantages of the partnership practice are the characteristics of taxation and liability (8,9). As discussed earlier, since the partnership is not considered a separate legal entity, it does not pay income taxes; therefore, all net income or losses become the responsibility of the partners. The partners must pay personal tax rates on this income and cannot receive the same tax benefits as they might obtain in a professional corporation. There are two potential liabilities to which the partners are exposed— professional and financial. Because each partner is liable for the acts and conduct of the others, a malpractice suit against one partner may be brought against all the partners as individuals. Similarly, since the partners are not employees of the practice but are co-owners, financial losses incurred by the partnership are the personal liability of each partner individually. Although these liabilities can be limited somewhat by the partnership agreement, the partners remain ultimately responsible for all professional and financial activities of the practice.

Professional Corporation

Beginning in 1961, every state has enacted legislation that allows the formation of professional corporations. Because corporations avoid the taxation disadvantages of partnerships, the Internal Revenue Service challenged the legality of professional corporations but lost in the courts and, since 1969, has conceded that professional groups could receive the tax advantages of other corporations. In addition to the tax advantages, physicians who practice in professional corporations avoid much of the professional and financial liability of partnerships. In large part because of these tax and liability advantages, by 1975, 61.1% of group practices in the United States were organized as professional corporations; partnerships accounted for only 27.2%, and other modes of practice accounted for 11.7% (2).

A professional corporation need not be a group practice, however. In fact, one or more professionals may incorporate so long as they are licensed in that state to practice that profession. State laws vary, but typically a professional medical corporation includes physicians who own all the shares of corporate stock and who are, at the same time, employees of the corporation. Physicians may be employed as nonowner employees, but only licensed physicians may own stock in a medical practice professional corporation. Therefore, the corporation must reacquire the stock of a deceased physician, since the members of his or her family, if they are not physicians, may not own stock in the corporation. Some corporations may issue no stock and are called "member corporations" [generally 501(c)(3) nonprofit corporations] (11). A board of directors is required for professional corporations and may include the same physicians who are owners and employees (7). In most states, the professional corporation must satisfy certain professional standards, and a physician who is disqualified to practice medicine in the state must terminate his relationship with the corporation. The legal physician-patient relationship is not affected by the corporate status of the practice.

In establishing a corporation, physicians should seek legal advice and carefully consider the appropriate state incorporation laws. If a corporation fulfills the state's requirements for professional incorporation, it becomes a *de jure* corporation; a corporation that has not fulfilled all the state's requirements may be considered a *de facto* corporation so long as an effort has been made to comply with the requirements. The *de facto* corporation's corporate status may be challenged, especially by the state, but it is usually treated by the law as a legitimate corporation. A partnership that converts into a corporation generally will transfer its assets, including property and accounts receivable, to the new corporation in exchange for stock. This transfer by the partners is generally not taxable. When a corporation is being established, the applicants must register the articles of incorporation with the state, describing the corporation's name (usually ending in "P.C.," for professional corporation, "P.A.," for professional association, "Ltd.," or "Inc.") and the names of the officers, directors, and initial shareholders (8,12).

A group of physicians will sometimes establish more than one entity to separate and protect their assets. For example, a professional corporation may be established for the management of the practice itself, and another corporation or partnership that owns the equipment or building and leases them to the first corporation may be established. In fact, even a partnership that is not incorporated may establish a corporation to hold its equipment and buildings.

The finances of a professional corporation include three principal elements—capital, employee benefits, and pay. Because corporate tax rates are lower than personal tax rates, physicians who incorporate may choose to invest part of their net income by purchasing capital, such as equipment or buildings. Since this portion of corporate income is never paid to the physicians as employee salaries, it is taxed only as corporate income. The investment in equity capital is made by the corporation on behalf of its physician owners.

Because the physicians are employees, their salaries and benefits are considered legitimate expenses of the corporation and are not taxed as part of the corporate taxation. As long as employee benefits are considered "reasonable compensation" by the Internal Revenue Service, they are not taxed as part of the physician's personal income as well. Therefore, these nontaxable employee benefits are an important aspect of a physician's participation in a professional corporation. Certain limitations exist regarding employee benefits; for example, nonphysician employees must be offered a similar benefits package.

The most important employee benefit is usually the professional corporation's pension or profit-sharing plan or both. According to the ERISA of 1974, a trust fund may be established by the corporation for its employees and given tax-exempt status so that the corporation is allowed to treat contributions to the plan as tax-deductible business expenses. The contributions and the earnings on them are not taxed to the employees until they are subsequently paid out from the fund. The most common plan usually permits an annual contribution by the corporation of 25% of the employee's pay or $32,700 (in 1979), whichever is less (12,13). Other nontaxable employee benefits of professional corporations may include life and disability insurance, death benefits, medical expenses, medical insurance, automobile expenses, and professional expenses. Retirement plans are discussed further in Chapter 7.

The principal advantage of the professional corporation lies in its special treatment regarding taxes. Since the Internal Revenue Service gave up its long-standing opposition to the formation of professional corporations by physicians in August 1969, incorporation has been popular, in particular because of the corporate tax advantages, especially those relating to deferred income and pension plans. If the corporation includes 15 or fewer stockholders, it may be treated as a Subchapter S Corporation, in which case it retains the corporate tax advantage and other advantages of incorporation but "passes income through" to the stockholders and attributes income directly to them rather than to the corporation (14). Also, Keogh limits regarding retirement plans would apply. Whereas the tax rate of a sole proprietor can be as high as 50% of his net income after deductions, the corporate tax rate is as low as 17%. Income in excess of $25,000 per year is unusual since most revenue is paid out as salaries (8). Expenses that may be deducted from taxable corporate income include all salaries, business expenses, and fringe benefits.

If a profit does occur after corporate taxes are paid, the corporation may either accumulate the earnings or pay dividends to stockholders. Income may be accumulated up to $150,000; income above this level either must be justified or is liable to an "accumulated earnings tax." If dividends are paid, they are considered personal income for the stockholder and, as such, are taxed again, already having been subject to a corporate income tax. In general, professional incorporation makes it easier to accumulate capital and pay for generous benefit packages because it decreases taxes, but it also causes take-home pay to decrease.

In addition to the tax advantages of professional incorporation, the corporate status reduces the liability of its physician members. Whereas in a partnership each partner is at risk for the professional and financial liabilities of any other member, in a corporation the potential loss is limited to the value of each physician's stock investment. For professional liability (malpractice), the physician is liable only for the misconduct of those over whom there is control and supervision (12).

Other advantages of professional corporations include the opportunity to establish an independent board of directors, which can relieve the physicians of some of their responsibility for management (8). The corporation need not dissolve itself every time a physician joins or leaves the practice: in contrast to partnerships, corporations have a life independent of the physician members of the practice. There is, however, the relative disadvantage of needing to assign a value to the practice for those leaving or buying into the practice. For example, the corporation's value might include its equipment, buildings, and accumulated earnings plus some portion of accounts receivable. To avoid the situation in which a former colleague continues to own part of the corporation, many practices require departing members to sell their shares. To avoid corporate taxation, this payment is sometimes described as separation pay.

Other disadvantages include the greater difficulty of dissolving the practice and the requirement to pay fringe benefits and unemployment compensation insurance (a corporate employer must provide fringe benefits for its nonprofessional staff as well as for its physicians) (12). Double taxation of dividends is a clear disadvantage. Corporations are exposed to more potential regulation than are other forms of practice (8). In addition, higher Social Security taxes usually have to be paid, and administration expenses are usually greater.

OTHER MODES OF PRACTICE

Although this chapter will not deal in detail with nonprofit and institutional practices, institutional practice may become more common as medical care becomes more complex, as physicians overcome their reluctance to work for large organizations, and as the population becomes more accustomed to turning to an institution for its care. Nonprofit practices are unusual and exist when all income beyond the physician's salary is donated to charity (8).

Institutional Practice

In institutional practice, the physician is an employee of a large organization, such as a government-sponsored or a hospital-based practice. Many physicians are employed by city, state, and federal governments, including the military. They are usually salaried and receive generous benefits. They exchange the advantages of job security and relief from administration for the loss of independence. Several specialty groups, such as radiologists and pathologists, are commonly employed by hospitals on a salaried basis. Other hospital-based physicians develop a contractual service agreement with the hospital and retain more independence. Some physicians are employed by universities as "salaried full-time physicians" and may be paid on the basis of a combination of salary and productivity. Other physicians are "geographic full time" and are responsible for their own income, although they practice in the academic center. Still other physicians work in industry, providing medical services to the industrial organization's employees.

Health Maintenance Organizations

The opportunities for practice described above do not exhaust the choices available to the physician. Included among the remaining alternatives are health maintenance organizations (HMOs) and independent practice associations. Although both types of organization have been part of this country's health care system for many years, their numbers are increasing rapidly. Because of their potential for controlling health care costs, they will probably assume more importance in the future. Therefore, physicians who intend to choose among future practice opportunities should look carefully at HMOs and independent practice associations to determine whether either type of organization fits their individual career plans. In the rest of this chapter, we shall review the organization of these forms of practice and examine the characteristics that might influence a physician's decision to join them.

Health maintenance organizations and independent practice associations are complex organizations, but the most important feature that distinguishes them from other practice organizations is prepayment for services. Instead of paying a fee for each service received, the patient makes a yearly payment, usually divided into monthly installments. In exchange for this single fee, the practice agrees to provide all the medical services the patient receives (provided that they are covered in the agreement), regardless of how much the services cost. In exchange for the advance payment, the practice transfers the financial risk of providing the patient's health care from the individual patient to the organization. The practice thus assumes one of the functions usually provided by an independent insurance company.

Health maintenance organizations and independent practice associations, therefore, can best be understood as organizations consisting of two component parts—the health plan is the component that insures the patient, and the medical practice is the component that provides services to the patient. Combining the health plan with the medical practice in one organization links the patient's financial and clinical interests and combines them with the organization's interests. The medical practices of most such organizations closely resemble the medical practices of other group or even solo practices.

Although both HMOs and independent practice associations provide health plans that require prepayment for services, the terms usually distinguish between two categories of organizations. Health maintenance organizations are commonly considered group practices that have one or only a few delivery sites. Independent practice associations commonly refer to less tightly organized groups of physicians who maintain separate offices and practices but who participate in a common health plan. Independent practice associations may also be referred to as "foundations for medical care." However, use of the terms has been complicated by the definition used by the Federal HMO Act of 1973. Either a prepaid group practice or an independent practice association can qualify as an approved HMO if it meets federal requirements. To avoid confusion, in the discussion that follows we shall use "prepaid group practices" and "independent practice associations" to refer to the separate organizational categories and HMOs to refer to both categories together.

The country's first prepaid group practice was started in Los Angeles in the late 1920s, and what is now the largest, the Kaiser-Permanente Medical Care Program, began in Washington State in 1938. Prepaid group practices developed slowly, at least in part because of restrictive state legislation and resistance from traditional medical organizations. In the early 1970s, when it was becoming clear that prepayment for services might slow the rapidly rising costs of medical care, the Federal HMO Act of 1973 was passed. This act authorized funds to develop HMOs. It required businesses to offer their employees the option of joining qualified HMOs, thus stimulating enrollment, and it eliminated much of the restrictive state legislation. However, relatively few HMOs became federally qualified because the act required comprehensive patient services, which made it difficult to offer competitively priced premiums.

The act was amended in 1976 to relax some of these restrictions, and the number of HMOs is now increasing more rapidly. As of April 30, 1979, there were 217 HMOs in the country, with a total enrollment of 7,891,000 patients; 91 of the HMOs were federally qualified (15).

Although a properly functioning HMO resembles many other medical practices in its day-to-day operations, there are important differences to be considered by physicians who are choosing practice sites. Perhaps the most important consideration is the arrangement made to reimburse physicians for their services. The HMO can either contract directly with individual physicians or it can contract with a separate organization composed of the physicians who supply medical services. Both organizational forms are common, but many physicians find it preferable to form their own independent organization and provide services to the HMO on a contractual basis (16). The advantages are increased flexibility in determining physician payments and a stronger voice in determining policy within the overall organization.

Whether or not physicians contract with the HMO individually or as a separate group, a variety of reimbursement plans can be used. Either the HMO or the physician group can hire physicians as salaried employees, and either can include the same production incentives that are used by other group practices.

It is also possible for either the HMO or the physician group to design a reimbursement program that transfers a part of the organization's financial risk to the individual physician. For example, the physician may receive a bonus or a reduction in yearly reimbursement, depending on the cost generated by the physician's patients during the year (17). Alternatively, physicians may be paid a fee for each service. If the overall practice provides health care for less than anticipated costs, physicians will share in the surplus that remains; if the overall practice spends all the premium money before the year ends, the physicians will receive a reduced fee for each service. Other arrangements can be made. Assumption of risk allows physicians to exert greater control over the amount of reimbursement they receive, although it obviously can produce reduced as well as increased reimbursement. Since no single reimbursement plan is used in all HMOs, it is necessary to determine the details of the organization's reimbursement plan when one is considering joining an HMO.

Because of their health plans and the resultant organizational complexity, prepaid group practices generally differ from traditional group practices in other ways. They are more heavily regulated. The state or the federal government regulates the health plan, and restrictions may be placed on benefits, marketing, and enrollment. However, few of these regulations directly affect the physician's daily medical practice. Prepaid group practices are often larger than traditional group practices since large numbers of patients protect the health plan from unpredictable changes in costs. Partly because of their large size, many prepaid group practices have developed professional administrative staff who support the medical staff in ways that may not be possible in smaller, more traditional groups. Marketing is also different. Most prepaid group practices conduct aggressive marketing campaigns to attract new patients into the program and maintain the large numbers of patients needed for financial stability.

Lower cost of health care is the single difference that has attracted the greatest public recognition. Prepaid group practices have the potential for reducing health-care costs by 10–40% when compared with the fee-for-service system, and many groups have achieved that goal (18). The reductions are produced almost entirely by a decrease in the number of hospital admissions. Hospital lengths of stay do not change, and the number of outpatient visits may even increase. The result is that more patient problems are managed in the office and that fewer are managed in the hospital, where care is more expensive. To the extent that they can be measured, there appear to be no differences in the quality of care, the availability of services, or patient satisfaction with care (19).

One reason for the reduced cost is that assigning financial risk to the organization and its physicians better aligns the objectives of the providers with those of the consumers of health care. Everyone benefits if the patient stays healthy or if the patient receives care in an efficient as well as effective manner. Other factors may contribute. The opportunities for peer review and for informal consultation with colleagues are greater in a relatively large group practice, and there are economies of scale made possible by concentrating the administrative and managerial functions in a professional support staff. Judicious use of the high-cost services provided by specialists is encouraged by the high ratio of primary to specialist physicians found in most groups.

How do these differences affect the physician's decision to join an HMO or to stay with one? One physician who is enthusiastic about his choice to work with an HMO is pleased about the flexibility to do more than provide patient care, the absence of administrative responsibility, the opportunity to continuously improve clinical skills, the comfortable salary, and his patients' continuous access to care (20). Another physician who is considerably less excited about his choice is concerned about the compromises he must make to accommodate the differing practice styles of his colleagues and the lack of continuity in patient care that results when patients cannot always see their own physician (21).

Since many HMOs are organized as group practices, the physician's decision to join involves the same considerations when any group practice, prepaid or traditional, is being examined; these considerations are reviewed in an earlier section of this chapter. However, it is important to remember that not all HMOs require the physician to join a group practice. Independent practice associations allow physicians to maintain separate practices in their own offices and require only that they participate in the reimbursement program of the health plan.

What are the special features of HMOs that might affect the physician's decision? For the HMOs that transfer part of the financial risk of care to the physician, the interested physician must weigh the benefit from increased control over personal reimbursement against the aversion that many have toward financial risk. Health maintenance organizations offer the physician an opportunity to deliver health care without considering each patient's ability to pay for each service (22,23). There is increased control over the full range of services that the patient receives, thus consolidating the physician's ability to supervise the patient's comprehensive health care (1). There are fewer billing statements for the patient and the organization to process. There may be a more egalitarian reimbursement structure that tends to equalize the payments given to primary-care and specialist physicians (24). Some physicians expect that practice in an HMO will shield them from the future regulation of medical practice (25).

In the past, some traditional medical organizations discouraged new recruits to HMOs by restricting membership in local medical societies or hospital staffs. This situation is changing. The courts have ruled against these restrictions, and local medical societies in some areas are now starting their own HMOs. These changes will no doubt be accelerated by the federal government's continued promotion of HMOs. The ability of HMOs to offer lower premiums than those of traditional insurance programs is expected to further encourage their acceptance.

Additional information about opportunities for practicing in HMOs can be obtained by writing to Group Health Association of America, Inc., 1717 Massachusetts Avenue, N.W., Washington, D.C. 20036, or by calling (202) 483-4012.

REFERENCES

1. Group practice: Guidelines to forming or joining a medical group. Denver, Colorado, Center for Research in Ambulatory Health, 1978.

2. Goodman LJ: Differences in group practice and prepaid group practice, in Henderson SR (ed): *Profile of Medical Practice.* Chicago, American Medical Association, 1977, p 31.

3. Henderson SR (ed): Physician work patterns, in *Profile of Medical Practice.* Chicago, American Medical Association, 1977, p 133.

4. Eisenberg B: Characteristics of group medical practice in urban and rural areas, in Henderson SR (ed): *Profile of Medical Practice.* Chicago, American Medical Association, 1977, p 47.

5. Beck LC, Kalogredis VJ: In forming group practice planning spells success. *Pa Med* 79:43, 1976.

6. Beck LC, Kalogredis VJ: Practical considerations of group practice. *Del Med J* 49:534, 1977.

7. Westcott CE: Organizational governance and the administrator, in Manning FF (ed): *Medical Group Practice Management.* Cambridge, Massachusetts, Ballinger Publishing Company, 1977, p 27.

8. Center for Research in Ambulatory Health Care Administration: *The Organization and Development of a Medical Group Practice.* Cambridge, Massachusetts, Ballinger Publishing Company, 1976.

9. Westcott CE: Organizational governance and the administrator, in Manning FF (ed): *Medical Group Practice Management.* Cambridge, Massachusetts, Ballinger Publishing Company, 1977, p 27.

10. Beck LC, Kalogredis VJ: Further considerations in establishing a group practice. *Del Med J* 49:589, 1977.

11. Allen SN: Productivity. *Med Group Manage* 22:20, 1975.

12. McCormick J, Rushing RL, Davis WG: *The Management of Medical Practice.* Cambridge, Massachusetts, Ballinger Publishing Company, 1978.

13. Beck LC, Kalogredis VJ: Professional incorporation and the Pension Reform Act. *Pa Med* 79:54, 1976.

14. Prager AJ, Hunter DM: Partnerships or professional corporations: A reappraisal. *Group Pract* 20:16, 1971.

15. U.S. Department of Health, Education, and Welfare: Plan update: One up, one down. *HMO Focus* 2(5):7, 1979.

16. Zelten RA: Alternative HMO models, Issue paper no. 3. Philadelphia, University of Pennsylvania National Health Care Management Center, 1979.

17. Moore S: Cost-containment through risk-sharing by primary care physicians. *N Engl J Med* 300:1359, 1979.

18. Luft HS: How do health maintenance organizations achieve their "savings"? *N Engl J Med* 298:1336, 1978.

19. Gauss CR, Cooper BS, Hirschmann CG: Contrasts in HMO and fee-for-service performance. *Social Security Bull* May 1976, p 3.

20. Engers MF: A Harvard plan internist: Practicing medicine, not business. *HMO Focus* 2(4):2, 1979.

21. Anonymous: Those cliches about big groups? Take it from me, they're true! *Med Econ* September 4, 1978, p 71.

22. Cook WH: Profile of the Permanente physician, in Somers AR (ed): *The Kaiser-Permanente Medical Care Program.* New York, Comonwealth Fund, 1971, p 97.

23. Gumbiner R: Recruiting and maintaining staff in the health maintenance organization: Putting it all together. St. Louis, CV Mosby Company, 1975.

24. Packer S: Physician remuneration, in *Proceedings of the 28th Annual Group Health Institute.* Washington, DC, Group Health Association of America, 1978, p 171.

25. Enright SE: I.P.A., the initials that may mean your future. *Med Econ* February 19, 1979, p 124.

2
Joining or Starting
a Practice

Vasilios J. Kalogredis

CHOICE OF GEOGRAPHIC LOCATION

One of the most important choices a new physician must make is where to practice medicine—a choice that will have long-range implications. It will have a direct impact on the physician's professional environment, social life-style, and economic potential. Because of the importance of this decision, the physician should critically evaluate the opportunities.

The physician should first decide which geographic area interests him or her the most. Many limit the choice to one community or state. Others are willing to locate anywhere within a larger geographic area, such as the Southwest or the Northeast.

In-depth research should begin once the initial geographic boundaries have been drawn. The AMA can be of assistance with its Physician's Placement Service, which aids about 3,000 physicians per year. The AMA Placement Service serves as a screening agent by introducing physicians to available positions. It provides useful information on each of the counties in the United States, and there is no fee involved. The state and local medical societies for the locales in which there is interest should also be contacted. Advertisements for available positions are often published in the periodicals of these societies.

The most rewarding possibilities are often not well publicized, and more work is required to uncover them. One method is for the physician to identify a favorable physician-inhabitant ratio for his or her specialty. For example, a good rule of thumb for primary care physicians is one physician per 1,500–2,500 inhabitants. One can write the appropriate state medical society and request a list of physicians, according to specialty and county, with each county's population figures and then calculate the physician-inhabitant ratio for counties that are possible practice locations. When the choices have been narrowed to three or fewer, the physician should write the chamber of commerce in each community for further information.

This process requires little more than some reading, letter writing, and postage. Before the final decision is made, it is necessary to visit the potential locations. During the visit, the physician should contact as many of the following people and organizations as possible.

1. *Local physicians.* Obviously, if a physician is contemplating joining another physician or group, he or she should meet with them. However, even if the physician is contemplating establishing his or her own practice, it is important to visit several local physicians (both within and outside one's specialty) to understand the medical community. Ideally, a visit should be arranged with a physician who has recently settled in the area. He or she is more likely to be candid in discussing the decision to locate there.

2. *Local health department.* The public health officer is often able to provide valuable information on per capita income, governmental services, and physician and specialty needs.

3. *Local medical society.* An officer of the local medical society usually has an excellent understanding of the area's professional needs. His or her attitude about a new physician will probably reflect the attitude of many other physicians in the area. Is he or she excited about the prospects of a new physician coming into town or not and, if not, why not?

4. *Local hospitals.* An appointment should be arranged with hospital administrators for tours of facilities. The physician should ask about potential office space, facilities available for practice, and the procedure for obtaining hospital privileges. Some hospitals in physician-shortage areas provide incentives to physicians considering locating in their areas. Some guarantee a specific gross income and provide facilities, personnel, supplies, or other items free or for a discount for a specified period of time; others help with financing of the new practice.

5. *City hall.* The physician should ask about taxes and municipal services, such as fire, police, water, sewer, garbage collection, and transportation.

6. *Real estate broker.* The broker can answer questions about neighborhoods, zoning policies, current purchase prices, and rental possibilities.

7. *Medical management consultant.* If there is a qualified medical management consultant in the area, an appointment should be arranged to talk to him or her. The consultant may know of problems in the medical community that other physicians or hospital personnel are reluctant to discuss with a newcomer. The visit with the consultant will also help the physician evaluate the consultant. If the consultant is knowledgeable and helpful, he or she may become a member of the new physician's advisory team.

After the visit, each area should be evaluated on the basis of three aspects— professional, personal, and economic considerations.

The following questions should be asked about each locale, and the answers should be compared with each other.

Professional Considerations

1. Have improvements recently been made in the medical facilities, and if not, should they have been?
2. Do general practitioners and specialists work together or compete with each other?
3. Do patients prefer specialists or generalists?

4. What professional standards govern the physicians, hospitals, and other medical care providers in the area?
5. Are there enough good pharmacists and pharmacies?
6. Are the laboratory and x-ray services satisfactory?
7. Are the new physician's skills needed?
8. What are the attitudes of the medical-society officer, the hospital administrator, the local physicians, the local lay people, and the medical management consultant?
9. Will coverage be a problem?
10. Is postgraduate education readily accessible?
11. Is suitable office space available?
12. Are capable house staff available in the hospital?

Personal Considerations

1. Will the physician's family be happy?
2. Are attractive residential areas available and affordable?
3. Are local taxes and assessments reasonable?
4. Are good schools available?
5. Are there satisfactory shopping facilities?
6. Are appropriate recreational opportunities available?
7. Will there be adequate social and cultural opportunities?
8. Are appropriate religious opportunities present?
9. Are the physician's attitudes and ethnic and family backgrounds compatible with those of the community?

Economic Considerations

1. What is the future of the area's population?
2. What is the local employment record?
3. How many people have health care insurance?
4. Are funds available from local lending institutions?
5. What has happened to the area's average family income?
6. Have physicians' fees in the area changed in proportion to other rising costs?
7. Will good advisors be available?

CHOOSING SOLO OR GROUP PRACTICE

Besides deciding on location, any new physician must decide whether to join a practice, buy a practice, or start a practice. Until recently, most physicians either bought an existing solo practice or started anew, but there is now an ever growing trend toward group practice. There are advantages to both solo and group practice that will have different appeal for different physicians. The following are some of the factors to consider. Further discussion of the choice of practice is found in Chapter 1.

Peer communication and review are a problem for many solo physicians, who lack professional relationships that help build and retain professional skills. These considerations are not as much of a problem for physicians in groups, whose colleagues may be from different training backgrounds and experiences.

Often the members of a group hire an additional physician to improve coverage, and in most instances, a group will provide better possibilities for coverage than will solo practice. A solo physician may not be able to find acceptable evening and weekend coverage, but a physician evaluating a group practice should critically examine the provisions for coverage. Will joining a busy group commit the physician to arduous work when he or she is on call? Will the volume of work be so heavy that anticipated time off does not materialize? For example, in a three-physician practice, one physician is usually on call every night, but a four-physician practice may be so busy that two physicians are really covering at all times—one as the primary and one as the backup physician on call. Sometimes, the larger the practice, the less free time the physicians really have. In such situations, adding a physician may help with coverage, but it is not always the best solution.

There is security in numbers. The physician's own sickness or disability is a cause for concern in solo practice. Income will stop once the receivables come in from work performed earlier. Some practice expenses, such as rent, will continue, and there is little chance of getting another physician to cover or purchase the practice on a timely basis.

More security is available in a group practice. If one physician in a group is too sick to work, the others can cover at least some of the extra work load. The sick partner can usually expect more continued income than he or she would have received in solo practice. In addition, the remaining partners are likely buyers if the sick physician must withdraw from the practice. It is in the best interest of all parties in such a situation to have an agreement prepared at the beginning of the partnership to cover any such eventuality.

There is no overriding economic advantage to group practice. Whether a physician is or is not part of a group does not mean that he or she earns more or less income. Income is still usually a function of productivity.

As groups grow larger than four physicians, overhead as a percentage of gross receipts often rises higher than does overhead in a comparable smaller group or solo practice. One reason for this situation is that the larger practice often needs a lay manager. Also, many larger groups purchase assets that smaller practices would not consider, such as expensive data and word processing equipment. A "group syndrome" often comes into play, as each physician values each purchase only in terms of what will come out of his or her pocket. In larger groups, that figure may seem relatively meaningless, and less than critical review of expenditures may result.

A solo practitioner has much more independence and flexibility than does a group physician. Other partners need not be consulted before practice decisions are made. A solo practitioner can shape the practice to suit his or her needs more readily than can the physician who is a member of a group. If the physician wants more vacation time, or if he or she wants to increase the work pace, either change can be made without group discussion.

JOINING A GROUP PRACTICE

This section provides guidelines for evaluating potential employers and for concluding a fair agreement benefiting the new physician and the existing practice.

Evaluating a Practice

A physician must decide what practice to join—a consultant can only advise. The physician is well advised to consider six aspects of the evaluation process that deserve separate listing.

1. *Professional considerations.* How does the practice care for patients? What procedures are and are not performed in the practice? Is the practice receptive to new medical developments? These and similar questions should be answered before the physician joins a practice—the quality of care and the attitudes of the senior physicians are important matters.

2. *Philosophical considerations.* A physician should feel comfortable with the way in which decisions are made about patient care. The physician should also judge if the physician members of the practice have compatible financial, family, and patient-care priorities. Unanticipated disagreements about philosophical considerations cause many groups to dissolve.

3. *Interpersonal considerations.* It is essential that physicians in a group relate comfortably and honestly to each other. If there is inadequate communication, serious problems often lie ahead. It is most important that personalities be compatible.

4. *Financial considerations.* Questions should be raised about the financial return the physician can expect in the future. The physician who recruits a new partner should be willing to share the financial statements of the practice with the prospective partner. A critical and fair evaluation of the financial future of the practice can only be made this way.

5. *Management considerations.* If a practice is operating efficiently, that is an excellent sign. However, if the practice is not running as well as it could be run, it does not necessarily mean that the physician should avoid the practice. If the practice is not being run well, the physician should ask if the senior physicians are receptive to change and then determine whether they have the skills to make the practice operate more efficiently. It is much easier to join a well-managed practice, but a new physician can introduce dramatic improvements in an existing practice if all the circumstances are right.

6. *Long-term and short-term considerations.* There are two important considerations any physician should keep in mind when evaluating a group practice. The first is to remember that the next year is not as important as the rest of one's life. The second is to ask oneself: "Am I being treated as a potential partner or as a one-year employee?"

Although many consultants normally recommend an initial one-year employment term, there should be an effort to create a long-term association. Both parties should be concerned about the prospects for an enduring joint practice. Such an undertaking involves possible lifetime earnings of $2,000,000 to $3,000,000 or more, and the question of a thousand dollars or two for the first year should be kept in perspective. Discussions should include future growth of the practice, sharing of duties, and opportunities for teaching and research. If a physician feels that the potential employer is unconcerned about his attempt to work toward an equal relationship in the future, he or she should strongly consider stopping the negotiations.

Questions for the Negotiations

Once the initial evaluation has been completed, many items remain to be negotiated. A sample agreement is included in this chapter as a guide (Exhibit 1). The physician who is being recruited often must react to the proposals offered and usually is presented with such a letter by the senior physician. Therefore, this letter should serve as a guide to the terms that must be covered in such an agreement. Inclusion of these terms will avoid future confusion and problems.

The question of partnership (or coshareholdership) should be fully discussed. Neither party should be obligated to a continuing relationship in the beginning, yet some understanding regarding this relationship should be reached (Exhibit 1, paragraph 1).

Physicians tend to become "partners" after one of two years of employment. Equal sharing of income tends to take anywhere from two to six years in most instances. One standard arrangement (assuming that one physician is joining another physician) for the first year of a partnership is to divide the income so that the senior physician receives 70% and the junior physician 30%. In the next year, the income is divided in a ratio of 60% to 40% and then 50% to 50%

Exhibit 1. Suggested Form of Letter Agreement (for the Letterhead of Medical Associates, P.C.)

N. U. Physician, M.D.
(Address)

Dear Dr. Physician:

As we have discussed, this letter is intended to set forth the proposal for your employment. I hope that it will be useful in making clear the suggested details of our relationship. If it meets with your approval, please sign one copy and return it to me at your earliest convenience. The details will, of course, be reduced to a more formal employment agreement, if you desire. They may have to be so drafted by our attorney to meet the corporate requirements. I am satisfied to let this informal but legally binding letter set forth our understanding. It will certainly determine the terms of any more formal document.

1. You will be an employee of my medical practice corporation for one year, starting approximately July 1, 19—. Although only a one-year relationship is herein set forth, we have discussed our intentions for the future relationship. No assurance can be made by either of us at this time, but if all circumstances are favorable to each of us, the discussed format will become our arrangement, starting July 1, 19—. We have agreed to start discussions on the topic after January 1,

Exhibit 1. (Continued)

19—, with a firm offer (if any) and decision to be made by April 1, 19—. In addition, we agree that either party may terminate this relationship by providing the other with 90 days written notice at any time.

2. As an employee, you will be involved full time in this practice of medicine, and you will not take any outside employment during this period.

3. Your first-year annual base salary will be $31,200, which is $600 per week for your year's employment. In addition, to the extent that the gross income of our practice exceeds $200,000 during the first 12 months of your employment, you will be entitled to extra "incentive compensation" of 30% of the excess. I am happy to share with you any such income over my "break-even" level.

4. The corporation will also pay the cost of your professional liability insurance, including "umbrella" insurance, your professional association or society dues, and hospital staff fees. However, other practice-related expenses, such as professional education, travel, entertainment expenses, and automobile costs will have to be paid out of your earnings during the first year. I estimate that the cost of those items to be paid by the corporation will be about $4,000 during your first year.

5. Because the practice is a professional corporation, you will also be entitled to certain fringe benefits. These benefits include the payment of Blue Cross/Blue Shield and major medical insurance for you and your family, reimbursement of all your and your family's medical, dental, optical, etc., expenses up to 3% of your salary, and your inclusion in both the pension and profit-sharing retirement plans. The usual contribution to the retirement plans would be about 20% of your salary, and we estimate that the entire package of fringe benefits will total about $7,000.

6. You will be entitled to two weeks of paid vacation and a one-week educational or professional society meeting absence during the first employment year. Arrangements for all absences must be made to assure that our practice is properly covered.

7. In case of absence due to illness or injury, your basic salary will continue for a period not exceeding four weeks. Absence in excess of that period of time would be without compensation. If I should become disabled for more than three months, I recognize the additional burdens you would have to bear, and I agree to raise your annual base salary to $36,000 for any such extended absence.

I hope that this proposal meets your approval, and I look forward to working together with you starting in July. If you agree to these terms, please sign one copy of this letter and return it to me. We will then each have a copy signed by the other, evidencing our agreement.

As mentioned, if you desire to discuss any parts of this proposal further, please give me a call at your earliest convenience.

Sincerely,

_____

Abel Doktor, M.D., President
Medical Associates, P.C.

Agreed and Accepted: _____

N. U. Physician, M.D.

Date: _____

afterward. In another standard arrangement, the new physician's income begins at 30% and increases by 5% increments each year until the income is split equally in the fifth year of partnership. In larger groups, the total income is often divided into equal shares according to the number of physicians in the group. A new physician might then expect to receive the same proportion of a share in the larger group as he would of the total income in the group of two physicians described above.

There should be no secrets about finances when the new physician is considered as a future partner. All financial data of the practice should be made available for review, including the records of past growth of the practice.

In addition, it is helpful to review the financial arrangements of the present members of the practice. For example, what growth in income has the practice experienced? What rise in income has the most junior member in the practice experienced? How long did it take for that physician to become an equal partner? A new physician will not necessarily receive the same income as will the most junior physician, but he or she may have difficulty obtaining a greater share since the other physician will feel slighted if a better deal is made. In addition, one should review the division of income of an existing group to determine whether productivity is a consideration.

It is better to negotiate for income percentages and the amount of time before partnership and before equal partnership than for items valued in dollars since future inflation may devalue the agreement.

If one is seriously interested in a group that does not provide such figures, the issue should not be forced, since it could scar the relationship before it begins. However, the new physician should question what existing members feel they have to hide.

It is most important to develop an understanding regarding the sharing of duties and coverage before joining a group. Usually, work schedules will be divided equally. However, a new physician may be asked to work more nights or weekends, and this possibility should be known beforehand.

Also, how might patients and work be distributed? It is sometimes difficult to get patients to accept a new surgeon. There can be no guarantee that a new physician will perform an equal amount of surgical procedures in a short period of time. What a young surgeon should realistically hope for and expect is a good faith understanding that he or she will perform a reasonable amount of surgical procedures.

A discussion should also include how patients will be treated. Will all patients be taken care of by all physicians, or will each physician have his or her own patients, with cross coverage only on weekends and evenings? If a young physician is expected to build his or her own practice, it can sometimes take time.

In primary care, base salaries start as low as $18,000 and go as high as $60,000. Generalizations should not be made about what is an appropriate salary. It is important to remember that the starting salary is only one item in the negotiated agreement. If all else is favorable, one should not be too concerned about a couple of thousand dollars in the first year. It is just not worth losing an opportunity to join a good practice. A low offer is usually not an indication of future problems. One must recognize that the hiring physician might be taking some serious risks. There may be a big drop in his or her income, particularly for the first year; patients and referring physicians may react negatively; or his established life-style may be threatened. These changes all could occur when the hiring physician is financially comfortable and committed to a certain level of income. Those couple of thousand dollars may seem more important to the hiring physician than to the new physician.

The base salary might be only part of what a new physician is actually paid. Many practices offer their newly employed physicians extra pay as incentive compensation to reflect increased work levels (Exhibit 1, paragraph 3). This approach is excellent and should be welcomed by most new physicians. It represents the following viewpoint: "We do not want to make money on you. We want you to join us, and we prefer not to lose money. If we can generate enough to keep our incomes where they are, we want you to share in the excess."

Exhibit 2 illustrates how the incentive might be determined. Note that this example bases the incentive figure on gross receipts (sometimes net income is used instead). It is preferable for the incentive to be tied to the growth of the practice. Some prefer to base the incentive on the new physician's own gross receipts. This system, in effect, encourages the new physician to develop his or her own practice within the group. This system is not as desirable since it establishes an individual instead of a group incentive.

There is no standard procedure for determining what expenses should be paid by the practice and what expenses should be paid by the physician. The important point is to make a written agreement describing what expenses the practice will pay and what expenses it will not pay (Exhibit 1, paragraph 4).

Obviously, a compensation package should be looked at as a whole. Whether a particular practice does or does not pay a specific expense is not as important as the value of the total package. Some employers prefer to pay a higher salary with no benefits; others pay a lower salary with more benefits. The important point is

Exhibit 2. Incentive Compensation Approach

1. Dr. N. U. Physician's salary	$31,200
2. Costs related to Dr. Physician:	
Malpractice insurance	$3,000
Dues, etc.	$1,000
One additional assistant	$8,000
Increased supplies and other costs	$6,000
Extra office space	$3,000
Fringe benefits for Dr. Physician	$7,000
3. "Normal" increase in senior physician's overhead	$3,000
4. "Normal" increase in senior physician's income	$6,000
5. Additional gross income needed for senior physician to "break even"	$68,200
6. Gross income before Dr. Physician arrives	$131,800
7. Gross income base for incentive compensation	$200,000

(Since senior physician runs at a 40% overhead, or 60% profit, he or she might divide the profit in half. Therefore, the formula could be that the new physician would receive 30% of gross income over $200,000.)

to describe clearly what expenses are to be paid by the practice. If the new physician is uncertain whether to submit bills to the practice, or if the employer has not anticipated certain expenses as his obligation, unnecessary problems will result.

The total dollar package should be determined first. Then, practice-related expenses should be determined. A reduction in salary is often appropriate, with the practice covering expenses up to a specified limit in place of salary. There is no preferential savings of taxes either way. If related to the practice, expenses are equally tax deductible for the practice or the physician. It is often a question of what the accountant prefers.

There is usually a difference between what fringe benefits a corporate practice and an unincorporated practice will offer a new physician. Generally speaking, unincorporated practices do not provide many fringe benefits for physician owners since they provide no great tax advantage. A corporate practice will generally offer generous fringe benefits to the senior physicians and, therefore, will be able to pass them along to younger associates during the first year of employment (Exhibit 1, paragraph 5). There usually is a preferential tax saving in this area.

Some provisions should be made in case the new physician becomes ill or disabled or in case the senior physician should be unavailable during an extended absence. In Exhibit 1, paragraph 7, note that the annual base salary would increase to $36,000.

The "buy-in" price method for partnership purposes should be made known from the beginning (although not necessarily in the initial written agreement itself). There are four major areas of value to consider in a practice.

1. *Real estate* is sometimes involved. In most instances, it is not part of the practice entity itself and therefore is handled separately. A good approach is to set the price at fair market value. There are several approaches—all parties agree to a price, all parties agree to abide by a single appraiser's valuation, or each party selects a licensed appraiser and agrees to take the average of the two appraisals.

2. *Tangible assets* of the practice, such as cash, equipment, and furnishings, are usually part of the sale price. The book value is often used (basically cost minus depreciation minus liabilities). In many instances, a modified book value is used (cost minus straight-line depreciation over a period of 10 to 15 years minus liabilities), which results in a higher and more reasonable price. Appraisals for these items are subjective and generally not helpful. The price for one physician's share of these assets is generally not more than $10,000 in most primary care practices.

3. *Accounts receivable* often have the largest value. Accounts receivable refer to the amounts owed to the practice by patients or insurers for services performed before the new physician became a partner. They should not be paid for in cash, but they should be recognized as a senior physician's right to higher income for a period of time. This system allows the new physician to purchase them with pretax dollars, while the senior physician is in the same position he or she would be in if the new physician did not buy in.

For example, suppose that a new physician joins a solo physician and the true value of the accounts receivable on the date the partnership would be effective is

$60,000 and the equipment is worth $10,000. The new physician should pay only $5,000 for the equipment to buy into one-half of the partnership. The new physician's income should be reduced, and the senior physician's income should be increased proportionately over a period of months to make up the $30,000 needed to buy one-half of the accounts receivable.

4. *Goodwill* is the fourth item of value and is usually related to the reputation of the practice. There is a serious question whether it exists at all in some practices. Most medical practices simply cannot be sold for more than their hard assets and receivables, but there are some practices with intrinsic, intangible monetary value. In most instances, one should be extremely dubious of a goodwill claim.

Some physicians have established a legal entity separate from the actual medical practice, although directly related to the practice. The most common is real estate. For example, a new physician may join a three-physician professional corporation that is leasing office space from a partnership in which the three senior physicians are equal partners. The new physician should be given the opportunity to buy into the partnership at the time he or she becomes a shareholder in the corporation. This approach helps avoid bad feeling on either side. Unless all the professional shareholders are also real partners, the shareholder who does not own real estate may feel that the rent is too high and that he or she is supporting a mortgage to help the other physicians, whereas the real estate owners may feel that they are charging too little rent for what they are providing. If an interest in such a related entity is not offered, it does not necessarily mean that a young physician should not join the practice. However, it is an important factor in the decision.

Arrangements regarding vacations and absences for meetings should be clearly described (Exhibit 1, paragraph 6).

Some senior physicians have pushed for restrictive covenants, which are provisions that limit where a physician may practice if he or she should terminate the relationship. Generally speaking, such provisions are not desirable. If they are not "reasonable in time and space," they are of questionable legality. A new physician should seriously question any practice that seeks to impose such restrictions. Restrictions may be appropriate if there are too many physicians of a specific specialty in an area, but that really holds true in an extremely small number of cases.

The final point is to make sure that everything is put in writing at the beginning to help avoid any unnecessary confusion and misunderstanding later on. That alone goes a long way toward avoiding many potential problems.

STARTING ONE'S OWN PRACTICE

For the physician who decides not to join an established practice, financing is often the major concern in buying or starting a practice. A new physician should buy and not lease equipment, furnishings, and improvements. By borrowing from a bank, a new physician will save money. Leasing is expensive. After all, the leasing company is a middle man and adds another level of profit.

Purchasing also has tax advantages, despite what the leasing company may say.

With depreciation, one can usually take larger tax deductions in the earlier years for purchased rather than leased equipment.

In general, a new physician should have little difficulty borrowing money from a local bank. Most banks will view a new physician as an excellent financial risk. For best results, one should contact several banks in an area. There is nothing wrong with shopping for the best deal.

Whereas it is preferable that a new physician purchase assets, it is just as preferable that he or she rent space when starting out in practice. Renting space may be the only economically feasible alternative for the new physician. However, even if the physician could afford to buy a building or condominium from the start, it should be discouraged. Buying real estate limits flexibility. When a practice is started, one cannot be sure how quickly it will grow. A dynamic, growing practice should not suffer from lack of space because the real estate is owned and is not easily disposable.

BUYING A PRACTICE

Practices are rarely sold today other than in situations where a physician has joined a practice and then bought out a senior physician. When a sale of a primary care practice does take place, there is little or no value from "goodwill" involved. Rarely after the sale of a practice will all the patients stay with the successor. In reality, the new physician could probably open up his or her own practice and do just as well.

3
Planning a Practice

Vasilios J. Kalogredis

Many factors are involved in establishing and maintaining a smooth and successful practice. The steps described in this chapter are important for planning a successful practice.

CONSULTANTS AND ADVISORS

Management Consultant

The first step for many physicians who are approaching the end of training and are beginning to plan a practice is to contact a medical-management consultant. To obtain the name of a qualified consultant, the physician should ask colleagues about their experience or contact the Society of Professional Business Consultants (SPBC), a national professional association whose members advise physicians and dentists exclusively. To obtain information about qualified medical-management consultants in a given area, one can write to the SPBC at 221 North La Salle Street, Chicago, Illinois 60601 or call (312) 346-1600. As a member of the SPBC, a medical-management consultant is subject to a strict code of ethics. The consultant serves only as an independent and objective advisor; the consultant does not sell equipment, supplies, insurance, or anything other than consulting services.

A medical-management consultant can assist physicians in many ways. Although each consulting firm differs somewhat in the services it offers, most are active in the following areas:

Practice Management

1. Personnel
2. Equipment needs
3. Billing and collections
4. Third-party insurance
5. Scheduling
6. Telephone handling
7. Patient relations

Facilities Management

1. Layout
2. Advice about financing
3. Advice about ownership versus leasing

Financial Management

1. Evaluation of practice operation
2. Supervision of bookkeeping system
3. Development of accounts receivable and cash-handling controls
4. Preparation of financial reports and budgets
5. Counseling about fees

Personal Financial Management

1. Objective coordination of short- and long-range planning
2. Objective advice about insurance, investments, and retirement planning

Tax Management

1. Development of systems for proper record-keeping
2. Assistance in tax-planning matters
3. Assistance in dealing with the Internal Revenue Service

Group Management

1. Advice about whether to go into solo, partnership, corporate, or expense-sharing practice
2. Assistance in forming a group
3. Assistance in income-division matters
4. Assistance in keeping the group together
5. Assistance in dissolving the group
6. Assistance in corporate compliance with requirements of the Internal Revenue Service

Most consultants charge on an hourly basis, generally in the $50–125 range. Several consulting firms supplement the above services by serving as a practice's accountant on a continuing-service basis.

A young physician about to enter the real world of private practice must critically evaluate what other advisory help may be needed. Three particularly valuable advisors are an attorney, accountant, and insurance agent.

Attorney

An attorney may be needed for assistance in buying a house, reviewing an office lease, preparing a will, and, possibly, reviewing an employment proposal. If the physician decides to incorporate his or her practice, the assistance of an attorney will be necessary. Almost no new physician should incorporate initially since plans are generally too unsettled and cash too tight. Further details about incorporation may be found in Chapter 1.

Accountant

A young physician will need someone to handle tax returns, to monitor office accounting, and to provide tax and financial advice. In many instances, the medical-management consultant will satisfy that role. In other cases, a local accountant or representative of a national firm knowledgeable in the medical-practice area is generally the best choice. It is crucial that the physician have the bookkeeping of the medical practice supervised and audited by an accountant on a regular basis. The accountant should preferably be a certified public accountant (C.P.A.).

Insurance Agent

It is important to develop a good relationship with a local insurance agent. For many types of insurance, such as automobile, homeowners, and office liability (liability, fire and theft, and excess liability), it is convenient and wise to select one reputable insurance agent who can coordinate all coverage. It is unsatisfactory to have different agents for each policy—one may not know whom to call if a problem arises, and there may be duplications or gaps in coverage. By contrast, life, disability, and medical insurance are costly items, and the physician should carefully select policies on the basis of price and coverage. A physician would be wise to have a trusted independent advisor (consultant, attorney, or accountant) review any insurance proposal before it is signed.

There are several important practice-related insurance needs that merit comment and discussion with the insurance agent.

Professional liability (malpractice) insurance has received much publicity during the past several years. Its cost has risen dramatically. Although malpractice insurance is expensive, most physicians have wisely retained the protection that it provides. In addition to the "basic" coverage (often $100,000/$300,000), most physicians should (and do) have excess professional liability insurance of $1,000,000 or more above the basic limits. Care should be taken in regard to the type of insurance coverage obtained. One type is *occurrence.* Under this coverage, so long as the policy was in existence on the date the alleged malpractice occurred (even if the suit is brought after the coverage has lapsed), there is insurance protection. Another type is *claims made.* This option is often initially less expensive than occurrence coverage. Claims made policies only protect the physician for claims brought while the specific policy is in existence, even if the policy existed when the alleged malpractice occurred. Under a claims made approach, *tail* coverage will be needed to protect oneself if the policy is dropped.

Automobile insurance is worthy of some discussion. Most physicians carry this type of insurance; some states require it. One should review appropriate coverages and limits with an insurance broker and trusted advisors. A separate facet of automobile insurance is important to practicing physicians. *Nonowner* automobile insurance protects the physician or his practice or both against liability if an employee becomes involved in an accident while driving in the course of employment (e.g., driving to the bank or to the hospital). This coverage is not expensive but it is important.

Office liability insurance is crucial. Accidents could arise in the office that have nothing to do with direct medical care. Here again, the physician should consult an insurance broker and trusted advisors to determine appropriate coverages and limits on the basis of need.

Fire, theft, and related types of insurance are often written with the office liability policy. Whether the physician practices in owned or leased quarters, comprehensive coverage is needed. For example, equipment, furniture, and other assets should be insured. There is a potential risk of substantial lost earnings if a fire interrupts the normal functioning of the office. Relocation costs could be high. Temporary quarters could be costly. In addition, the proceeds of an insurance claim might offset some lost earnings until a satisfactory facility is found.

Accounts receivable insurance can also be valuable. The ledger cards and financial records that document which patients and third-party insurers owe the practice are an important practice asset. A practice should develop systems whereby it can show an insurance company what the receivables were worth when the records were destroyed. Without some evidence of value, accounts receivable insurance is not worth as much.

Any physician should have excess, or "umbrella," coverage. This type of insurance provides additional protection over and above that given by the liability policies. Typically, $1,000,000 of extra coverage is obtained. The cost of such coverage is relatively low and should be obtained (personally and professionally).

Workmen's compensation insurance is required to cover an employee's occupational injury. If a physician incorporates, the policy should reflect this change. Incorporation causes a physician to be added to the payroll as an employee. Therefore, he or she will have to be covered.

Others

Depending on the circumstances, a physician may need the services of a real estate broker, investment counselor, or other advisors early in private-practice life. If the physician has a sound advisory team (consultant, attorney, accountant, or all three), they can help direct him or her to competent persons in these other areas when the need arises.

Selecting Advisors

The following criteria should be used when selecting advisors. The criteria will help one hire competent, experienced advisors.

1. Clearly define the problem or problems needing resolution.
2. Match the qualifications of the potential advisors with the problems needing resolution.
3. Employ an advisor with experience in the specific area in question.

4. Check references about the specific services needed. Check them by telephone; people are less candid in writing. They should be asked: "Did the advisor do a good job? Would the person retain the advisor again if the same or similar circumstances arose? If not, why not? What were the advisor's weaknesses?"

5. Determine in advance the fees to be charged. Determine the method used to compute fees, and set a maximum dollar limit.

6. Seek out qualified advisors who are personally compatible with each other and with you.

7. Determine if the advisor is able to perform the task in a reasonably prompt fashion; many otherwise competent advisors work slowly.

8. Finally, hire a person with special talents to handle specialized tasks. For example, a physician would be best served by retaining an attorney specializing in professional corporations to handle incorporation. Most likely, the work will be done more competently and, in many instances, less expensively.

HOSPITAL AFFILIATIONS

In selecting a hospital affiliation, the physician should determine which hospitals need his or her services in the area where he or she has chosen to practice. The physician should determine if the hospitals in an area have good or bad reputations among the residents of the community. Whether warranted or not, people's attitudes toward a hospital will carry over to the physicians active on its staff. This attitude could affect how a practice grows.

A physician may attempt to affiliate with many hospitals because of uncertainty. This desire is understandable, but it can be a serious mistake. By trying to maintain visibility and quality care in too many institutions, the physician may end by doing a bad job in all of them. It is generally preferable for the new primary care physician to concentrate his or her efforts in one or two hospitals. By use of this approach, the new physician may be a little less busy at the beginning, but it is the best approach in the long run. The consolidated approach will produce a more efficient practice and increased visibility at the physician's principal hospital.

Another important factor in selecting hospital affiliations is whether the hospital is a teaching institution. Many new primary care physicians enjoy teaching as part of their professional lives. If it is important, the physician should consider the availability of teaching when choosing hospitals.

The availability of coverage from other physicians in the same specialty who have privileges at the hospital is another critical factor. No physician wants to be on call seven days a week, 24 hours a day, all year. The presence of capable house staff who can manage acute emergencies in hospitalized patients may also influence the choice of hospital.

Coverage of the emergency room is important. Is it adequate? Does a primary care physician on the staff have to rotate through the emergency room? In many nonmetropolitan hospitals, rotation is the rule, and this possibility should be clarified at the outset.

OFFICE LOCATION

Flexibility is most important for the physician starting out in practice. The future of the practice is uncertain. The practice may grow rapidly and require additional space, or the physician may decide to move elsewhere. Because flexibility is so important, the physician should avoid purchasing or constructing an office when beginning a practice. Such a step commits the physician to permanent and inflexible facilities and requires a lot of money. It is preferable to wait several years to determine how the practice develops before considering office ownership. The physician also avoids the problems of trying to sell the building if the arrangement does not work out well or if the practice grows so quickly that a move is required. A short-term lease is desirable, and one to three years is ideal. Rental costs can run anywhere from $3.00 to $15.00 or more per square foot per year. Location, building age, and availability of alternatives all help to dictate the price. The best barometer for evaluating whether a practice is paying reasonable rent is to compute it as a percentage of gross receipts. The normal range is between 4% and 7%.

Home Office

The office should not be located in or adjacent to the physician's home. Although some older physicians (many of them in primary care fields) have such office locations, there are many problems when the office is so close to home. The physician's professional development is often hindered because there is less communication with his or her peers than would be the case in a professional building. Also, the home-office arrangement can cause problems if the physician decides to have an associate join the practice. The new partner will usually have great difficulty establishing independence since the physician who owns the house will appear to control the practice. Also, it is difficult to establish safeguards to protect the new partner if the senior physician should leave the practice. Many home-office arrangements exist because special zoning rules allow business use when the physician lives in the home. Many zoning laws do not allow a nonresident physician to also practice in the house.

Last, having an office in the home greatly reduces the physician's privacy. Some patients may take unfair advantage of the situation "since the doctor lives right next door to the office anyway" and assume that they can visit at any time.

Health Care Professional Building

The preferred location for a physician starting out in practice is to locate the office in a medical building limited to health care professionals.

Such a location can be of particular importance to a new physician. The building lends an aura of professionalism to the practice. Patients who are in the building may notice the physician's sign and decide to try his or her services for convenience, since they are accustomed to going to that building and may want to centralize their health care.

Family practitioners, general practitioners, general internists, and pediatricians sometimes think that close proximity to the hospital is not important. Depending on the community, the geographic distribution of similar specialists in the area, the location of area hospitals, and the physician's emphasis on hospital versus office work, this attitude may or may not be wise. There is no question that close proximity to the hospital can save otherwise wasted travel time. This factor should not be ignored by a physician with a reasonable hospital load, especially if there is much emergency work.

Furthermore, other physicians may more readily consult the physician who is close to the hospital, believing that their requests are more likely to be satisfied promptly.

Multioffice Arrangements

A physician should start by opening only one office. Rarely will a primary care physician be better served by a multioffice arrangement. The inefficiencies should be enough to discourage a physician from having more than one office. Overhead tends to be higher; it is harder to find charts; billing is more complicated; and there is much wasted time. There must be serious overriding factors before the multioffice step is considered.

HOW TO GAIN AND RETAIN PATIENTS

There is no one factor that makes one physician more popular, busier, and wealthier than another. There are many. However, the four "A's" (availability, accessibility, affability, and ability) are important.

Availability

Many primary care physicians believe that they will have little trouble making themselves available, since they often fear that they will not be busy enough. But what does availability really mean, and how can a physician have it work to his or her advantage?

A good first step is to contact other physicians in the same specialty and express a willingness to cover for them. This approach gives work to the new physician and provides the other physicians with an opportunity to see him or her in action. In many areas, new primary care physicians are welcomed. If the new physician does a good job, the established physicians may refer patients whom they are too busy to handle, especially new patients.

The new physician may also provide some different services to attract patients. For example, if the other pediatricians in town have only weekday office hours, a new pediatrician may decide to try night hours or Saturday hours to attract patients. Also, if other physicians in town take Wednesdays off, a new physician may attract patients on Wednesdays. The disadvantage of such an approach is that the physician may be locked into these sessions when his or her practice gets busy later.

Although it may be difficult at times, a new physician should respond enthusiastically when called by his patients for a night or weekend problem. It is not always enough to care about patients' well-being; it must also appear to other physicians, nurses, and patients that one sincerely cares.

Accessibility

Office location is the most important factor for ensuring accessibility. Convenience to public transportation may be important in some areas, and the physician should study public transportation routes. Free parking is helpful. Available parking is essential. Any practice site should have safe parking that is available during practice hours.

Being accessible by telephone is also important. A primary care physician's practice can flourish or die depending on how the telephone is managed (see Chap. 5). Patients, physicians, and others should be able to easily reach the office, and an answering service is essential for times when the office is closed.

Affability

It may be obvious, but it merits repeating—people prefer to deal with those whom they like. Being concerned and interested in patients is important. Doing a good clinical job is important. However, in many instances, the impression that a physician makes has nothing to do with any of these things. Was the physician friendly? Was he or she more concerned with money than anything else? Was he or she abrupt, rushing to get to the next patient? Was the physician on time? If not, did he or she apologize or explain the delay or do both?

People care about these questions, and the answers to them go a long way toward determining how people feel about their physician.

Ability

Last, the clinical ability of the physician determines to a great extent how active and successful he or she will be. Patients often may not be able to judge the clinical competence of a physician. However, other physicians can. Also, nurses and other assistants in the hospital and in the office can and often do judge the physician. Word can spread quickly when the physician is not doing a good job. The staff's apparent competence is also important and reflects on the physician.

Patient Information Booklet

A well-prepared and friendly patient information booklet is particularly useful for a new practitioner. It can provide a feeling of permanence. A patient information booklet should clearly set forth a practice's policies, both in business-related matters (collections, insurance, and billing) and in clinical matters (e.g., what to do in case of emergencies).

Medical-management consultants have estimated that the number of incoming telephone calls can be reduced by 25–30% by use of such a booklet. Although the reduction might not be that high in all practices, proper use of such a booklet will reduce unnecessary telephone calls.

The booklet should be given to all patients. If there is time, it should be mailed to patients before they come in for a visit. The A.M.A. has an excellent booklet on this subject, entitled "Preparing a Patient Information Booklet."*

Referral Lists

A new physician may benefit by being included in referral lists. Some local medical societies operate a system that will circulate a new member's name, background, and specialty to all other members. Many societies also have a rotating referral list to answer requests for physicians from the general public.

Many hospitals have emergency-room referral services. Most of them have rotating referral lists that favor the new physician. If an emergency-room patient asks for a private physician for continuing care, names from the referral lists are provided.

Introducing Oneself

Once a physician has obtained an office location, telephone number, and hospital affiliations, announcements should be sent out. The announcements might include the physician's specialty, credentials, the official opening date of the practice, and office hours. This announcement should be sent to other physicians in the community, allied health professionals, pharmacists, chiropractors, podiatrists, and opticians. The county medical society should be contacted in regard to ethical guidelines for announcements.

The potential role of pharmacists should not be discounted. The pharmacist is often the patient's entry point into a community's medical-care system. If a patient's condition has not been relieved by over-the-counter remedies, the pharmacist is often asked for the name of a physician.

Although written announcements are helpful, personal contact with local physicians and other health-care professionals is even more important. It is useful for the new physician to give other physicians an opportunity to get to know him or her well. Making rounds when other physicians normally do, eating in the hospital cafeteria, using the hospital medical library, and getting involved in hospital-staff activities all help. If a new physician will be practicing near his or her medical school or training program, the physician should tell those involved in his or her training about the opening of the practice.

Much has been written and argued about advertising physician services. Few physicians have actually advertised in the press or on radio or television. Most who have were scorned by their fellow physicians. It still is not a generally accepted mode of attracting patients for the physician (whether legal or ethical or not), although the situation may change in the future.

Retaining Patients

Being available, accessible, affable, and able not only help a new physician gain patients but also help retain them. Retaining patients requires effort, particularly

*The booklet can be obtained by writing to Department of Practice Management, Order Dept. OP-40, American Medical Association, 535 North Dearborn Street, Chicago, Illinois 60610.

for primary care physicians. Unlike most medical specialties, primary care practices are built from long-term patient relationships. Good scheduling practices, proper handling of the telephone, fair billing and collecting policies, and open and honest communication with patients are among the features of the practice that keep patients coming back. If another physician or someone else refers a patient, a letter describing the patient's disposition will encourage future referrals.

Outside Activities

Some new physicians have found religious and fraternal organizations to be excellent vehicles for increasing visibility in the community. However, nominal affiliation will generally do little good—active involvement is a must. The physician should not join purely for professional advancement—it will show. In the end, the physician will then be hurt more than helped by the involvement. However, if the physician is sincerely interested, active participation will add patients to his or her practice as a bonus.

The physician should work to lead a balanced life. Much of what the physician sincerely does for pleasure (hobbies, sports, artistic pursuits, and social activities) will contribute to professional contacts. In addition, the physician should allow enough time for his or her spouse and children. Inevitably, the physician's personal happiness will contribute to professional success.

How to Refer

A physician should consult with other physicians frequently. If a patient seems dissatisfied or unconvinced, the physician should suggest that another opinion be obtained. The patient should be given the name of a well-qualified specialist in the field. This approach is better than waiting for the patient to suggest another physician or, worse yet, have the patient look up another physician's name in the telephone book. Several principles can be helpful in referring patients:

1. If possible, speak with the specialist personally and explain the reason for the consultation.
2. Send a summary letter and photocopies of important laboratory data in advance.
3. Ask the patient to carry important x-ray films and pathology slides or mail them in advance.
4. Inform the patient of the purpose for the referral.
5. Refer the patient only to physicians who send prompt and complete letters to you as the referring physician and who will continue to involve you in important clinical decisions.
6. Try, when possible, to match the patient's personality to that of the consultant.

4
Financial Office Management

Vasilios J. Kalogredis

For many physicians, one of the most difficult aspects of practice is financial management. Few physicians have been trained in accounting, health insurance, or collection systems, but knowledge of these disciplines is crucial to a financially successful practice. In this chapter, I shall review the principles of financial management. This chapter is designed to help the physician deal with these issues and to communicate more effectively with financial advisors.

FEES

One of the first questions a new physician asks when establishing a practice is: "What should my fees be?" Although a medical-management consultant can offer help in this regard, it is still a difficult matter. There is no one right answer. Fees vary so widely from community to community (and, at times, even among physicians in a community) that a single answer is inadequate. However, certain important guidelines relating to fees will be described below.

Relative-value Scales

In the past, a convenient method for creating fee schedules was to secure a copy of a relative-value scale from the physician's national specialty society or other source; for example, the California Medical Society had an excellent one. The relative-value scale was not a schedule of fees; it was a guide for practitioners to set fees. The relative value provided a means of determining the comparative worth of various services and procedures. It reflected the complexity, skill, and time involved. A uniform conversion factor could then be applied against the unit value to arrive at the appropriate fee.

Even though relative-value scales are not in themselves fee schedules, the federal government believes that they constitute "price-fixing" and has barred their use. No practice should now be quoting its fees as a multiplier of a relative-value scale.

Medicare Profile Information

The Medicare fiscal intermediary in every state (Blue Shield, in many states) maintains a profile of fees charged by each specialty. The profile will generally show the 75th percentile of the range of fees for each service charged by all practitioners of a specialty in that general area.

A physician should make a written request for profile information for his or her specialty. This information is valuable to the physician (even though it may be more than a year old in some instances). Generally speaking, if this "prevailing area charge" is higher or the same as what the doctor is charging, it indicates that the physician's fees are actually lower than others since the Medicare "profile" data are not usually up to date.

In reality, even though its legality can be argued, most physicians seem to set their fees on the basis of what the competition is charging. For example, depending on the circumstances, it is not unusual for a new primary care physician to set basic fees (particularly for office visits) a dollar or two lower than those of the highest priced competitor. The rationale is that patients may "shop around" to determine office-visit fees and perhaps try the new physician if his or her fees are lower. In other instances, the physician may have determined that he or she should charge the highest fees.

It is too easy to raise fees indiscriminately, and fee restraint should be exercised. If spiraling health care costs continue, increasingly stringent price controls, and perhaps even rollbacks, may be called for by the federal government. However, there is a dilemma for many physicians who have kept their fees down for years. When these physicians finally raise their fees in response to inflationary pressures, they often have found themselves locked into low reimbursements from Blue Shield, Medicare, and other plans, thus inducing them to drop out of participation. Their profiles just were not high enough to allow the increased fees. This situation has caused some physicians to continually raise fees to keep their profiles high so they will always be eligible for the highest reimbursement allowed.

For a new physician starting out in practice, it is important to develop a specific written fee schedule. Such a schedule helps maintain consistency in fees charged and makes billing much less confusing for patients and the staff. In addition, it helps give the physician the appearance of being removed from the collection process since he or she does not have to write the fee down in front of the patient. Merely recording the services performed is sufficient to set the billing and collection process into operation since the staff can record the fee from the written fee schedule.

BILLING SYSTEMS

Before deciding what sort of a billing system to adopt, a physician should focus clearly on exactly what a well-run system should provide. The more important aspects of an ideal billing system include:

1. A method of communicating information about the services provided (from the physician or other provider to the staff responsible for billing and collecting)

2. A method of recording the charge and payment on a patient's account
3. A method of recording the charges and payments on a daily transaction summary (sometimes called a "day sheet")
4. A method of acknowledging and recording the patient's payment
5. A method of preparing a bill to send to the patient
6. A method of rebilling a patient for any unpaid balance

For an office to work effectively and efficiently, it is important to select a system that accomplishes all these tasks with the least duplication, cost, and employee time. Several systems are reviewed, including pegboard systems, accounting machines, and computer billings.

Pegboard System

For almost all new physicians starting practice, the pegboard system is ideal. Basically, the pegboard system requires that information be written only once. In a single step, the receptionist can prepare a bill, receipt, and patient account (ledger) card or day sheet for a particular transaction. By using carbon paper, the receptionist can prepare all three forms simultaneously. This approach reduces duplication, thereby saving time and money. It is easy to train even an inexperienced employee to use it. It forces the assistants to complete all entries on a daily basis, whereas without such a system, some employees develop the lazy habit of delaying posting to the ledger cards, which may result in errors and does result in a loss of control. The pegboard system also helps avoid errors. Through this approach, transposition errors are avoided, and there is reasonable protection against embezzlement. The receptionist is the key to the pegboard system.

A physician starting out in practice should get in touch with a representative of one of the pegboard supply companies and select a system to fit the expected needs of the practice. Calling in a salesman gives the physician an opportunity to review systems implemented by other physicians in similar fields and can help avoid misuse of the pegboard. Some offices have instituted the pegboard and have not used it properly because the staff were not trained in its use.

The top companies' products are similar, so a pegboard system is often selected on the basis of the quality of the representative. The best sources for capable representatives in the area are the local medical-management consultants or accountants and local physicians who use the pegboard system.

With a pegboard system, billing is easy. Before billing, patient ledger cards will have already been prepared (through duplication at the time of writing). The cards with outstanding balances (which should be kept in a separate active file tray) should be run through a duplicating machine and then stuffed into stamped, windowed envelopes.

A new physician (particularly in high-volume specialties) should use the pegboard system from the beginning. More expensive accounting machines or computer billing approaches generally will not be efficient at the outset. Active practices of one to five physicians are generally served best by the pegboard. It is only with larger practices that one of the more mechanized approaches might be appropriate.

Accounting Machines

As a practice grows and the burdens at the reception desk become overwhelming, a more automated system may be required. An accounting machine (sometimes called bookkeeping machine or mechanical posting machine) is one alternative. Although they are becoming more expensive, accounting machines are generally less expensive than are most computers.

Companies that provide excellent accounting machines for medical office use include Burroughs, Monroe, and National Cash Register (NCR). The initial outlay can run into the tens of thousands of dollars. If an accounting machine is purchased, a full-time operator will usually have to be hired. In addition, staff must be trained to back up the primary operator to help retain efficiency.

The accounting machine takes a burden from the receptionist. The receptionist collects the fee slips from office-visit patients and routes them to the machine operator (usually in the back office) for mechanical posting to patient ledger account cards.

Computer Billing

Another alternative billing system for the office that has outgrown the pegboard system is computer billing. Under present circumstances, rarely will a practice with fewer than three physicians be better served by a computer system.

There are three basic computer-related alternatives.

1. *Outside billing service.* Unfortunately, most outside billing services do not handle the billing and associated needs of medical practices satisfactorily. The first rule is that the service must deal only with medical practices. Some outside computer billing services with which physicians have dealt have not fully appreciated how a medical practice's needs differ from those of commercial enterprises. Second, a list of all the company's medical customers over the past several years should be requested. References should be checked thoroughly before any selection is made. Also, a physician should talk to physicians he or she knows who have considered this approach. Medical-management consultants, attorneys, or accountants who are actively involved with medical practices may have valuable input about any alternative under consideration. One problem with the outside computer billing service is loss of control. No ledger card is readily available as part of the system. If a patient calls regarding the status of a bill, the most recent summary sheets from the service may be a week or more old, thereby causing uncertainties concerning what has transpired in the interim.

2. *On-line computer.* This alternative requires either a data terminal in the office or a telephone connection with the main computer, allowing for relatively easy retrieval of information on a timely basis. Costs can vary dramatically (both for the actual leasing or purchase of the hardware and for the monthly charges for billing). This approach generally provides less control than does the pegboard approach. However, instant retrieval of account balances is usually possible. Many of these systems will also prepare insurance forms automatically. Of the three computer alternatives available, the on-line approach has generally been the most successful in the medium-sized medical office.

3. *In-house computer.* The cost of an in-house computer generally limits its use

to clinic-sized practices. It is not unusual for the initial cost to be $40,000–50,000 or more. Developing proper programs and systems ("software") is the key to a successful in-house computer. For it to work well, a tremendous amount of time and effort is required-of the physician or office manager. Unless that time and effort are committed, great problems will arise.

The following are general comments about computers.

· Rarely will a computer system reduce personnel costs. Usually, the same amount of help is needed. Additional help is often needed, particularly during the transition period.

· Any computer system should be able to prepare insurance forms automatically. A system's ability to do so indicates that some thought has been given to applying a computer to the needs of medical practice.

· Patient recall systems are part of many excellent computer systems.

· Some argue that the added costs are justified by all the financial and management information a computer can provide. In some instances, this contention is valid; in others, it is not, particularly if the information received is not necessarily the information desired by the physician. Usually, less mechanized systems can provide the information that the physician wants with less effort.

Handling of Office Charges

One of the main purposes of any billing system is to avoid lost charges. If a charge is lost, it is never recorded on a patient's bill, and the physician will not get paid. Therefore, in developing any system, the physician should seek to make it as "loss proof" as possible.

The key to proper handling of office billing is the fee slip (sometimes called the route slip or charge ticket). Regardless of the type of billing system selected, a fee slip can be made a part of it. When properly used, the fee slip keeps everyone informed about what has transpired and also helps to get the patient to the receptionist for collection.

Normally, the fee slip, which includes the patient's name, previous balance, and, in some instances, other information, is attached to the patient's chart before the examination by the physician. When the physician has completed the work in the examination room, he or she can mark down on the slip what services were provided. This slip should then be given to the patient and the patient instructed to give it to the receptionist.

In this fashion, the physician can tell the receptionist what services were performed. The patient will go by the reception desk and give the slip to the receptionist, who can then record the fee and request payment from the patient. Without the slip, the receptionist could only guess about the services provided. In addition, there might not be a reason for the patient to stop by the desk.

In general, physicians should not purchase a prepackaged fee slip. The physician should use suppliers' samples to design a fee slip to fit his or her practice. The fee slip should list primary office procedures and should contain proper coding.

In addition, the fee slips should be prenumbered, which will allow for a check of the slips at the end of the day for a gap in numbers. Perhaps the physician forgot to complete the slip, the patient left with it, or the receptionist threw it away, attempting to hide an embezzlement. Without prenumbering, it would be more difficult to detect these problems.

Superbill

In developing a fee slip for a practice, serious thought should be given to the "superbill." In effect, the superbill is a more extensive fee slip that contains space for the pieces of information needed to complete an insurance form.

The appropriate procedure codes, spaces for the diagnoses, the patient's signature, and the physician's signature are all on the superbill. Commercial insurance companies must accept this form; Blue Shield plans in more and more states are accepting it, as are various Medicare intermediaries.

The superbill saves time for office visits that are covered by insurance. By completing the superbill during the visit (which merely requires a few checkmarks and a couple of signatures), the physician does almost all the insurance form work. In most states, all that need be entered on the actual insurance form is the patient's name, address, and some other information at the top of the form. The middle and bottom parts of the form can be replaced with the superbill by printing "see attached slip" on the insurance form. The superbill can then be attached and submitted with the original insurance form. Many practices have used the superbill for hospital work as well.

Retrieving Hospital Charges

Many practices have difficulty billing for services provided to hospitalized patients. Billing for such patients requires the cooperation of the physician (unless one has the luxury of a physician's assistant, nurse practitioner, or other assistant in the hospital). Recommendations in this area are intended to keep the practice from being overly dependent on the hospital for discharge summaries, operative reports, and other information for billing or completing insurance forms. Insurance companies are slow enough in paying physicians without adding to the delay by waiting for the hospital.

Because of this potential delay, the physician should keep a specific card for each hospitalized patient. Many hospitals will provide a stamp with relevant information about the patient, for example, name, address, age, and insurance numbers. A simple coding system might then be developed for use by the physician and staff. For example, F might mean first day hospital services; I might mean intermediate hospital visits; C might mean cardiac-care unit visits; D might mean discharge day. The important point is to record exactly what services were provided on which days so that the physician is properly paid for what has been done.

In many instances, Medicare and Blue Shield audits of physicians have looked to the hospital chart for entries to confirm that services were provided. Accurate billing can avoid embarrassment in the event of such audits.

At least once a week on a specified schedule, such as every Friday morning, the physician should turn in the cards to a responsible person in the office. This employee should then transfer the information from these cards to a separate notebook or card box and return the cards to the physician so that further charges can be recorded.

COLLECTION SYSTEMS

In these inflationary times, physicians face increasingly difficult business decisions. On the one hand, their costs are rising dramatically, and, on the other, they are being pressured to hold down health care costs. Since most physicians find it undesirable to increase their fees indiscriminately, they must become increasingly critical of their collection procedures to assure that sufficient receipts are received.

There are certain charges that should not be collected. Practices participating in Blue Shield or accepting Medicare assignments will obviously have some write-offs due to insurance disallowances. In addition, write-offs for the accounts of patients who truly are unable to pay cannot be avoided. In light of this problem, it is important to collect the accounts of all other patients effectively and professionally.

When deciding to refer an account to a collection agency or small-claims court, one must determine whether there is the possibility of a malpractice claim. If such a claim is possible, a critical evaluation should be made about whether the overdue account should be pressed.

In reality, success in collection requires implementing systems to assure prompt payment by patients (or their insurers) who can afford to pay. Patients who are unable to pay for medical services should, in many instances, be excused from payment and continued as patients of the practice.

Collection at Time of Service

The surest collection of all is the collection that is made at the time of service. Collection at the time of service avoids the increased cost involved with billing (postage, supplies, and personnel costs). In addition, by receiving payment at the time of service, the resources required for collection can be reduced dramatically.

By collecting at the time of service, cash flow will accelerate, which is important for a newly established practice. There are some real advantages for physicians starting out in practice. Patients will be more likely to accept collection at the time of service than they might if the physician joined a practice where patients had not been expected in the past to pay at the time of the visit. A new practice with new rules will be easier for a patient to accept. It is not unprofessional to have the physician's assistants request payment when the patient is leaving the office. So long as the staff is courteous and consistent in making the request for payment, there should be no problem. In addition, an immediate request for payment might turn up legitimate payment problems. It is far less embarrassing to learn about such a problem early than to discover it after several dunning efforts. Immediate payment removes financial tension between a patient and a physician.

It is important that goals be established regarding collection at the time of service. Primary care specialists should collect at least 50% of their office charges at the time of service. Some primary care practices collect in excess of 80% of charges at the time of service. For a physician starting out in practice, a patient information booklet can be an excellent method for describing one's collection policies.

Including the following comments in the booklet might be helpful:

"Inflation is growing for everyone, including this medical office. We are confronted with ever-increasing costs for almost every supply and service used in rendering professional care to you.

"In an attempt to keep our fees at their present levels (while recognizing that we may have to raise them from time to time), we are asking your help in a cost-cutting plan. We will ask you to pay for your office visits at the time of service. With your help, we can substantially reduce the cost of billing and bookkeeping.

"We understand that occasions may arise when it will be necessary for you to request a statement rather than to pay immediately. We also recognize the need to set up payment plans for patients who require extensive treatment. These needs will be accommodated as they arise.

"We are sure that you understand our concerns, and we look forward to working closely with you to continue to provide you with the best professional care at the most reasonable cost possible."

The real key to good over-the-counter collections is the receptionist. This person must understand the importance of collection and must be able to talk with patients in a professional way. Some offices even have signs in the waiting room that announce the practice of over-the-counter collection.

For example, when a patient arrives at the desk with a fee slip, the receptionist should say, "That will be $15 for today, Mr. Smith." Nothing more need be said. This statement forces the patient to respond. If the patient does not have the money at that time, the fee slip can then be given to the patient with a self-addressed return envelope as the first bill.

The fee slip itself is important to the success of collection at the time of service. Without it, the receptionist will not know exactly what to charge, and the patient might not even stop by the front desk.

In designing the office, it is important to locate the receptionist, who will be the collector in most offices, at a control point that the patient must pass on the way out of the office.

Use of Bank Credit Cards

The use of bank credit cards (such as Master Charge and Visa) has not been recognized as ethical by medical societies. Moreover, their use in the health care setting has generally not been well accepted by patients. Therefore, most practitioners are well advised not to get involved with them. Where they have been used, the problem of opening a separate bank account tied into the bank that offers the credit cards has often not been worth the availability of the credit card. In addition, a percentage of the physician's collection goes to the bank. Although it varies, in most medical practices, this fee to the bank ranges from 3% to 5%. Practices for which bank credit cards are the most useful are those with a large number of transient patients. For example, physicians in resort areas have found them useful since they may never see the patient again.

Budget Plan

A physician's office should be willing to cooperate with patients who make a good faith effort to pay off their bills. If patients cannot satisfy all their bills in one lump sum, a payment plan should be established. For the physician to be protected from federal and state governmental regulations regarding truth in lending, a written payment plan should be instituted. It is especially important that the plan be in writing since it reaffirms the patient's obligation. Before developing a specific written budget plan, the physician should check with a local attorney to assure that the plan meets local legal requirements.

Delinquent Collection

There is usually no valid excuse for failure to collect at least 90% of the physician's charges after insurance disallowances. The Society of Professional Business Consultants (SPBC) indicates that the average collection ratio ranges from 93% to 95%.

To assure a high collection rate, it is important to develop a specific follow-up procedure for collections. The important points are to develop a schedule, put it in writing, and follow up on the accounts in a standard fashion. Nothing is gained by merely sending out bills for several months or sending out some mild-mannered reminders that are disregarded by patients. Too often, direct contact with the patient begins with dunning by a collection agency. Early efforts should be more direct to resolve the problem before conflict arises.

The most effective collection procedure consists of letters and telephone calls. Form letters are not as effective as those that appear to be individually typed. They can be typed on the office typewriter and then sent to a local offset printing company for reproduction. It is important to delegate responsibility for collection follow-up to specific staff, who should be given the time and privacy to do their job well. In a busy primary care practice with office hours every day, it is not fair to expect good collection follow-up from an assistant who is constantly at the reception desk. Notices should be distributed throughout the month, with follow-up notices sent on a regular basis. A reminder box with dates will help the collections staff send out the letters on time.

A practice should be its own collection agency, if possible; if office collection procedures work well, few accounts will have to be sent to outside collection agencies. It is preferable for a practice to be in touch directly with the patient to obtain payment, work out an extended payment schedule, or write off the account than to send the account to a collection agency.

Last Resorts

No matter how good a job an office does on in-house collection, some accounts will remain unresolved and will require further action. Several possible alternatives are available.

Collection Agency

A collection agency is an independent entity that will receive a percentage (often, 50%) of whatever it collects for a client. Before selecting a collection agency, the physician should obtain a list of all the prospective agency's medical clients. The physician should then communicate with these clients to determine if they are happy with the service. It is important to use a collection agency that deals exclusively with medical and dental clients. If one uses an agency that deals with other types of client, that agency may not fully appreciate and understand the need for professionalism in dealing with the patients of a health care practice. In addition, it is important that regular and timely reports be received from the collection agency on at least a quarterly basis. Even if no money was collected during that quarter, a written report should be sent to the practice.

Collection Letter System

Some physicians have found collection letter services effective. For a fee, a series of letters is sent out on the collection system's stationery. The collection letter system differs from the collection agency in that the fee is paid whether the money is received from the patient or not. In addition, the patient is instructed to pay the physician directly, whereas a collection agency receives the money itself.

Small-claims Court

An excellent approach being used by more and more physicians is small-claims court. This approach involves an actual legal action, generally not requiring the services of an attorney or even the physician. If many instances, one of the staff assistants can go to the local courthouse and file a complaint, which a court official will help complete.

In most instances, the patient does not appear in court, and a default judgment is obtained. The physician can then pursue one of two courses. In most instances, a judgment lien is filed in the county courthouse, whereby the patient cannot sell any real estate in that county without satisfying the obligation to the physician. In other instances, a physician may decide to "execute the judgment," whereby the patient's assets can be taken away to satisfy the debt.

The small-claims court approach will usually influence people of means. In addition, the cost is usually quite small (usually no more than $25 or $30) and can be recouped from the defendant if the physician wins the case.

Federal and State Laws Directly Affecting Collection Policies of Medical Practices

There are a variety of important legal considerations about collections. Some of the key ones are explained below.

Federal and most state laws prohibit a creditor (a physician or practice, in this situation) from threatening any action against a person that the creditor does not, in fact, take or intend to take. For example, an assistant might call a patient and say, "If we are not paid by the end of the month, we will sue you." If the office did not intend to follow through with that threat and did not, in fact, follow through with it, a practice could be found to have violated a federal regulation that expressly forbids telephone calls that falsely threaten a debtor with legal action.

Although it is admittedly rare, there have been defamation of character legal suits brought against creditors. Several creditors have been sued on such grounds and have lost. Even when the creditor prevailed, the publicity and embarrassment of the trial offset any gains from the original action.

The Federal Trade Commission has adopted rules to curb scare tactics. They forbid deceptive representations or deceptive actions intended to collect debts or to obtain information for the collection process. The Federal Communication Commission has also entered the field, primarily to prevent the misuse of telephones "for a call or calls, anonymous or otherwise, in a manner reasonably expected to frighten or torment another." The Federal Communication Commission also bans nuisance calls at late or early hours, unjustified calls to the debtor's employer, relatives, or friends, and calls falsely threatening court action.

Many state laws, in New York and Massachusetts, for example, expressly prohibit communication or threatened communication of a debt's existence to the debtor's employer. Massachusetts law goes even further, prohibiting the communication or threatened communication to anyone without the express written permission of the debtor. The same Massachusetts law states that the use of language on an envelope indicating that the communication relates to the collection of a debt is equivalent to communicating the debt.

In many areas, credit bureaus will compile lists of bad credit risks. Some physicians have been asked to provide the names of their nonpaying patients. Providing the information is not in and of itself illegal, and in some situations it may help others avoid deadbeats. However, involvement with a credit bureau can have some serious legal and practical implications. Under the Federal Fair Credit Reporting Act, if a patient named as a "bad debt" is denied credit because of the credit information, he or she may obtain the names of those who supplied that information, thus exposing the physician to a possible damage suit. So long as the information supplied was truthful, the physician should not be liable for supplying it. However, the physician should clear matters with his or her attorney before forwarding information to a credit bureau. There are other state laws as well as federal laws in this area that can have far-reaching implications.

Sometimes, a patient will deliver a check marked "payment in full," even though it is for less than the balance actually owed. If the physician is, nevertheless, determined to collect the whole fee and recognizes the patient's ability to pay, the check should not be deposited. Courts have generally held that the cashing of such a check is an acceptance of the debtor's words—his "offer." Thus, the balance of the account would not thereafter be legally collectible.

Some have recommended that physicians merely cross out the words "payment in full," cash the check, and bill the patient for the difference anyway. However, this unilateral action may not be enough to keep the balance collectible. If a physician wants to consider such a step, he or she should ask an attorney about the specific situation.

One might instead return the check (unendorsed) with a certified letter to the debtor stating that the check sent (listing the amount) was not "payment in full" and requesting payment of the specified full amount. This approach may result in noncollection of the previously mailed amount.

Another, and perhaps better, approach involves holding the check marked "payment in full," but not cashing or even endorsing it, while a certified letter is sent to the debtor. The letter could confirm the total balance, say that the check is being retained, and state that the physician does not intend to cash the check until the debtor remits the balance owed.

The federal bankruptcy laws are complex and extensive. A physician encountering a bankrupt patient should contact an attorney to determine the best way to handle the patient's debt. However, in general, if a patient enters bankruptcy, payments will be made out of whatever assets exist to those who have filed valid claims. A claim form can be obtained from the bankruptcy section of the local federal district court, filled in by the physician, and returned to the court. When notice of a hearing arises, the physician need not attend. Such action may result in only partial payment, depending on the assets and debts involved, but it is usually worth the effort.

If a patient has filed for bankruptcy and the physician did not know of the action, the physician might still be able to collect after the bankruptcy action as an "unlisted creditor." In some situations, the physician may then be able to collect in full since the "discharged" debtor may be in better financial condition than previously.

There are often difficulties in collecting for services to a spouse or child involved in a separation or divorce. The physician should avoid being placed in the middle of squabbles over which spouse owes the fee. The physician should insist on its payment by the parent or other family member with whom he or she is directly involved. Any question about the ultimate responsibility between the husband and wife should be resolved between them after the physician has been paid.

BOOKKEEPING AND ACCOUNTING

Because physicians generally have little difficulty generating income, their tendency is to pay scant attention to practice management, in particular to bookkeeping and accounting. However, more careful financial management could enable the physician to increase income or free time or even to reduce fees. The principles of accounting practice will help the physician operate a more efficient practice.

Monday Morning Report

Every week, the physician should receive weekly information on the practice's important financial figures. A sample of a "Monday morning report" is included (Exhibit 1). Space is provided for eight weekly summaries. Many physicians have found it useful to punch holes in these sheets and place them in looseleaf notebooks for easy reference and comparison. This system will help a physician and his advisors spot trends and ward off difficulties before they become more serious. Too often, the problems inherent in a practice go unnoticed for a long period of time because weekly or monthly financial reports are not prepared or made available to the physician and his or her advisors. When the problem does surface, it is a crisis and much more difficult to resolve.

Exhibit 1. Monday Morning Report.

	/ /	/ /	/ /	/ /
CASH IN BANK AND ON HAND	$			
ESTIMATED RECEIPTS (WEEK)				
TOTAL	$			
ACCOUNTS PAYABLE:				
PAYROLL FOR WEEK	$			
INSTALLMENTS OR LOANS				
OTHER CURRENT				
TOTAL	$			
TOTAL ACCOUNTS RECEIVABLE				
INSURANCE FORMS PENDING				
_____				
_____				

	/ /	/ /	/ /	/ /
CASH IN BANK AND ON HAND	$			
ESTIMATED RECEIPTS (WEEK)				
TOTAL	$			
ACCOUNTS PAYABLE:				
PAYROLL FOR WEEK	$			
INSTALLMENTS OR LOANS				
OTHER CURRENT				
TOTAL	$			
TOTAL ACCOUNTS RECEIVABLE				
INSURANCE FORMS PENDING				
_____				
_____				

The sample Monday morning report lists the cash in the bank and on hand as of the beginning of business on Monday morning and estimates the receipts for the coming week. In addition, bills payable should also be summarized. It is helpful to attach a separate list of the bills outstanding. The physician can then establish a payment priority list in light of the estimated income for that week and the cash available.

An accounts receivable figure is also included on the sample Monday morning report. By putting the figure in front of the physician on a weekly basis, any unusually large increases or decreases in receivables will be clearly noticeable, and necessary corrective action can be taken in a timely and informed fashion.

A tally of insurance forms pending is also an important category. Included within this list are the number of forms to be completed, the date of the oldest forms, and the approximate value of pending insurance forms.

The Monday morning report might also include other information. Some practices like to keep track of the number of new patients, the number of people admitted to the hospital, and the number of different types of visits.

Monthly Accounting Statement

Unfortunately, many medical practices receive financial statements only on a quarterly, semiannual, or annual basis. To make matters worse, those reports often end up in the physician's hands many months after the fact. They are of little help as an effective management tool. This situation should be avoided; even a physician just starting out in practice needs to be kept informed on a regular and timely basis.

Most accountants prepare formal financial statements for medical practices. They generally provide a "balance sheet," which lists the practice's assets and liabilities, and an "income and expense statement," which shows the financial progress during the period in terms of profit and loss. Although they are helpful, too often these formal statements do not contain the information most useful to physicians and their advisors for ongoing business decisions. They are less than optimal because they are infrequent, delayed, and too lengthy. Therefore, formal accountants' statements should be augmented by less official, more relevant, and more timely internal reports.

Monthly financial statements should be prepared in the office by all practices. In most instances, these statements are best prepared by the practice's bookkeeper, who should prepare an informal monthly statement with useful and timely financial information for the physician. The bookkeeper should be required to provide this statement within the first few days of each month (usually by the 10th day). In group practices, the physicians should hold regularly scheduled monthly meetings to discuss practice management and financial matters. Such a financial statement can serve as an important agenda item at each meeting. In addition, a copy of the monthly report should be sent to the accountant, medical-management consultant, and attorney each month as a useful method of keeping them informed so that they can better serve the practice as advisors. By allowing its advisors to review the statements, a practice is able to take advantage of their experience and capacities for the physician's benefit.

Virtually all the information necessary to prepare an in-house monthly financial statement is already produced by most practice bookkeepers. The accountant or medical-management consultant of a practice usually trains the bookkeeper to summarize all receipts and to categorize all expenditures.

If an office has a computer service that provides reams of paper breaking down charge, receipt, and expense items into many categories, it is still advisable for the bookkeeper to summarize on a single sheet the more important items from that computer printout. One of the problems with computer printouts is that the physicians often do not have the time or the interest to go through the many pages of summaries the computer sheets provide and make sense out of them. A simple reference sheet would be much more practical and useful to the physician.

Exhibit 2 is a sample in-house monthly financial statement. It will be referred to throughout this section. The specific categories and format of this statement need not be used by each practice. However, the basic concepts can and should be used.

Relevant Financial Information

Charges are an important management tool. Unfortunately, they are not normally provided in reports prepared for physicians by accountants, since most accounting reports are geared to preparing tax returns and therefore ignore the charges. Charges are necessary to compute the collection ratio and to keep a running total of the accounts receivable of the practice.

The sample monthly financial statement breaks down charges among Hospital 1, Hospital 2, the main office, and the satellite office. In addition, it breaks down the charges among the two physicians and ancillary personnel who produce income.

Other practices may decide to categorize productivity into different categories. The important point is for each practice to decide what charge information it wants and then provide for it. More and more group practices are dividing income among physicians at least partially on the basis of productivity. In those instances, it is most important that the charges be assigned to the specific physicians involved.

Receipts are summarized in all accounting reports. They should be broken down between "office receipts" (meaning money received at the time of service) and "mail receipts" (which would include all other receipts). The "time-of-service" collection ratio is computed by dividing the office receipts by the office charges. In primary care, 50% is a minimum goal; some primary care physicians collect more than 90%.

Most practices have no idea what their collection ratios are, although they are not difficult to compute. Practice receipts are divided by practice net charges (meaning charges reduced by Blue Shield, Medicare, and Medical Assistance disallowances, for which the patient cannot be billed). Note that the suggested monthly report has room for the Blue Shield, Medicare, and Medical Assistance disallowances (for the month and year to date) as well as for the collection ratio for the month and year to date.

Accounts receivable often are not provided by accountants in accounting statements. The sample report provides space for listing the accounts receivable and keeping a monthly summary.

Practice expenses also should be summarized. The monthly financial statement sample breaks down the overhead into several categories, including retirement-plan contributions, medical benefits, and insurance benefits. This expense information can be gathered easily from a check register, which provides columns for the breakdown of expenditures within a practice.

The overhead ratio of the practice is calculated by dividing all expenses (excluding physicians' expenses, as defined above) by the receipts. Note that on the sample, there is room for the overhead percentage, both for the month and the year to date, for determining trends. In addition, these figures are readily available for comparison purposes with other similar practices.

There is also space on the report for the checking-account balance and the

Exhibit 2. Statement for _____, 19___.

	This Month	Year-To-Date	Ratios; Comments	Budgeted for Year
TOTAL CHARGES (per p. 2)	$	$		$
RECEIPTS:				
Office:	$	$		$
Mail:				
TOTAL RECEIPTS	$	$		$
EXPENSES:				
Lay Payroll (Gross)	$	$		$
Payroll Taxes				
Rent				
Prof'l Supplies				
Prof'l Insurance				
Office Supplies & Expenses				
Total Overhead	$	$		$
Doctors' Expenses:				
Salaries				
Pension				
Profit Sharing				
Medical Expense Plan				
Insurance				
Total for Doctors	$	$		$
TOTAL EXPENSES (except depr. & interest)	$	$		$
NET INCOME	$	$		$

Supporting Information for _____, 19___.

CHARGES:	This Month	Year to Date
Hospital #1	$	$
Hospital #2		
Main Office		
Satellite Office		
Dr. M.		
Dr. E.		
Ancillary Personnel		

Checking balance at month-end $ _____

Savings balance $ _____

   Special Savings earmarkings:

Large bills due soon:

Overhead percentage for month   _____%

Overhead percentage year to date   _____%

Accounts Receivable–Beginning Balance $ _____

PLUS: Charges $ _____

      Recoveries   _____

LESS: Receipts   _____

      Write-offs   _____

Accounts Receivable–Ending Balance $ _____

	Month	Year
Overall Collection Ratio	_____%	_____%
Time of Service Collection Ratio	_____%	_____%
Blue Shield Disallowances	$ _____	$ _____
Medicare Disallowances	_____	_____
Medical Assistance Disallowances	_____	_____

Other Information or Comments:

savings-account balance. In addition, if any of the savings funds are specifically earmarked (e.g., retirement-plan contributions or malpractice-insurance premiums), they should be so designated. In addition, large due bills should be listed on this report.

There is also room for special comments from the bookkeeper or office manager. This feature of the report is useful and provides room for important observations; for example, the lease may be up for negotiation or a malpractice-insurance premium may be due in a month.

Notice that everything is broken down for "this month" and for "year to date." Ratios (e.g., payroll as a percentage of gross receipts) can be listed. The final column provides room for the budgeted figure for each item. This column will allow regular comparison of the actual and budgeted figures.

Budget

More and more practices are preparing a budget and finding it useful. Exhibit 3 is a sample budget.

A little thought and common sense are all that is involved. By looking at the figures of the year before and predicting expected growth, inflation, and fee increases, a physician can project a budget, which is especially helpful in making major decisions, such as whether to hire a new physician, raise fees, or incorporate.

EMBEZZLEMENT PROTECTION

Since physicians are generally preoccupied with patient-care matters, and since they often ignore good accounting-control principles, physicians' offices are prime targets for employee theft. In this section, I shall discuss some of the areas of exposure, the symptoms and the prevention of theft and embezzlement in medical offices.

Exposure

Theft and embezzlement characteristically occur in certain areas. Undoubtedly, the most obvious is the pilfering of patients' cash payments. In a loose system, a receptionist or other employee who handles cash could embezzle with little difficulty. Therefore, a sound cash-control system is required.

Checks are another potential source of embezzlement. There are several potential problem areas. (1) An employee asks the physician to sign a blank check "to save time." Once a blank check has been properly signed, the employee can easily cash the check. (2) Checks made to "cash" are easily negotiable and should be avoided, if at all possible, since it is difficult to trace the payee. (3) The forged endorsement of a check by an unauthorized employee can be a problem. (4) Occasionally, there may be insurance overpayments, usually because a patient paid more than the correct share of a bill. In those instances, there is some risk that an employee might embezzle the excess over the amount owed to the physician. The patient would not be suspicious since he or she would no

Exhibit 3. Sample Practice Budget.

	Last Year Actual	This Year Budget	Monthly Average	January 1 through June 30 Year to Date Budget	Year to Date Actual
Services rendered					
Institution	$ 48,000	$ 54,000	$ 4,500	$ 27,000	$ 27,000
Dr. M	115,000	126,000	10,500	63,000	60,000
Dr. E	90,000	108,000	9,000	54,000	56,000
Totals	$253,000	$288,000	$24,000	$144,000	$143,000
Receipts					
Patients	$180,000	$204,000	$17,000	$102,000	$ 99,000
Institution	48,000	54,000	4,500	27,000	27,000
Totals	$228,000	$258,000	$21,500	$129,000	$126,000
Expenses					
Lay payroll (gross)	$ 22,000	$ 24,000	$ 2,000	$ 12,000	$ 13,000
Payroll taxes	2,800	3,000	250	1,500	2,300
Rent	14,000	14,400	1,200	7,200	7,200
Professional supplies	2,800	3,000	250	1,500	1,700
Professional insurance	3,000	3,600	300	1,800	3,600
Office supplies	3,600	4,200	350	2,100	2,200
Professional fees	2,000	2,400	200	1,200	1,400
Medical-expense plan	4,000	4,800	400	2,400	2,000
Professional salaries	140,000	162,000	13,500	81,000	81,000
Pension	16,000	18,000	1,500	9,000	9,000
Profit sharing	15,000	18,000	1,500	9,000	0
Totals	$225,200	$257,400	$21,450	$128,700	$123,400
Balance	$2,800	$600	$50	$300	$2,600

longer be receiving bills. The physician's office might not become aware of the embezzlement since the bill had been fully paid. (5) Petty cash can sometimes allow theft that is not so "petty." Offices sometimes have about $50 available in petty cash, and a programmed and regular embezzling from this account by a determined employee can be costly. Therefore, it is important that there be a review and audit of petty cash periodically by someone other than the persons who handle it on a regular basis. (6) The last problem involves an overstated payroll. In small medical practices, there would be great difficulty in having "phantom employees," but this deception may be easier with large employers, such as municipalities and, possibly, hospitals.

Money is not the only valuable item that can be stolen from a medical practice. Drugs, supplies, and other office materials can be easily taken from an office, particularly if the physician is not often in the office at closing time. The physician should therefore make someone responsible for ordering drugs and other supplies and should also have an independent party, such as another physician or an office manager, review the records from time to time.

There have been instances in which an employee in a medical office has conspired with someone outside of the practice. One example involves an office employee and a salesman. The salesman could charge the practice much more than is reasonable for a specific item and split the profits with the employee. Again, it is important to have someone overseeing the ordering of supplies and drugs to detect major discrepancies.

Symptoms

There are various symptoms of embezzlement that can sound an alarm. The first is a declining collection ratio (receipts divided by net charges). If there is not another logical explanation for the decline, there should be real concern about embezzlement. If there is an unexplained and unusual cash-flow problem in a practice, this sign also should cause concern. Unexplained trends in accounts receivable can also be a warning. For example, if the accounts receivable are dramatically increasing while productivity is relatively constant, one must wonder why collections have not kept pace. Dramatic increases in drug and other supply costs without any other reasonable explanation might also be an alarm.

No one should simply assume or directly suspect an employee of dishonesty without reason. However, an overly conscientious assistant may be the prime candidate for an embezzlement. For example, if a bookkeeper maintains unduly long working hours, never taking time off for illness or vacation, and keeps all financial responsibilities to himself or herself, that person may be covering up an embezzlement. The bookkeeper may be trying to keep everyone else away from the books. Such a person would characteristically resist anyone else's review of the bookkeeping, fearing discovery. Of course, most assistants who fit such work patterns are in reality honest and loyal.

Employees who show unusual emotional stress or who experience personal financial difficulties are other potential candidates. Although it may seem extreme, another symptom would be a dramatic increase in an employee's standard of living.

Constant discrepancies in accounting can signal a problem. Constant difficulties in balancing the checkbook or tallying the "day sheet" so that deposits equal cash and checks also can be warning signs.

A final symptom is a progressively disrespectful attitude of an employee, who may begin to feel so smart having taken so much advantage of the practice, that it may begin to show in the employee's attitude toward work and toward the physicians.

Preventive Measures

There is no foolproof system that can guarantee an employer that the practice is embezzlement free. However, conscientious application of the principles described below go a long way toward preventing theft and embezzlement. Application of these principles makes it more difficult for someone to steal.

A practice should hire well and seek good employees (see Chap. 6). If the physician has done a good job in hiring, there will be less theft and embezzlement. Good hiring procedures require a conscientious follow-up on references and a thorough interview. Once a practice has hired qualified employees, it is then important to cultivate loyalty among them.

All employees who are in any way involved with handling funds should be bonded. One of the key questions to ask on an employment application is whether the prospective employee would refuse to be bonded. If a person refuses to be bonded, he or she should not be hired. Such a refusal probably indicates a past experience that would be on record with the bonding companies.

Also, during the reference check, previous employers should be asked whether that employee was bonded at the previous job. This questioning, can also lead into a discussion of whether the employee handled cash or other valuables and whether the previous employer thinks that the employee did a good job in those areas.

Another preventive measure is to keep control of accounts receivable. Too many practices have no idea what their outstanding accounts receivable are at any given time. A system should be established for computing the accounts receivable on a regular basis.

The increased emphasis on "collection at the source" in medical practices does increase the amount of cash available for theft. Therefore, there is an increased need to assure that a system for recording office charges and collections be as foolproof as possible. One of the outstanding features of a pegboard billing system is embezzlement control. Each office patient would be handed a slip showing the charges incurred and the payments received that day. The receptionist's record of this information would be duplicated simultaneously on a day sheet and the patient's ledger card.

Computer and accounting-machine billing systems can have similar safeguards built into them. A common approach is to have a two- or three-part fee slip with carbon paper on which the entries are copied through to the other forms. The top copy could be handed to the patient as a receipt.

Day sheets should be totaled each day and reconciled with the cash and checks received during the day. In many cases, the receptionist should be expected to handle this closing-out process each day, thereby making that person accountable for the work. However, the bookkeeper or office manager who receives the materials should review the books and deposit the receipts.

Another preventive measure requires outside, periodic surveillance of the books and records, which should be performed by the accountant or medical-management consultant of the practice. This surveillance would not necessarily require a full-scale audit of the books of a medical practice. Letting one's staff know, however, that an outside expert will be reviewing the books periodically on an unannounced basis should prove to be a good preventive measure itself.

No matter what system might be established and how good the physician's outside advisors might be, often the most effective audit control is the physician's own attention. This concern might involve only an occasional few minutes of time in informal and irregular audits. According to no particular schedule, a physician should check isolated portions of an assistant's work. This checking might be coordinated by the accountant or medical-management consultant so that guidelines can be established. For example, the physician might ask the receptionist if he or she can compare each name on the appointment book for a specific date to the names on that day's summary sheet and to the entries on the patients' ledger cards.

Testing should follow no predictable pattern. The major goal is to deter rather than discover theft. An assistant who knows that efforts to steal might be caught by this random process may decide not to risk being caught. For this reason, this "audit" should be performed in the presence of the employees involved. It should be explained to them that it is being done for the physician's and the assistant's protection on the accountant's or consultant's recommendation.

Except for clinic-size practices, a physician should sign every check. This practice helps to discourage a bookkeeper from writing unauthorized checks. In addition, it has the advantage of keeping the physician informed about where the money is spent.

The bookkeeper should be required to fill out each check completely and to attach the bill or invoice for the physician's signature. It is important that incomplete checks never be signed, including blank checks, and that the physician be critical of checks made out to cash or checks made out without an invoice, with incomplete invoices, or with a confusing invoice. The fact that the bookkeeper knows that the physician is signing the checks and will be reviewing the invoices can help serve as a deterrent.

Checks ready for the physician's signature should be placed in a special file, which might be an unusually colored plastic folder so that he or she will readily recognize it. The physician can sign a batch of checks in a few minutes and look at each invoice to see where the money is going.

In group practices, any one of the physicians' signatures should be sufficient for routine expenditures. A policy in which each physician signs checks for a designated period of time (perhaps three months) is desirable. It helps prevent the bookkeeper from avoiding inquiry by spreading similar checks among signers and gives each physician a better feel for the expenses of the practice.

Last, an employer should avoid the possibility of extortion. The two most common situations in which this problem can arise involve tax evasion and personal relationships. This possibility may seem obvious, but it is a problem in too many practices. In cases where extortion has arisen, the physician can be powerless to act against a known embezzler.

5
Organizing of
the Office

Vasilios J. Kalogredis

In this chapter, I shall review the efficient and effective organization of a medical office practice. Space needs and the layout of the office are discussed, as are techniques for scheduling patients and developing telephone and medical records systems.

SPACE NEEDS AND THE PHYSICAL LAYOUT OF THE OFFICE

Plan for Growth

Selecting or designing too small an office can be disastrous to the growth of a practice. The new physician should think in terms of not only what his or her space needs are today but also what they will be in the future (at least during the proposed lease term) before contracting for office space. If the wrong decision is made initially, one may be locked into inadequate space to the detriment of the practice.

In primary care, a solo physician should generally have between 1,200 and 1,500 square feet. Two primary care physicians practicing together should generally have 2,000 square feet, and three should have approximately 2,700 square feet of space.

The term "reception area" is preferable to "waiting room" since it is expected that patients will be seen reasonably on time. Even so, sufficient space must be made available. Having sufficient seating space in the reception area is imperative for good patient relationships. Leaving patients standing (perhaps even in the hallway) should and can be avoided by providing adequate space from the beginning.

In primary care practices, there should be space to accommodate seating for up to three times the number of patients who might be seen in the physician's busiest hour. The exact number of seats needed is primarily a function of the physician's ability to keep to a schedule and the number of people who tend to accompany the patients. Particularly in pediatrics, obstetrics and gynecology, and geriatrics, the numbers of nonpatient visitors in the reception area can be high.

Business Area

Too often, physicians tend to slight the business area when laying out an office. They often underestimate the volume of business and clerical activities and therefore underestimate the amount of space necessary to support these activities. A solo practitioner should provide for a minimum of 200 square feet of business space. This space should be contiguous to the reception area to allow the receptionist to communicate with patients as they enter and leave the office.

A more private space should be made available within the business area, or contiguous to it, for an assistant to handle bookkeeping, collection matters, and other office work.

In most offices, the patients' charts and records are kept in the business area. Because the number of charts continues to increase in any practice, they require considerable space.

Examination Rooms

There should be at least three examining rooms for each physician who has (or is likely to have) office hours in the facility at any one time. A physician may choose to have only two examination rooms at the start, feeling that he or she cannot afford more, but frequently will find that productivity and efficiency thus become limited as the practice grows.

In determining the number of rooms to provide, the physician should consider the current and projected use of assistants. For example, space may be needed for persons other than the physician to handle history-taking, injections, electrocardiograms, dressings, and instructions for the patients.

The sizes of the examination rooms depend only on the physician's individual preferences. Primary care physicians most commonly select rooms that are 8 feet by 10 feet or 10 feet by 10 feet. Important considerations include what the physician is accustomed to and comfortable with and space requirements for equipment, changing clothes, plumbing, and seating for relatives.

To maximize efficiency, all examination rooms should be similarly laid out, equipped, and supplied for basic patient-care purposes. A uniform examination room layout will make things easier to find and will facilitate patient care. Most physicians prefer to have their examination tables away from a wall to enable them to walk around the table. Equipment and supplies should be easily reachable, requiring a minimum amount of movement. The layout depends to a large extent on the physician's work habits.

Nursing Station and Laboratory

A nursing station can be extremely useful to the physician and the nurse. It gives the nurse space where charts can be reviewed, chart entries made or dictated, instructions given, and telephone calls handled. This station usually takes up a small amount of space convenient to the examination rooms being served. One popular arrangement is to design the nursing station as the center of a module that includes several examination rooms surrounding the nursing station.

Laboratory space is also important (even if little diagnostic testing is performed at the office). In some practices, the nursing station and laboratory occupy the same space. This area may also serve as an important medical-supply storage area.

Storage Facilities

Since supplies should never be stacked in hallways, examination rooms, or lavatories, a storage closet is a necessity. In addition, carefully designed cabinets and shelving in space otherwise not being used (e.g., over doors) can provide additional storage space.

Consultation Room

Each physician should have a private office that will serve as a consultation room. Not only is it a place to consult with patients but it should also be available for dictation, telephone calls, paperwork, and personal business. A consultation room need not be large. In most instances, it is not efficient use of space to have a consultation room larger than 12 feet by 12 feet.

Office Appearance

One should be interested in the physical appearance of the office. This consideration is particularly important to a new physician, since the impression he or she makes can be affected by how the office looks. An attractive and tasteful office will influence patients' and other physicians' views of the physician. It can affect the morale and happiness of the staff. It can have a tremendous impact on the physician's attitude. Pleasant surroundings help patients feel more comfortable and make it easier for the physician and staff to work.

Most physicians have little time to master the fine points of design. Yet, physicians often decide to design their offices to save money, since interior designers can be expensive. To help with the design, it is well worth a new physician's time to visit existing offices and local furniture stores and suppliers to get ideas. Whichever approach one follows, it is important that the office reflect the attitude and style of the physician.

Additional Basic Principles of Layout

1. Allow a private entrance and exit for the physician so that he or she does not have to go through the reception area.
2. Keep the entire office on one floor.
3. Place the examination rooms and consultation room(s) near each other (keeping the doors as close to each other as possible to save steps).
4. Make the office square in shape—it is the most efficient layout.

5. Provide separate "public" and "private" bathrooms.
6. Keep the distance from the reception counter to the medical areas as short as possible.
7. Have the reception desk visible from the office entrance.
8. Provide a single "control point" so that the receptionist can monitor patient flow, check in patients, see them as they leave, and conveniently collect money from them.
9. Visit similar medical practices and gather layout ideas from what others have learned. Many management consultants have copies of clients' layouts that are worth reviewing.

SCHEDULING

Although a new physician may initially be more concerned with gaining patients than with how he or she will see them, it is most important that sound scheduling procedures be established from the start. One important scheduling principle should be remembered—develop a schedule that fits the reality of the practice—do not try to have the practice fit a rigid schedule. A schedule should change as the practice patterns and demands change. It should not be stagnant.

Practice Profile

Although it may not be as important initially, as time goes on it will be necessary to know information about the practice profile. With this information, the physician will be able to effectively apply the scheduling principles described below.

The following information should be gathered and periodically examined.

1. *How many cancellations and "no-shows" are there?* Putting a single line through these patients' names in the appointment book when they are identified will make it easy to count them later on. Patterns are important. What types of patients are not showing up—new patients, annual-checkup patients, others? By reviewing this information, the physician can detect and then correct problems as they arise. For example, if many of the no-shows are annual-checkup patients, the problem may be that they are scheduled too far in advance.

2. *How many emergency or walk-in patients are there?* Are there any apparent patterns? Are there more walk-ins on one day of the week or among patients with a similar problem? The physician can keep track of such patients by entering their names in the appointment book with a colored pencil (e.g., red if black lead is used for the others). This system makes the information easier to tabulate.

3. *How much can be done by a nonphysician (e.g., electrocardiograms, blood pressures, injections, and history-gathering)?* The physician may do some or all of these things at the beginning. However, as he or she gets busier, ancillary help can perform many of these tasks and free the physician for matters that require a certain level of training and experience.

Keeping on Time

A major problem in many medical practices is the physician's failure to arrive at the office on time, thereby causing lengthy and unpleasant delays. It is important to establish priorities early. The first priority is obviously the emergency patient. However, it is a mistake to ignore the obligation to the regularly scheduled patient.

In many instances, the patients' major complaints are not about the fee or the quality of care. Instead, patients frequently complain that they were not treated properly in the office because they had to wait an inappropriate length of time to be seen. This situation creates the feeling that the "doctor does not care about my time. I am losing time from work and paying a baby-sitter when I come to the office." These delays do little to foster patient goodwill.

At the same time, it is important to recognize that the practice will grow. As it grows, the starting time for office hours may have to change. For example, if a new physician has been able to start office hours at 9:00 A.M. but becomes busier at the hospital and is never able to return to the office before 9:30 A.M., there is no reason to continue to schedule patients for 9:00 A.M. This example illustrates how the schedule can be changed to fit the practice instead of attempting to fit the practice into the schedule.

Wave Versus Stream Schedules

There are two basic methods of scheduling in a medical office. The first method is the stream schedule, for example, one patient at 10:00 A.M., one at 10:15, one at 10:30, and one at 10:45. The second method is the wave schedule, which would schedule all four patients at 10:00 A.M.

There are definite advantages and disadvantages to either approach. The stream schedule may minimize waiting time for patients but may be inefficient for the physician. For example, if the 10:00 patient does not show up, the doctor has 15 unproductive minutes. If that patient is 10 minutes late, the doctor is 10 minutes behind schedule. Also, the stream system assumes that each patient's visit will be exactly the same duration, which is not realistic.

The theory behind the wave schedule is that by scheduling all patients at the beginning of each hour, unexpected changes will average out, so that the doctor will tend to finish on time at the end of the hour (which is also good for the patient). For example, if one patient shows up late, another can be seen instead. Although a short visit may become a longer visit, some of the scheduled longer visits may end up being shorter than expected. The wave schedule does have problems. Patients in the waiting room may become upset when they find that they all have the same appointment time, especially when some wait and others do not.

Many practices use a modified wave schedule that serves as a workable compromise between the stream and the wave approaches. For example, a physician who sees four patients per hour may schedule two patients at 10:00 A.M., one at 10:30, and one at 10:45. This system is a popular version of the modified wave schedule. Half of the patients are scheduled at the beginning of the hour, with the other half spread throughout the second half-hour.

Exhibit 1. Methods of Scheduling.

	Name	Stream Schedule Telephone Number	"N" If New
10:00			
10:15			
10:30			
10:45			
	Name	Wave Schedule Telephone Number	"N" If New
10:00			
10:00			
10:00			
10:00			
	Name	Modified Wave Schedule Telephone Number	"N" If New
10:00			
10:00			
10:30			
10:45			

A physician should be willing to experiment with different modifications of the wave schedule. Each physician's practice is somewhat different, and the physician must determine what best fits his or her work patterns. However, some application of the wave approach is well worth exploring. One important concept to keep in mind when working with a wave schedule is never to schedule more patients for one block of time than one has examining rooms to handle. For example, if the physician has three examination rooms, no more than three patients should be scheduled at once, so each patient can wait for the physician in a separate room. Exhibit 1 illustrates the three approaches.

Grouping Procedures

It is a well-known principle of management that one is more efficient and effective when performing one task repetitively during a specific period. Patients who require a common procedure should be scheduled together. This practice should be reviewed from time to time as the physician develops a schedule that is most suitable.

Other physicians find it useful to group different procedures together. For example, an internist who is involved with numerous routine physical examinations may find that he or she can perform two or three short follow-up visits at the same time as the routine physical examination by having ancillary personnel perform parts of the routine examination.

In summary, give serious throught to how one works best, continue to experiment with various approaches, and prepare a schedule that best fits one's own needs.

Open Times

In primary care, open time slots in the appointment book are important since they allow time for unexpected tasks, such as telephone calls and emergency patients.

These open times can be staggered throughout the work week, designated on the basis of information gathered in the practice profile. For example, most primary care physicians find that Monday mornings are the most hectic, with many unscheduled patients needing to be seen that day, often in the afternoon. If the physician is working under these circumstances, more open slots should be available on Mondays than on other days. It is generally preferable to set aside open time slots in the next to the last hour of the day. Assuming a 9:00 A.M. to 5:00 P.M. day, this approach would entail leaving open the slots between 3:00 and 4:00 P.M. This practice allows time to fit people in but does not lock the physician into an unduly extended day.

Designing the Appointment Book

Too many practices simply purchase a printed appointment book and use it uncritically. In many instances, the appointment book does not fit the practice's needs. Since printing is relatively inexpensive, the physician should design his own appointment book, giving thought to the various scheduling principles discussed in this section. In addition, by using loose-leaf notebook pages, one can develop an appointment book that will be easy to update and change from time to time as the practice develops and changes. The physician should color code the appointment book. The easiest way is to have an assistant in the office pencil in the appropriate colors in the appropriate slots. The color coding will indicate what types of patients should go into what types of slots (see Exhibit 2).

Exhibit 2. Sample Appointment Book.

G. T. Anderson, M.D., General Medicine			
	Name	*Telephone Number*	*"N" If New*
9:00 Physical examination			
9:00 Checkup			
9:15 Checkup			
9:30 Checkup			
10:00 Checkup			
10:00 Checkup			
10:00 Checkup			
10:30 Checkup			
10:30 Checkup			
10:45 Checkup			
11:00 Emergency			
11:00 Emergency			
11:00 Checkup			
11:30 Call-back time			
11:45 Checkup			
11:45 Checkup			

TELEPHONES AND PAGING DEVICES

Once a physician has selected the office location, a telephone number and a notice in the business directory under his practice specialty should be arranged with the local telephone company.

Many physicians find it helpful to have their new telephone lines hooked up at least a month before the actual starting date of the practice. By so doing, potential patients and referring physicians may speak with either the office assistant or the answering service regarding possible appointments and other matters.

An answering service is a necessity in a primary-care medical practice, but it is sometimes difficult to find a good one. The best approach is to ask other local physicians if they have been satisfied with the service they are using. Several answering services should be contacted and their services evaluated before a decision is made. It is preferable to obtain a service with numerous medical clients. A desirable service is one that understands the requirements of the practice for patient care (particularly emergencies). Costs vary dramatically from area to area. The most important point is to select a service considered excellent by colleagues.

Some physicians use answering machines instead of answering services. In general, such machines are not as well received by people as a good answering service. However, they do provide an acceptable alternative if a good answering service is not available.

A solo practitioner, just starting out in practice, generally should arrange for two incoming telephone lines, one of which is listed and automatically transfers a call to the second line if the listed number is busy. The physician should also arrange for one private or outgoing line. The telephone is important to the success of a practice. If the office cannot be reached, patients may be lost, care may suffer, and problems may arise. More than one line is worth the cost because the result is easier access to the physician's office.

Push-button telephones are preferred over dial telephones because they consume less time and cause fewer mistakes.

The telephone company provides other services that are often free. One is a busy-signal check. The telephone company will record the number of busy signals received during specific periods of a specific test week. This can help the physician determine whether additional telephone lines are needed. A busy-signal check should be run at least once a year. Another service is the peak load test. The telephone company will record the number of incoming telephone calls made to a telephone number during specific times of a given test week. This service can help the physician determine how to assign responsibility for telephone-answering among the office personnel. Neither test breaches the confidentiality of the telephone conversations.

Answering the Telephone

It is important that telephone calls be answered promptly. In addition, no person should be kept on hold for more than 30 seconds. As a practice grows, it is important to have a primary telephone answerer and a designated back-up answerer who can take over when the primary answerer is busy.

Staff should be trained to answer the phone politely and pleasantly. A telephone caller's first impression of a physician's office is influenced by the voice, attitude, and friendliness of the person who answers. Telephone etiquette makes a difference. The receptionist should not answer the telephone by saying, the telephone number (e.g., "Hello, 3456"). Each call should be answered with the physician's name and the receptionist's name, for example: "Dr. Jones's office, Chris speaking." Most callers find an impersonal response unpleasant and unprofessional. The telephone answerer should always give the caller an opportunity to explain whether an emergency exists.

Staff should be trained to handle questions and comments that commonly arise. Common responses should be written down so that the telephone answerer will be able to answer them easily. For example, policy regarding payment at the time of service and questions regarding insurance and how long the first visit might take could all be handled in this fashion.

Screening Calls

It is important that the physician establish a system for screening telephone calls so that only calls that require a direct response by the physician are forwarded. A physician just starting out may choose to handle many of these calls personally because the practice often is not busy and there may be limited help. However, as the practice grows, it will become important for calls to be screened well.

A telephone priority listing should be prepared. The following categories are appropriate:

1. Must get through to the doctor immediately.
2. Must interrupt the doctor for evaluation and instructions.
3. Doctor will return the call after the present patient is seen.
4. Call can be transferred to nurse or other assistant.
5. Doctor will return call during his or her normal call-back time.
6. Hold for doctor's instructions and operator's call back.
7. Receptionist may handle.

The physician, working with the staff, should continually examine which calls are to be assigned to each category. A separate notebook page listing examples should be established for each category. This list is not intended as a reference book for the receptionist to use while on the phone. There will be no time for that. However, it will help educate new employees before they begin, and it will help assure consistency. Some calls will have to go through to the physician out of medical necessity. However, the physician should not forget the relative priorities of the emergency and the regularly scheduled patient.

Telephone Hour and Call-back Times

Many primary care physicians find a telephone hour helpful. Some schedule the hour at the beginning of the day and find that it reduces the overall number of calls, especially during normal office hours when the lines are most in use. Patients must be instructed to call during the telephone hour.

Call-back times are also helpful. By being told that the physician will call during a designated time period, for example, between 3 and 4 P.M., the patient will not have to stay home all day waiting for the call, and the physician will find the patient home when the call is made.

Call-back Lists

Call-back slips or a call-back list can help the physician make patient calls during the day. Many physicians prefer a combined list to individual slips, since all the patients' names and telephone numbers are on a single piece of paper. The physician can more easily judge whom to call first. With the slips, there is always the possibility that a particular message might be lost. In either case, it is important for the staff to pull the medical record for the physician before any call is made so all the information necessary to make a fully informed decision will be available.

Buying Telephone Equipment

It can be financially advantageous to buy telephone equipment instead of renting it from the public telephone company. However, most physicians starting out in practice should delay purchasing telephone equipment until they need five or more pieces of telephone equipment and they are certain of their needs. Only then should they evaluate private telephone systems and consider purchasing one.

The most important considerations are the service that the private telephone company will provide and the company's viability. Present users of the systems under consideration should be asked about their experiences with the company. In evaluating the cost, the physician should note that the top line of the standard telephone bill, "equipment and service," is the fee that will be reduced by buying equipment. In most instances, the monthly payments for a four- or five-year loan will approximate the service and equipment charges that are being paid to the public telephone company.

Beeper Services

Many physicians find that a long-range paging device ("beeper") is an invaluable tool for ensuring their accessibility to patients. Beepers can be either purchased or leased. As electronic equipment such as these long-range pagers becomes less expensive, purchase of beepers becomes preferable.

If a beeper is purchased, a physician can expect to spend about $200. The physician would then have to lease access to a transmitter, which would cost approximately $10 per month. However, the radius that a purchased beeper covers may be smaller than that of a leased beeper, so the physician should check the beeper's range with the distributor of the device.

Generally speaking, companies offering beepers are listed in the "yellow pages" of the telephone book under "radio paging and signaling service—common carrier." Companies that list telephone-radio communication usually have beepers as well. The Federal Communications Commission licenses companies to offer beepers and public utility commissions regulate prices for leasing beepers and broadcast time.

A leased beeper can cost between $20 and $30 per month, depending on its range; the price usually includes insurance coverage and battery replacement. The physician should investigate companies in the local area and speak with other professionals to determine whether leasing or buying a beeper will be most beneficial.

Two types of beepers are generally used: voice and tone. The voice beeper is usually more expensive and allows a verbal 13-second message. It is limited, since only those who know the number can call. Often, the physician will have a secretary or hospital operator call him. A tone beeper usually signals the physician to call the office or answering service for a message.

Many beepers are tied into computer systems that activate the beeper tone. Some beepers have dual-address systems. With this system, a short beep may signal a physician to call the office, and a long beep may signal a call to the hospital. Beepers may also have a memory component that allows the physician to turn the beeper off and activate the memory at a later time to determine if there have been messages.

Beeper systems may also offer short-range, long-range, and itinerant service. A short-range beeper often covers an area of one city. A long-range beeper covers an average radius of 35 miles. Itinerant beepers may cover a number of cities in different states. This system works when beeper companies agree to form integrated systems and allow one company's system to tie into another.

MEDICAL CHARTS AND RECORDS

Designing Preprinted Charts

The physician must remember that the real purpose of a medical record is to document the patient's medical history. Serious thought should be given to the information that the physician desires most and how it can best be recorded and stored. It is a serious mistake merely to buy plain manila folders, put plain white pieces of paper in the chart, and consider that effort a sufficient medical record.

A physician should design personal medical charts and records so that they suit individual needs and style. The folders should thus be preprinted with space for such information as allergic reactions, key historical data, a problem list, and a check list for preventive care. In addition, the inside pages of a medical record might also be preprinted. Some pediatricians use charts with inner folders that are color coded according to the patient's age; for example, birth to one year might be pink; one to three years might be yellow, and so on. Each of these color-coded inner folders is also preprinted, with space for the important diagnostic laboratory and radiologic results usually ordered for patients of that age.

Although many physicians consider the problem-oriented medical record approach (POMR) too complex for office practice, many have simplified and adapted the problem-oriented format for their own preprinted charts.

Financial information should not be placed in patients' medical records. This practice helps to keep the charts thin and simple.

It is preferable to use medical records that measure 8½ by 11 inches. Smaller records will not easily accept standard-size letters and reports without folding. It is often useful to set aside a full-size sheet of paper inside the folder for laboratory results. Many physicians make this sheet a distinctive color, different from that of the other sheets in the folder, and tape the laboratory results on the sheet chronologically for easy reference. Others create a ruled table, or flow sheet, and list successive determinations of each test as a row of results in chronologic order. Either method is preferable to throwing the laboratory reports into the folder, where they become disorganized and occasionally lost.

The most efficient filing system for practices with less than 10,000 charts is an alphabetical rather than a numerical system. With a numerical filing system, an extra step is involved. An assistant has to take the patient's name to an index file and look up the patient's chart number before going to the record file. If the index card is lost or not available, it will be almost impossible to find the patient's chart. When patients' charts are filed alphabetically, there are no intermediate steps. In addition, most people are more comfortable with alphabetical systems because they are more familiar with them.

Color Coding

Color coding is useful in chart filing. It is aesthetically pleasing and prevents misfiled charts. Charts should be color coded by the first and second letters of a patient's last name (or in a numerical system, by the first and second numbers). Since most misfiling is done according to the second letter of the last name, it is important that both the first and second letters be color coded. If a chart is misfiled, it can be easily noticed because the color(s) will not match the adjacent charts.

In addition, the physician should color code according to the year that the patient was last seen. For example, the first time a patient comes into the office, a color tape specific for that year should be placed on the chart. Nothing more need be done until the following year. If the patient comes in the following year, that year's color tape should replace the original color tape. Several years later, when filing space is limited, inactive charts can be recognized by color and pulled from the active files for long-term storage elsewhere.

There are two major methods of filing the standard-size chart. One is in drawers, and the other is on open shelves. Open shelves are preferable. They provide a larger file capacity in less floor space. The standard five-shelf cabinet is 3 feet wide and 1 foot deep and requires 3 square feet of floor space. Stacked above those 3 square feet of floor space are 15 square feet of shelf capacity. Standard five-drawer files are generally 27 inches deep and 14 inches wide. To open the drawer, one needs an additional 24 inches of floor space. Floor-to-ceiling shelves should be used to take advantage of the available space. The middle sections of those file shelves are the ones used for the active files. The bottom and top shelves can be used for storing inactive files.

Charts should be divided into three major categories: active, inactive, and dead. No specific time defines how long a chart is active. It is a function of the practice's space, specialty, volume, and continuity. One rough guideline is to remove charts from the active file when there has not been a visit for three years or more. However, in some practices charts are removed every six or 12 months.

Inactive charts should be kept in the office if there is space, for example, at the bottom or the top of the floor-to-ceiling files. They might also be kept in the basement of the office building or in the physician's house.

Dead charts do not necessarily refer to dead patients but to patients that have not been seen for many years (10 years is often used as a guideline). The dead charts often are stored somewhere other than in the office. To maintain access to the dead file, one can keep the patients' account cards and place a black mark on them to indicate that they are in the dead file. Dead charts are often kept in inexpensive warehouse space. This system is generally preferable to microfilming, which is too expensive and complicated for the great majority of practices. Medical records should be kept forever. Although statutes of limitation restrict liability in some cases, there are exceptions. The safest approach is indefinite storage.

Several other office rules should be established for medical charts.

1. Charts should be refiled daily, including laboratory reports, radiology reports, and correspondence. It is important to designate one person in the office for this task and see that it is performed regularly. Charts that are not filed cannot be found quickly when needed.

2. There should be only a small number of designated chart locations in the office. For example, one should be in the physician's office, where charts ready for refiling can be placed, and one should be in the business office. In addition, there should be designated chart locations where charts that are still being used for typing purposes or billing can be placed so that assistants know where to look for them if they do not find them in the record file.

3. Charts should always be visible. If they are kept in desk drawers or in closets, they will easily become lost.

4. Medical charts should not leave the office.

6
Managing Office Personnel

Vasilios J. Kalogredis

Nothing is more vital to the efficiency of a practice than good office personnel. A physician can experience a great deal of aggravation and dissatisfaction if the office is staffed by employees who are either unsatisfactory or who have not been well trained. In light of this possibility, personnel management merits the time and energy of the physician.

RECRUITING AND HIRING OFFICE ASSISTANTS

New assistants must be conscientiously and methodically recruited. Hiring should never be approached casually. A specific procedure for employing new assistants should be established and should never be bypassed, even if a promising applicant has been identified.

Recruiting

Recruiting, the search for capable applicants, is the first step. The goal should be to attract as many satisfactory applicants as possible, since the physician can never be sure where the right employee will be found. The larger the applicant pool, the better the chances of finding an excellent employee.

One reliable approach is to advertise in area newspapers. In suburban areas, advertisements should be placed in the city newspapers as well as in local suburban papers. A physician should create an attractive advertisement. For example, the following advertisement will not attract much interest: "Med. Sec. sought by med. off." The following advertisement has a much better chance of attracting talented candidates and standing out among others in the newspaper:

A YOUNG AND GROWING PRIMARY CARE PRACTICE SEEKS A MEDICAL ASSISTANT FOR FULL-TIME WORK. SALARY OPEN.

Note that the starting salary for the job is purposely left vague. The absence of a specific salary in the advertisement is preferable, especially for smaller offices.

73

Employment agencies are another source of applicants, although experiences with them are often disappointing. Generally speaking, any person recommended by an employment agency should be put through the same screening processes as other applicants. In addition, the physician should be aware that a commission is charged when someone is hired from an employment agency, but that does not mean that one should not hire through an agency.

Physicians often offer a position to someone already employed at another medical office or at the hospital. Too often, physicians conclude mistakenly that someone whom they have seen from time to time working in the hospital would be ideal for their own practice. Unfortunately, this casual knowledge of the person often causes the physician to bypass the planned recruiting and hiring procedure. Because this casual approach often results in problems later on, it is important that the recruiting and hiring process never be cut short just because of personal knowledge of a person.

Some educational institutions have excellent programs for training medical assistants and can serve as a source of applicants. Moreover, many of them have work-study arrangements, which allow physicians to observe student applicants at work.

Screening

Other than applicants for office manager, persons interested in a position should be required to make a telephone call so a preliminary screening can be conducted. In an established practice, it is preferable that someone other than the physician handle this preliminary work. This person might be the office manager or the senior assistant. For a new physician who is just starting out in practice, the physician or the physician's spouse would be the best person to handle this preliminary screening.

One can determine a lot about people over the telephone. Do they have a pleasant voice on the telephone? Do they appear to have the basic qualities needed to handle the specific job? What about their personalities? These initial reactions often need to be verified, but they do help to eliminate people who should not be called in for a personal interview.

Although a new physician will probably not have this opportunity, it is helpful to have an assistant handle the initial recruiting. One reason is to spare the physician's time. Another is to get the assistants more involved in the success of the office. New employees will be most valuable if they are accepted by the rest of the staff. Employees will spend more time working together than they will spend working with the physician. Because of this consideration, it is important that a compatible staff be developed.

Initial Interview

In an office where there is already an employee who can help in the interviewing process, it is preferable for the initial interview to be scheduled when the physician is not present. The initial interview could be set for a time when the staff is less busy than usual or during nonoffice hours. The major purpose of the initial meeting with the staff is to allow them to evaluate the applicant's personality. In addition, it gives the applicant a chance to see what the office is like. For a new physician with no employees, it is obvious that he or she will have to conduct the initial interview. However, the second person hired might be interviewed by the first person hired.

Before the first interview, the applicant should fill out a preprinted application form (see Exhibit 1). The form need not be extensive. It should merely provide basic information for discussion and for checking references. It is important to ask the reasons for leaving previous jobs and what was liked and disliked about them. These answers are useful for testing the applicant's employment history and honesty. It is helpful if the written application requests information about outside interests, the last book read, and other personal questions. The application should ask what salary the applicant hopes to receive. It is easier to evaluate what to offer when one knows what the other person is seeking.

It is important for the interview to be a two-way discussion. The interviewer should determine the applicant's experience for the position and get a sense of the applicant's personality.

Skill Testing

Whenever possible, an applicant should be given a brief skill test to determine ability; it may also help to test for honesty. Many employers are surprised when persons who claimed to be excellent at certain tasks actually begin work and are not able to handle the job.

A short test of typing skill is rather simple. For example, a tape can be dictated for each applicant to transcribe. Copy typing should be part of the skill test if it is needed on the job. One can determine an applicant's accuracy, neatness, and speed rather easily. A bookkeeping test can also be quite helpful.

Second Interview

Anyone sincerely interested in a position should be willing to come in for a second interview. Usually, only a few need return for a second visit. This interview always should involve the physician. People often look very different the second time they are seen, and favorable first impressions may be quickly deflated during the second interview.

The second interview should involve a discussion about the applicant's thought patterns, previous work experience, previous employers, what was liked or disliked about the jobs, reasons for leaving earlier jobs, and reasons why this position is attractive. In addition, the physician should be sure that the job description, personnel policies, and benefits are understood so that the applicant can more clearly evaluate the job. Although no offer should be made during this interview, all details (including the initial salary offer, if all else goes well) should be discussed to determine if they would be acceptable.

This interview need last only about half an hour. Several interviews should be scheduled in succession to make best use of the physician's time. When the second interview has been completed, the applicant should be thanked for returning and given assurance of notification about the outcome within five to seven days.

Exhibit 1. Application for Employment.

DATE _____

NAME _____   TELEPHONE # _____

ADDRESS _____   SOC.SEC. #_____

_____DATE OF BIRTH_____

IN CASE OF EMERGENCY NOTIFY: _____
                                                (Name)

_____
              (Address)   (Telephone #)

EDUCATION-Please list schools attended, years attended and fields of concentration.
List any degrees received.

WORK EXPERIENCE-List the names and addresses of all your former employers,
beginning with the most recent. Please indicate your starting and leaving salary,
the reason you left and the name and phone number of your immediate supervisor
at each position. Continue the list on the reverse side, if necessary.

What Salary Would You Expect for This Position? _____per_____.

How Would You Get to Work?_____.

Date Employment Can Begin_____. Would You Object to

  Being Bonded? _____.

Outside Interests, Activities, Etc. _____

_____

_____

Book Last Read: _____

76

Even if one of the applicants clearly stands out, the position should not be offered at that time. No one should be hired until references have been checked after the second interview.

Reference Checks

No applicant should be hired without checking references. At the very minimum, the physician should communicate with the two previous employers. Reference checks should always be made by telephone and never by letter. Written references are generally worthless. People are hesitant to make derogatory comments on paper.

An applicant may request that references not be checked, since the present employer is unaware of the search for new employment. These requests should be respected until it is time to offer the position, but a physician should never hire without checking references. Prospective applicants must be told that their references will have to be checked before they are hired. The physician must insist on the right to protection provided by checking references.

By checking references using telephone calls, one can detect hesitations, inflections, and enthusiastic comments that would not be as noticeable on a piece of paper.

The reference check should include the following specific questions:

1. How long was the person employed by you?
2. What was the starting and ending salary?
3. When did the person begin and end employment?
4. Why did the person leave?
5. What did the job involve?
6. Were these duties performed to your satisfaction?
7. Was the person punctual?
8. Was absenteeism a problem?
9. Did family or personal matters affect work performance?
10. Did the person handle money for you? Was the person bonded?
11. What were the person's best and worst qualities?
12. Would you rehire the person?

These questions should lead to other questions. In some instances, the answers to these questions can be compared with the applicant's answers for accuracy.

Reference checks might only take a few minutes, but they are important minutes, since they reduce the chances of making a serious hiring mistake.

Hiring

If the reference check provides satisfactory results, the position can be offered on the terms discussed at the second interview. If the applicant accepts the job, the remaining applicants should be notified and thanked for their interest. Information on these applicants should be kept on file since several of them may be excellent prospective employees for future positions.

RECRUITING AND HIRING FOR A NEW PRACTICE

Physicians starting a new practice should follow the basic procedures described above. However, there are some additional guidelines that are helpful in a new practice.

In many primary care practices, the first person hired should handle the reception desk, the telephone, billing, and bookkeeping. This person need not be a nurse. In most instances, this person should be hired on a full-time basis. If this person is working full time, he or she can help provide appropriate coverage for the telephone and the office. Full-time workers help the new physician to be available, which is important for developing the practice. It is important to hire the right person to get the practice off to a good start. When hiring this person, the physician should keep in mind that this employee is likely to become the manager of the practice after others are hired.

In many primary care practices, a part-time nurse, who may be a licensed practical nurse or lesser trained person, will be needed to work some or all of the office hours with the physician. This person may not be needed at the beginning, and the original full-time employee may be able to help enough for some time.

Many physicians consider asking their spouses to assist in the office at the beginning to save money. In many instances, the spouse employee is a serious mistake. Even if not necessary for the first month or so, within a short time another employee will be needed in the practice. As this time approaches, the spouse and the physician have to make serious decisions. It is difficult for other employees to work comfortably with the physician's spouse. It then becomes necessary for the spouse to be less actively involved in the practice. When this situation arises, it is often a traumatic experience for the spouse, who now feels less needed and therefore unhappy about the change. Because of this possibility, it is generally preferable to hire another person from the start and avoid what otherwise might become a difficult situation.

A physician starting off in solo practice should recruit this full-time employee several months before starting practice. This person can begin working a month or so before the practice is ready to open. The assistant could help with many of the start-up functions, such as telephone hook-up, answering the telephones for appointments, and setting up and coordinating furniture and equipment.

Most such employees have some medical-office experience. Age is not as important a factor. Experience is the key ingredient. After all, most new physicians have little or no practical knowledge of how to manage a practice and need a capable employee for assistance.

Six criteria are particularly important for any employee. Many of them are subjective. They are, in decreasing order of importance:

1. Loyalty
2. Stability
3. Enthusiasm
4. Judgment
5. Intelligence
6. Technical ability

Many are surprised that the most important characteristics are the most subjective. Others are surprised that intelligence and technical ability rank at the bottom of the list. The low level of ranking these characteristics is in no way intended to demean employees in medical offices. Medical-office employees must have a certain level of intelligence and technical ability to get the job done. However, once that basic level is present, the employee's performance depends more heavily on intangible factors. It is much more important to hire a pleasant, conscientious, loyal, and efficient person than the world's fastest typist, who may have a terrible personality or attitude.

Assigning Responsibilities

At the beginning, the question of dividing duties among the staff may not be a problem, since only one employee may be involved. However, once a second employee is hired, it is important to put down on paper in a job description exactly what each employee's responsibilities are. Jobs tend to get accomplished in a more efficient manner when they are specifically assigned to employees. This system allows the physician to discuss problems in specific areas with the people responsible. In addition, it gives the employee involved a chance to develop some expertise and satisfaction in the job.

Job descriptions should not encourage the syndrome of "this is not my job." In medical offices, it is important that there be at least some ability for staff to cross cover each other during vacations, illness, or other times. For this reason, it is important to describe primary, secondary, and tertiary responsibilities for all employees, including on everyone's job description "all other tasks as may be needed from time to time within the office."

Nonphysician Practitioners

Much of what a physician does really could be done by someone else. The difference between an efficient and an inefficient practice often is a direct result of the physician's intelligent use of other personnel. For example, in handling the telephone, a good screening process will allow nonphysician staff to answer some telephone calls. Having capable employees to handle some history-taking and injections can also greatly assist the physician.

At the beginning of the practice, the physician may do all these things. Unfortunately, this practice often creates bad habits that may be difficult to change later on. The physician's use of ancillary personnel often depends on his or her philosophy. Medical-management consultants urge that the physician critically evaluate what could be done by others so that he or she can concentrate on activities appropriate to training in medical school.

The use of nurse practitioners and physician's assistants is growing, although not as swiftly as some would like. A new physician starting from scratch would be ill-advised to hire a nurse practitioner or a physician's assistant until he or she is certain that such an employee is affordable. However, as volume increases, the physician should consider using a nurse practitioner or physician's assistant. The physician must be careful to check the state laws as well as the policies of the local hospitals. Some hospitals limit what they allow a nurse practitioner or physician's assistant to do. Chapter 12 contains additional information about nurse practitioners and physician's assistants.

PROBATIONARY PERIOD

Even with all the efforts described above, the physician can never really be sure how well a person will work until that person is an employee. Because of this uncertainty, it is important that a probationary period be established, preferably for a 90-day period. This probationary period ensures evaluation of the employee's performance and a meeting with him or her to discuss job performance.

The probationary period is an integral part of avoiding having marginally satisfactory employees. Without this evaluation, many employers would allow the marginally satisfactory employee to continue by default. By establishing a definite time for reviewing performance, both sides are aware that there will be an evaluation and that the employee might be terminated if performance is not satisfactory. The use of a probationary period does not obligate the practice to employ the person for three months. If it is obvious early on that performance is unsatisfactory, the employee can be terminated.

COMPENSATION

Retaining good employees is so important that the physician should be willing to pay generous salaries to keep them. There is no "right" salary for all employees in each position. In many well-run offices, several key employees might be overpaid in comparison with others. However, they are often worth their salaries because they contribute to the efficiency, atmosphere, and productivity in those offices.

There are ways of helping determine what fair starting salaries might be for positions in a medical office. Among the sources are the local employment bureau, local hospitals, and other physicians. In addition, the physician's advisors (medical-management consultants, attorneys, or accountants) are often excellent sources. Most fringe benefits have little or no desirable impact on employees. The most important benefit is medical and hospitalization insurance.

Regular review and evaluation of staff performance is most important. These aspects of employment help motivate employees and allow the employer and employee to discuss problems. It is important that review and evaluation be done at least once a year and that they be tied in to the salary adjustment period.

It is important that these review meetings be called "performance review" and not "salary review" sessions. They can be used to discuss raises, but it should be stressed that they are held to discuss performance.

It is generally preferable that reviews be conducted at the same time every year for each employee, for example, in December for January 1 raises. A single review date for all employees helps avoid forgetting someone. Some offices use the anniversary date of the employee's hiring. This system can work well, but it increases the odds that some review sessions will not be timely.

By having the review sessions at the same time for all employees, the physician can take best advantage of the motivational aspects of salary raises. Raises should be given on the basis of merit. If two employees are working side by side and not doing equally good jobs, the more satisfactory employee should get a larger raise. If both employees get the same raise, even though they are not performing equally well, the better employee might lose a motivational incentive.

An employer's evaluation should be made clear. During the discussion with each employee, the physician should state that this year's raise is an excellent one since an excellent job has been done or is low since there is some dissatisfaction with performance.

The important point is to establish a policy, communicate it to the staff, and follow it. If the policy is followed, the physician can avoid requests for raises throughout the year by saying "your fine performance will be reflected during the next raise period."

Bonuses to staff employees should be avoided, including Christmas bonuses. Bonuses are not really appreciated but become an expected part of compensation. For example, a Christmas bonus given in the spirit of the season soon becomes expected compensation in succeeding years. It would be more meaningful if small gifts were given to employees at Christmas time.

A new physician can establish this policy from the beginning. A practice that has been paying Christmas bonuses can drop them if the matter is handled appropriately. For example, if bonuses have been paid every Christmas and a practice wants to stop that policy, it will be important to pay the Christmas bonus for the upcoming December. At or shortly after that date, the practice should inform the staff that there will be no further bonuses but that a salary adjustment will be made for each employee in the following year. This approach is fair to the staff and should make the announcement more acceptable.

Federal and state laws require that overtime pay must be provided for medical-office employees who work over 40 hours in any week. There are state and federal exceptions to this rule, few of which will apply to a new solo practitioner's office. It is thus important that specific time sheets or cards be kept for each employee listing the hours that they work, even if they are salaried employees. Although there have not been many labor audits, there have been some, and they can be difficult and painful to a practice that is deemed not to have paid for overtime work.

Since the federal and state laws in this area constantly change, the physician should check frequently with his or her advisors.

OFFICE STAFF MEETINGS

Office staff meetings should be held regularly, at least once a month, even if there is only one employee and one physician. It is important to keep the lines of communication open. As a practice grows, it becomes even more important to communicate with the staff in regular meetings. Office staff meetings make employees more loyal to the practice, and they provide ideas and information for improving the practice.

OFFICE POLICY AND PROCEDURE MANUALS

It is important to set specific policies and rules for the staff and to write them down in an office-policy manual. Exhibit 2 is a sample office-policy manual. Having such rules in writing can help avoid problems. It is better to make policy for anticipated problems before they arise than to make decisions once the problem develops. For example, it is easier to determine a fair policy for extended sick leave in advance than to wait for an employee to have a prolonged illness.

A procedure manual should describe how specific tasks in the office are to be handled. Procedures for screening telephone calls, completing insurance forms, and collecting bills should all be written in a procedure manual. One advantage is to prevent the practice from being overly dependent on any one employee. The procedure manual also helps train new staff, and it may prevent mistakes by the regular staff. The procedure manual need not be fancy—typed pages placed in a notebook are sufficient.

PERSONNEL MOTIVATION

Staff motivation is important. In this section, I shall discuss the principles of personnel management that affect motivation. Further discussion of personnel management may be found in Chapter 14.

The Golden Rule

For management purposes, the Golden Rule should be interpreted: "To manage as you would want to be managed and to supervise as you would want to be supervised." The best leaders are those who follow management's Golden Rule.

Motivation

Motivation is a complex process. Each person has changing psychologic and physiologic needs that affect how he or she responds to supervision and direction. One person may not be able to motivate another, but a manager can call upon the employee's internal drive by creating alternatives that appeal to his or her needs. There are several basic concepts that allow managers to provide the best leadership and motivation for their employees.

Praise should be given when appropriate and as often as possible. There is no better way to make a person feel important than to give sincere compliments. A compliment is recognition that the other person has done something worthy of praise.

"Thank you" are two of the most powerful words in the English language. How simple they are to say for a job well done. Unfortunately, they are too seldom said.

A physician or office manager should be available for frank and unhurried discussions of staff problems and complaints. More and more practices name an office manager to fill this role. This approach should not mean that the physician does not get an opportunity to listen to the staff's ideas. However, it does delegate much of the preliminary work to someone who can devote time to it on a daily basis.

Staff members should never be publicly criticized. This statement is a basic principle of human relations that is too often ignored. The physician must be sensitive to the feelings of the staff. To publicly criticize some staff members belittles them in the eyes of the others and patients who may be present.

Involve employees in their work. They should have some say in how things are done. Involve them in office meetings, and give them an active role in the decisions that affect them; for example, what type of calculator, pegboard, or typewriter would they prefer?

Discuss basic operating policies with staff members before putting them into effect. This approach will help gain the employees' commitment to the policies. People are fearful of change, often because they have not been involved in planning the change. Even if the final decision conflicts with the employees' ideas, more staff cooperation will generally result than if no staff input was sought.

Much good information can be learned from the staff. They know the office because they work there every day. Too often, office employees are not given the opportunity to express their opinions and make recommendations. Every office should take advantage of the employees' suggestions.

An office should review performance at least once a year at the time of salary reviews. There is no better way to convince an employee that the employer is interested in his or her progress than to spend time systematically reviewing work performance. All employees want to know how well they are doing. People like to know how they compare with others and what supervisors think of them. A review also gives the employee the opportunity to privately express personal views about the job.

A written office-policy manual is an important part of personnel management. A copy should be given to each present and new employee. The manual should be kept up to date and should reflect any changes in benefits or responsibilities. Too many employees know nothing about personnel rules or benefits. One example is the employee in an unincorporated practice with a Keogh plan who knows nothing except that "there is some sort of a retirement plan." A medical office that provides such a benefit should explain it to the employees so that they will understand the full advantages of the compensation plan.

Not having written policies can create feelings of discrimination and inconsistency. For example, when employees do not know the policy regarding vacation and sick pay, this situation can cause confusion and embarrassment.

Each office should have written job descriptions for each employee, clearly setting forth their primary and secondary responsibilities. Generally speaking, job descriptions are best written down by the office manager.

A written operations manual for all the procedures in the office is also helpful. The use of such a manual is another way that the physician may convince the staff that he or she is interested in their welfare—the office is trying to make it easier for them to do well so that their efforts will be better recognized by the physicians, patients, and fellow staff members. It is not difficult to develop an operations manual. One way is to ask each employee to list his or her tasks from the job description and then explain how each task is performed. The operations manual consists of a collection of these explanations. The office manager or, in

Exhibit 2. Office Policy Manual

1. WORKING HOURS. Our basic hours are 9:00 A.M. to 5:00 P.M. on Mondays through Fridays. Part-time employees will have different hours by prearrangement. We expect all employees to be on time each day. We try to close the office on time each day, but there are occasional times when one or more of us will have to arrive earlier or stay longer to meet a special need. When those occasions arise, we expect you to contribute as needed.

2. LUNCH HOUR. One hour is provided for lunch for all full-time employees, to be arranged among us to assure proper coverage of the office. Part-time employees are entitled to a lunch break of shorter duration.

3. PROBATIONARY PERIOD. All employees are hired for a 90-day probationary period. An employee is not considered to be on permanent status until having successfully completed this period of evaluation. There will be a review and discussion with each employee as he or she approaches the end of the 90 days. If an employee does not seem to fit into our work patterns and relationships, we feel that it is preferable to both parties to terminate the employment by the end of the probationary period; if the relationship appears to be satisfactory, we would prefer to openly say so and discuss the job.

4. TERMINATION. We will generally provide at least two weeks' notice or two weeks' salary (as separation pay) if dismissal of an employee should be necessary. You are similarly expected to give at least two weeks' notice in case you decide to terminate your employment, to enable us to seek a suitable replacement or coverage. Please note that unused vacation and/or sick leave days are not normally paid for upon termination. Any gross violation of our work rules or dishonesty could, of course, result in immediate discharge without notice or separation pay.

5. CONFIDENTIALITY. The work for our patients is by its nature quite personal. *You must, therefore, keep any information about our patients, their problems, and their relationships absolutely confidential.* Nothing would be more embarrassing to us than a discovery that information has been divulged, even casually, by any one of us to someone outside. *This rule is perhaps the most important one, and we must insist that you respect it.*

6. COMPENSATION. All employees are paid every two weeks, on every other Friday, unless other arrangements have been made. Each employee's work performance will be reviewed once a year, during the month of June. This review will include a discussion of your personal strengths and weaknesses as we see them and of your suggestions for our improvement. The review will also result in an annual salary adjustment, which is effective on each July 1. Please do not ask for or expect salary raises at other times of the year. Salaries are adjusted only on the basis of merit and not on the basis of seniority or cost of living. Furthermore, we do not pay bonuses (including Christmas bonuses) in the belief that your good work should be reflected in your salary.

7. HOLIDAYS. We close the office for the following paid holidays: New Year's Day, Washington's Birthday, Good Friday, Memorial Day, July 4, Labor Day, Thanksgiving Day, Christmas Day. If any of these holidays should fall on a weekend, we will be closed on the nearest weekday. Part-time salaried employees (those working regular hours and paid by the week, rather than by the hours worked) will be entitled to pay for absence on holidays falling within their regular working days but not for holidays falling on days that they are not usually working. Other part-time employees will not receive pay for holiday absences.

Exhibit 2. (continued)

8. VACATIONS. Each full-time employee is entitled to vacation during each calendar year as follows:

a. Two weeks (10 working days) in each calendar year, provided that full-time employment began before July 1 of that year, but no more than one of those weeks may be taken until after three months of full-time employment.

b. Three weeks (15 working days) in each calendar year, provided that there have been five years of continuous full-time employment by July 1 of that year.

c. Four weeks (20 working days) in each calendar year, provided that there have been 10 years of continuous full-time employment by July 1 of that year.

Part-time employees are entitled to proportionately less vacation time, depending on the number of days and hours regularly worked and the length of service. Other part-time employees are entitled to no paid vacation. Vacations may be taken at any time during the calendar year, but proper coverage of the office will be considered before any vacation request is granted. To properly schedule all vacations and office coverage, we expect all requests for vacation to be made at least one month in advance. It is preferred that vacations be taken in blocks of at least one week, but vacations of lesser periods will be granted if possible.

9. SICK LEAVE. Each employee is important to our overall success, and his or her presence on the job is thus similarly important. Although sick leave is provided, it is to be used only when absence is unavoidable because of illness. It is not a "right" to additional time off, it is not cumulative from year to year, and it will not be paid for if unused. Indiscriminate use of sick leave will be a factor in measuring an employee's annual salary increase. Each full-time employee can use the following paid sick leave:

a. Ten days in each calendar year, provided that there have been 12 months of full-time employment. An employee is entitled to no sick leave until he or she has been employed full-time for six months, and he or she is entitled to only five days' sick leave until so employed for 12 months.

b. Fifteen days in each calendar year, provided that there have been five years of continuous full-time employment by July 1 of that year.

c. Twenty days in each calendar year, provided that there have been 10 years of continuous full-time employment by July 1 of that year. Any additional absence because of illness or injury must, unfortunately, be treated as time off without pay.

Part-time salaried employees are entitled to proportionately less sick leave, depending on the number of days and hours worked regularly and the length of service. Other part-time employees are entitled to no sick leave. To be properly granted sick leave, you or a member of your immediate family must call the office with information concerning the illness each morning promptly at 9:00 A.M..

10. OTHER ABSENCES. If there is an emergency, it will be treated on an individual basis upon advance discussion, if at all possible. Any absences from work, other than those permitted by our rules, will be without pay. Unless such absences are approved in advance, they may be cause for termination.

11. EMPLOYEE INSURANCE PROGRAM. We have a group insurance package covering all full-time employees who have been employed at least two full months. Part-time employees are not included in this insurance package. Each employee will receive information on this insurance program when he or she becomes eligible. In addition, we have a profit-sharing plan for those over age 25 with one year of employment.

smaller offices, the physician can review the explanations and write a more detailed operations manual. This approach promotes communication.

Each employee should have as much status as aptitude and interest will permit. Each person in the office should be convinced that his or her job is important.

The best possible physical working conditions should be provided. Few offices cannot be improved, especially in the business area, which often has inadequate space.

Often, employees are assigned to use the telephone to collect delinquent accounts without adequate privacy or space. An employer who agrees to provide more privacy shows the employee that the job is important enough to merit good working conditions.

The physician should provide the best possible equipment. This need is often ignored. Inefficient filing systems, typewriters, calculators, adding machines, and telephone systems can hurt morale. Assistants who feel that they are working with awkward or outdated equipment may begin to believe that their employer does not consider their work important enough to merit efficient equipment.

It is important that an office's pay plan be understood and that it be competitive for the community. Merit raises are more important than uniform cost-of-living increases. Unfortunately, most medical-office employees have no real understanding of office policy on pay raises—often because there is no policy. Pay raises should be directly tied in with the performance review. Unfortunately, too many offices give all their employees the same raise, a practice that destroys employee motivation.

The physician or office manager should know the community pay scales. If the physician wants superior performance, he or she must pay superior salaries. Unfortunately, more ill-will can be generated by handling a pay plan poorly than by anything else.

Managers should delegate as much authority and responsibility as possible. It is a mistake for the office manager to try to do everything. What often happens is that the most capable person in an office becomes the office manager, having "worked up the ranks." Since this person "does everything better than everybody else," there will often be problems with the delegation of duties. This situation is not a healthy one. The manager cannot possibly do everything, and by refusing to delegate tasks, the manager demeans the other employees' abilities.

One important part of delegating responsibility is to encourage employees to expand their capabilities by offering them tangible assistance for education. An office should send people to practice-related seminars and courses and encourage formal training. If employees learn more, they will be better able to work in the office. Employees should also have access to a good library of books, magazines, cassettes, and other learning aids.

A leader's expectation affects the performance of subordinates. People often behave as others expect them to. Effective leaders are able to create high performance standards for subordinates by expressing confidence in their abilities. Leaders who fail to develop positive expectations allow subordinates to accomplish less. A important point to remember is that subordinates will not be influenced by the leader's expectations unless the expectations seem reasonable and realistic. Goals that are too high or too low will have little impact. The best way to lead is by example.

7
Financial Planning

Michael T. Walsh
Frank Caliri, III

Financial planning may be defined as the orderly development of a person's goals with an eye toward financial security. The proper coordination and implementation of savings, insurance, investments, and retirement, together with tax planning, are vital in achieving the objectives of financial planning.

In focusing on the different objectives of one's financial future, each person should examine personal idiosyncrasies and needs. The person should consider various questions: How risk oriented am I? What are my liquidity needs? Can I sacrifice any current income for long-term growth? How much money would my family need if I died or became disabled? At what age do I expect to retire?

INVESTMENTS

In investigating the different investment opportunities, it is assumed that a sufficient portion of one's funds has been set aside in a savings account as well as in life insurance for emergencies and other contingencies. Common stock, mutual funds, corporate bonds, and real estate offer greater potential returns than do the guarantees of savings accounts and life insurance for any funds not so used. Although there is the possibility of greater returns with such investments, there is also a greater amount of risk and sacrifice of liquidity.

Common Stock

Common stock distributes the ownership and profits of a corporation among numerous people. Owning common stock entitles the shareholder to many rights, among which are:

1. Right to vote for directors.
2. Right to receive dividends declared by directors.
3. Right to transfer ownership.
4. Right to inspect corporate books.
5. Preemptive right to purchase additional shares in proportion to one's present holding in the event that the corporation increases the amount of stock outstanding.

6. Right to share in distribution of cash or other assets if liquidated. However, the common shareholders bear the greatest risk because they are last in priority upon dissolution of the corporation.

In analyzing the investment merits of a particular corporation, an annual report can be of invaluable assistance. These reports can be obtained from the respective company at no charge or may be found in a business library. The annual report will contain audited financial statements (income statements, balance sheets, and statement of changes in financial positions). Normally, a letter from the president describing the past year and the coming year is also included. In addition to annual reports, consideration should be given to both the broad economic and the specific industry outlook, the earnings potential and stability of the company, the management, and dividend yield. For more in-depth information, a 10-K report (required by the Securities and Exchange Commission) can also be obtained from the company. The advice and assistance of a competent broker employed by a reputable brokerage house are invaluable, especially for someone like a physician who may not have the time or inclination to pursue intensive personal evaluation and research on each investment.

The selection of the stockbroker is thus an important task. Asking colleagues for a referral may be helpful in the selection process. Before any trading, the stockbroker should know and understand the physician's investment objectives. The amount of risk, capital, available time (long term or short term), and desired return (dividend income versus capital appreciation) should be thoroughly discussed. The stockbroker can provide additional reports and recommendations from the brokerage's in-house research department. The costs of such transactions involve commissions, which can be negotiated and usually run about 2.5% to buy and another 2.5% to sell plus state or local transfer taxes or both, which are minimal.

Bonds

A bond is a long-term promissory note that promises to pay a stated amount of interest (coupon rate) per annum and the face amount (par value) at a fixed date (maturity). Bonds are purchased in denominations of $1,000, and the interest is usually paid semiannually. Bondholders have priority over stockholders in both earnings and liquidations but have no voting privileges, unless it is provided for when interest is in arrearage.

The principal use of corporate bonds in financial planning is to supplement current income with higher-yielding interest payments. Three important criteria in selecting bonds are yield, rating, and maturity. Current yield is determined by dividing the annual interest payment into the price of the bond. There are two independent agencies that rate the quality of the bonds being issued. *Standard & Poors* rate bonds from AAA (highest quality), AA, A, BBB, BB, B, CCC, CC, C, to D (in default). *Moody's* also has a similar rating: Aaa, Aa, A, Baa, Ba, and so on. The higher the rating, the less risk involved, and therefore a lower coupon rate. These two publications are generally available in business as well as large public libraries. Maturities can run up to 40 years. Although the bond can be sold to others before maturity, the risk of price fluctuation can affect the bondholder. The price of bonds is inversely related to current market interest rates. As interest rates tend to rise, bond prices fall. A decline in interest rates engenders higher bond prices. For this reason, bond prices will fluctuate to make the current effective yield close to that of current interest rates. In periods of rapidly rising interest rates, short-term notes are a good investment because of their proximate maturities. When interest rates are peaking, it may be a good time to buy long-term bonds.

Bonds normally have call provisions. This provision allows the corporation to buy back the bond before maturity at a stated price above par value.

There are also convertible bonds, which can be converted into the issuing company's common stock. Convertible bonds have more price volatility than do nonconvertible bonds. The price of the convertible bond tends to move more in harmony with that of the common stock.

Municipal Bonds

Municipal bonds are similar to corporate bonds in that there is a stated interest rate and a fixed maturity date. However, they have one extremely attractive feature—interest on municipal bonds is tax exempt from federal income tax and normally from any state income tax in the state where issued. Because of this special tax treatment, municipalities issue bonds with substantially lower interest rates. Persons in high tax brackets will find that the tax-exempt nature of these bonds can generate higher after-tax returns than can corporate bonds. Municipal bonds are also rated by *Standard & Poor's* and *Moody's*.

There are different types of municipal bonds. The physician should procure a prospectus and examine it thoroughly before investing. The more secure type of municipal bonds are general obligation bonds, since they rely upon the broader state tax base. Revenue bonds often run into difficulties because they are tied to specific projects.

Preferred Stock

Preferred stock is a hybrid class of security somewhat between common stock and bonds. It is preferred because it has claims ahead of common stock but behind bondholders in the case of the company's liquidation. Preferred stocks have a stated dividend, normally a percentage of the par value (nominal face value of the stock). The preferred dividends must be paid before common dividends can be paid. Preferred dividends are usually cumulative, so arrearages must be made up before any other dividend can be paid. There are generally no voting rights attached to preferred issues.

Preferred stocks are purchased for their greater income-producing ability and not for their capital appreciation, since there is no significant appreciation. In comparison to common stocks, they have higher yields and smaller price fluctuations. An exception to this rule is convertible preferred stocks. The price of convertible preferred stocks is volatile and moves in parity with that of the underlying common stock.

Mutual Funds

Instead of selecting individual common stocks, some people prefer to buy into a mutual fund. Mutual funds offer professional management and diversification, which should translate into lower risk.

There are essentially two types of mutual funds, open-end funds and closed-end funds. An open-end fund is held open in terms of the number of shares outstanding. The purchase and redemption of the shares are from the fund itself at the net asset value (assets per shares). Open-end funds are offered on a load or no-load basis. A load fund has a commission added up front to the purchase price, whereas the no-load fund has no extra charges. The commissions paid to the salesman on the load fund have no effect on the actual management of the fund.

Closed-end funds are fixed in terms of the number of shares outstanding. These funds are not purchased or redeemed but are traded on a stock exchange. Because they are traded on an exchange, the price is determined by the demand and is not tied to the net asset value.

Mutual funds have been designed to match most financial desires. There are growth funds, income funds, dual funds, and bond funds. Prospectuses of each fund will describe the fund's objectives and the fees.

Real Estate

The purchase of a house is typically the first real estate investment people encounter. In the past several years, real estate has been one of the few investments that has outpaced inflation. The advantages of home ownership are the tax deductibility of mortgage interest and real estate taxes, as compared with rent, which is not tax deductible, unless it is a business expense.

Nonowner-occupied real estate offers even greater tax benefits. In addition to the deductibility of interest and taxes, depreciation and current expenses can also be offset against the rental income. The objective of real estate investments is to generate tax deductions in excess of cash outlay, which creates current income tax savings, while at the same time the appreciation of the property will be taxed favorably at capital gains rate upon disposition.

The rate of return determines both the ordinary income tax savings together with appreciation over time. The rate of return in real estate has been attractive because of these tax savings.

Tax Treatment

Common stocks, preferred stocks, bonds, mutual funds, and real estate are considered capital assets for federal tax purposes. All interest, dividends, and rental income are taxable as ordinary income, with federal rates ranging from 14% to 70%.

If such an asset is held for a period of one year or longer before disposition, gains or losses are considered long term; otherwise, they are short term. Short-term capital gains and losses are included with ordinary income. For long-term capital gains, a taxpayer may exclude 60% of the gain and then be subject to ordinary income tax on the remaining 40%. Long-term capital losses are first used to offset capital gains, with any excess being deductible up to $3,000 per year after the 60% exclusion is applied. Any balance not deducted is then available to be carried forward for up to five years on future tax returns subject to the same limitations.

LIFE INSURANCE

Life insurance is sold by two types of insurance companies—stock companies and mutual companies. Stock insurance companies are owned by the stockholders, who assume the ultimate risk and share in the profits. The control of the stock company naturally lies with the shareholders. Stock companies primarily issue nonparticipating policies, which have a fixed annual premium, normally lower in the initial years than that of a participating type of policy. Should actual experience be adverse, the losses will be borne by the stockholders. If experience is better than anticipated, the profit margin will be allocated among shareholders and surplus.

Mutual insurance companies have no stockholders. In theory, the policyholders as a group own the company. However, in actuality, the management controls a mutual company due to the dispersion of ownership among a large number of policyholders. Mutual companies only issue participating life insurance. With participating insurance, the premium is fixed at an amount higher than that which will be needed for the cost of insurance. Should the actual experience be favorable, the policyholders would receive the excess in the form of a dividend. Dividends from mutual insurance companies are a return of the excess premium charged. These dividends should not be confused with ordinary corporate dividends; they are nontaxable because they represent a refund. Dividend illustrations in policies are not guaranteed. Theoretically, participating policies should attain greater equity among policyholders, but this expectation is not always borne out.

There are essentially two types of life insurance: term and ordinary life. The common feature of these contracts is the obligation to pay a fixed principal sum to the beneficiary on the death of the insured.

Term Insurance

A term policy can be defined as insurance protection for a limited number of years. If death occurs within the limited number of years, the face value would be paid; otherwise, nothing would be paid in the case of survival beyond this period. A term policy essentially provides temporary insurance. Policies can be issued for one, five, or 20 years. Most companies offer term policies to age 65 or 70. (In some states, annually renewable term to age 100 is offered.)

Some of the provisions that can be found in a term policy are convertibility and renewability. Convertibility offers the insured the privilege of exchanging the existing term policy to a whole-life contract without any evidence of insurability. Renewability gives the policyholder the option of renewing the term plan for the same period, also without furnishing evidence of insurability. These two provisions are important parts of any term insurance contracts.

Common reasons for purchasing term insurance are:

1. Maximum insurance is needed, but premium paying ability is limited
2. The need for the protection is for a short period of time
3. To guarantee the repayment of a mortgage or other fixed-term obligation

Term insurance can be well suited for a specific need. Sole reliance should not be placed upon this type of insurance because of its limited life and prohibitive costs in later years, as well as the risk of future uninsurability.

Ordinary Life Insurance

An ordinary life policy provides insurance protection for a lifetime. The premiums are payable for the life of the insured. However, the policyholder is not obligated to continue payments, should he or she desire to terminate or surrender the policy for either cash or some other option.

The difference between ordinary life and term insurance is that ordinary life offers lifetime protection and also provides a savings element (cash value). The savings element stems from the fact that in the early years of the contract, the premiums are more than adequate for the cost of protection. The excess premiums are accumulated along with interest to offset premiums in later years, when the cost of insurance actually exceeds the premium charged.

Nonforfeiture Values

All ordinary life insurance policies are required to have nonforfeiture values. These values arise from the savings element described above. There are three types of nonforfeiture values:

1. Cash-surrender values
2. Reduced paid-up life insurance
3. Extended-term insurance

These options are available if and when the insured decides to stop paying premiums. When the cash-surrender option is selected, life insurance protection ceases. No further payments are required, and the policyholder receives the amount of the savings element. The reduced paid-up option is an alternative to taking the cash-surrender value and terminating all insurance coverage. Under this option, the policyholder exchanges the cash value for a reduced face-amount policy on which the premiums are paid up. The extended-term nonforfeiture option will automatically go into effect if the insured does not make an election. With the extended-term option, the cash value is exchanged for a term policy with the full face amount. The duration of the policy is determined by the amount of cash value available to purchase the term insurance.

Contract Provisions

Insurance contracts have various standard provisions of which the policyholder should be aware. These provisions include the incontestable period, the grace period, policy loan provisions, automatic premium loan, assignment rights, beneficiary designation, and reinstatement clause.

The incontestable clause is a provision that states that the policy will be incontestable after a given period of time (usually two years), even if the insured concealed or misstated facts or otherwise erred in the application's completion.

The grace period is the period during which a life insurance policy stays in force after the premium has become due but has not been paid. The grace period is 31 days.

The policy loan provision gives the policyholder the right to borrow the cash value of the policy without surrendering the contract. Interest is charged on the loan at a rate stipulated in the contract. (Interest rates can vary among companies but are generally lower than market rates.) Policy loans do not have to be repaid; however, if the insured dies, the policy loan will be deducted from the face amount.

The automatic premium loan is a provision that protects life insurance from lapsing in the event that the premium is not paid. The premium is paid out of the policy loan value, provided that there is sufficient loan value to cover the premium payment.

Life insurance contracts are assignable. An absolute assignment transfers all the ownership rights to another. A collateral assignment transfers certain rights when the policy is used as security for a loan.

The owner of the policy has the right to name the beneficiary who is to receive the insurance proceeds. The owner can also change the beneficiary at any time, provided that the previous beneficiary designation was not irrevocable.

The reinstatement clause enables a policyholder to reinstate a policy that has lapsed due to nonpayment. Evidence of insurability together with back premium payments are required.

Dividend Options

Policyholders who own participating insurance contracts are entitled to dividends. Dividends can be applied in five different ways:

1. Cash dividend
2. Dividends applied toward future premium
3. Dividends left with company to accumulate at interest
4. Dividends used to purchase paid-up additional insurance
5. Dividends used to purchase one-year term insurance.

Settlement Options

Life insurance proceeds can be paid in several different methods upon election by the owner or beneficiary. A lump sum is the most common form of settlement. The other options are the interest option, the fixed-amount option, the fixed-period option, and the life-income option.

The interest option pays a guaranteed amount of interest on the proceeds left with the insurance company. The interest rate paid can be higher than the guaranteed rate and often is. The interest option provides the greatest amount of flexibility in that the beneficiary may be given the right to change to other settlement options.

The fixed-amount option pays a stated dollar amount each month until the proceeds are exhausted. The monthly payment is composed of interest and a partial return of principal.

The fixed-period option pays the proceeds out over the period of time fixed by the owner. Interest also constitutes a portion of each payment.

The life-income option provides monthly payments for the lifetime of the beneficiary. Should the beneficiary die shortly thereafter, payments would cease. To circumvent this problem, the life-income option can have a guaranteed number of payments. The age of the beneficiary, the minimum number of payments, and the amount of insurance proceeds would determine the monthly payment.

Insurance proceeds received by virtue of an insured's death are not taxable income. The interest received is taxable as ordinary income. However, $1,000 a year of interest on insurance proceeds is tax exempt if it is paid to a surviving spouse by the insurance company.

Settlement options are a valuable tool in planning for financial needs after the insured's death. These options can be used to make sure that the proceeds paid to a beneficiary are not squandered.

Riders

Life insurance policies can be modified to meet certain individual needs. Riders provide an easy way to add to the basic benefits of a contract. The most common riders are accidental death, guaranteed insurability, and waiver of premium.

Accidental death riders double the face amount of life insurance should the insured die by accidental means. There is little economic justification for accidental death riders because the financial needs of the insured should not be based on the manner of death.

The guaranteed-insurability rider gives the insured the option to purchase additional life insurance at ages stipulated in the contract without providing evidence of insurability. This rider is a valuable addition to any insurance contract.

Waiver of premium releases the insured from paying the premiums if he or she becomes disabled for a period of six months.

Insurance Comparisons

Life insurance policies and costs can differ substantially. Because of the complex nature of insurance policies the insurance industry devised a simple method for appraising insurance costs for similar contracts.

The interest-adjusted method helps the consumer to quantify the differences between premiums, cash values, and dividends. An interest factor is used to discount the timing differences in the flow of payments and values. The interest-adjusted index is shown as a per $1,000 amount of insurance cost and is found on most proposals or can be requested.

The interest-adjusted method should not be relied upon as a panacea for the consumer. Policy features and settlement options often differ and are not computed in the index. Dividends are not guaranteed and can deviate from expectations. These deviations can have a positive or negative effect on the true cost. The service of the agent and the company is an intangible benefit that may compensate for a higher cost.

Disability Insurance

The need for income replacement when the breadwinner is disabled is an integral part of financial planning. Disability-income insurance provides cash benefits to replace earnings lost during periods of incapacity due to a sickness or accident.

The definition of total disability is the most important provision in a disability contract and will vary among companies and policies. The most favorable definition for total disability is "the inability of the insured to perform the duties of his regular occupation." A lesser definition would be stated as "gainful occupation for which the insured is reasonably prepared by education, training, and experience."

The importance of the definition is best illustrated with an example. Dr. John Smith lost the use of his right hand in an accident. To support his family, he took a position in a medical laboratory. Under the regular-occupation definition, Dr. Smith would receive disability payments since working in a laboratory was not his regular occupation. With the gainful-occupation definition, Dr. Smith would not receive benefits since he is reasonably fitted for that position.

The elimination period is that span of time at the beginning of disability during which no benefits are payable. Elimination periods range from one week to one year. The shorter the elimination period, the higher the cost of coverage.

The benefit period, or payment period, is the time span during which disability income will be paid. Benefit periods can extend from six months to age 65. However, benefit periods of at least five years are most common, with elimination periods of 30 days. The applicant's main concern should be long-term disability, but longer payment periods increase the cost of protection.

The applicant's earned income determines the amount of disability for which he qualifies. Benefits are limited to 40% to 65% of earned income, depending on the company.

Noncancelability and guaranteed renewable clauses are important provisions in a disability contract. Noncancelable means that the insurer does not have the right to refuse to renew the policy. Guaranteed renewable assures the insured that his premium cannot be adjusted on an individual basis.

Pricing of disability policies varies. Terms and benefits of the contract are important considerations when comparing policies and prices.

The need for disability-income insurance parallels that of life insurance, and no financial plan is complete without disability insurance.

Agent Selection

The selection of an agent is the foundation for a well-structured insurance portfolio. The agent's knowledge and ability to advise clients regarding amounts of insurance, types of policies, and options available are invaluable in dealing with such a specialized financial product.

In choosing an agent, there are many different qualities to evaluate. What is the agent's background and experience? Does the agency represent more than one company, or is he or she forced to place all business with one company? What are his or her professional qualities?

One indicator of an insurance agent's technical skills is the "chartered life underwriter" (C.L.U.) designation. The C.L.U. is achieved by demonstrating proficiency in a series of insurance and business examinations. However, there are many highly skilled brokers who do not possess this designation, and the lack of such a designation should not necessarily be a deterrent to working with any agent.

Colleagues can also be of assistance in referring the physician to an agent who they feel is qualified. Confidence and trust in an agent should be the determining factors.

BUSINESS ENTITIES

There are three classes of business entities: the sole proprietorship, the partnership, and the corporation. In this section, we shall review the retirement plans and other financial benefits available in each class of business entity. Modes of medical practice are discussed in greater depth in Chapter 1.

Sole Proprietorship

A sole proprietorship can be described as an unincorporated business owned by one person. The physician in solo practice is a sole proprietor. Sole proprietors are eligible to create their own retirement plans. They have the choice of contributing to an H.R. 10 (Keogh plan) or an Individual Retirement Account (IRA).

The H.R. 10 is a qualified plan that enables the sole proprietor to deduct an amount from current income up to the allowable level of contributions. During the accumulation period, the interest earned on the contributions to the plan is also tax deferred.

One of the provisions of an H.R. 10 plan is that no withdrawals can be made before age 59½, and none can be made later than age 70½. Upon distribution, the proceeds are taxed as ordinary income. If a lump-sum payment is taken, the recipient can elect a special 10-year income-averaging rule. Should the retiree take the distribution as an annuity, the proceeds would be spread out and taxed in each year as received.

Self-employed persons may contribute up to 15% of earned income or $7,500, whichever is less. Employees working over 1,000 hours per year with at least three years of employment must be covered under the plan for it to be tax qualified. Employees must have the same percentage of their salary contributed by the employer. All plans must be 100% vested from the inception.

Funding vehicles for the H.R. 10 are annuities, savings accounts, retirement-income life insurance, and special government retirement bonds. One plan that is widely used is the "split-funded" plan. In this plan, the insurance or trust company holds ordinary life insurance policies plus a "side fund" of either an annuity or a savings account. The amount of assets invested in life insurance premiums cannot exceed 50% of the total contribution into a participant's account. At retirement, the life insurance policies can be converted into an annuity.

When life insurance is used in an H.R. 10 plan, the Internal Revenue Service realizes that there is some economic benefit passing to the participant. To compensate for this benefit, the government established an imputed income table (P.S. 58), which the participant must declare on his tax return. This table measures in essence the life insurance protection afforded as though it were term insurance.

The other tax-qualified retirement plan available to sole proprietors is the IRA. Individual retirement accounts are available to all persons not covered by a qualified pension plan, profit-sharing plan, or H.R. 10 plan.

The IRA is similar to the H.R. 10 in that contributions are tax deductible and accumulate tax free. Withdrawals cannot be made without penalties before age 59½ and later than age 70½. The maximum contribution to an IRA is the lesser of $1,500 or 15% of earned income. The same funding instruments as those available for an H.R. 10 can be used. An employer is not obligated to include employees in this plan since the employer is contributing on an individual basis. Congress has expanded the concept of an IRA under the Revenue Act of 1978 by allowing an employer to contribute the lesser of $7,500 or 15% of an employee's compensation to an individual IRA so long as the employer does not discriminate against other eligible employees. Although these limitations are similar to those of an H.R. 10 plan, this "simplified pension plan" is easier to administer.

Partnership

The Uniform Partnership Act defines partnerships as "an association of two or more persons to carry on as co-owners a business for a profit." Most professional partnerships are created by solo practitioners joining with someone with similar expertise to provide better service as well as ongoing service to the clientele. In most situations, few tangible assets are contributed; instead, each partner contributes his or her services. Partnerships are discussed further in Chapter 1. Partners are eligible for either an H.R. 10 plan or an IRA.

Professional Corporations

The advantages of incorporation accrue from the tax deductibility of the various prerequisites to the employees, as described in Chapter 1. The professional is now a stockholder employee and as an employee is eligible to participate in these programs. The following fringe benefits are deductible by the corporation and not taxed to the employee:

1. *Adoption of a qualified pension or profit sharing plan.* Corporate retirement plans offer much greater benefits for the owners of corporations than does an H.R. 10.

2. *Tax-free group term life insurance up to $50,000.* Premiums paid for group term insurance are deductible from the corporation's income and are not included as taxable income to the employee.

3. *Tax-free death benefits up to $5,000.* This amount is paid by the corporation to the deceased shareholder's beneficiary and is deductible by the corporation. It is not taxable income to the beneficiary.

4. *Disability-income insurance.* Premiums paid for disability insurance are tax deductible. However, the proceeds are taxable income. (An income exclusion for employees disabled for 30 days or longer is allowed to the extent of $100 a week.)

5. *Medical-expense plans.* Premiums paid for medical insurance for employees are tax deductible and are not considered compensation to the employee.

6. *Ability to defer compensation.* This benefit is also available in qualified plans. Although not deductible to the corporation, such plans defer present income to a future date, when an employee expects to be in a lower tax bracket.

7. *Long-term capital gains and losses.* These benefits are available to the stockholder when he or she sells shares in the corporation after holding them for one year or more.

Since most corporate income will be paid out as either compensation or fringe benefits, there should be little income if any to be taxed at the corporate level. However, should there be any left after such expenditures, the corporation tax schedule is applied as follows:

17% on the first $25,000
20% on the next $25,000
30% on the next $25,000
40% on the next $25,000
46% on the excess over $100,000

Any income left after the application of the corporate tax rate is then subject to ordinary personal income tax rates if paid out as a dividend; thus, the so-called double tax would be encountered.

Qualified corporate pension plans differ substantially from H.R. 10s in rules and eligibility. With a corporate plan, all employees must be eligible after they have worked one year and reached 25 years of age. The one-year period can be extended to three years if the plan immediately vests 100% of the benefits to the employee. Seasonal and part-time employees must be included if they work 1,000 hours or more. The Internal Revenue Service can disqualify any plan that is discriminatory in operation, for example, if it favors high-pay employees over low-pay employees.

The maximum contributions to a qualified corporate pension plan are substantially higher than those allowed under an H.R. 10 plan. Under a defined contribution plan, the maximum deduction allowed for an individual is $32,700 (adjusted annually for the cost of living) or 25% of earned income, whichever is less. With a defined-benefit plan, the maximum benefit that a person could receive at retirement in 1979 is $98,100 (also adjusted annually) a year or 100% of average salary during the highest three consecutive years of employment, whichever is less. A special rule exists in which a combination of plans can be used but not to exceed 140% of the benefits of a single plan. In general, defined-benefit plans allow for larger deductions for persons in their mid to late forties and older, due to the shorter period existing to accumulate the retirement dollars. Defined-contribution plans usually generate a greater deduction for persons in their early forties and younger.

All valid contributions to a qualified pension plan are tax deductible to the corporation. If the plan is funded with life insurance, the employee must recognize the economic benefit of the insurance—P.S. 58 costs (discussed earlier). Life insurance death benefits must be incidental to the plan's main purpose of providing retirement benefits. (The use of life insurance in a pension plan can have estate tax advantages. Insurance proceeds in addition to the balance of other plan assets paid to a named beneficiary other than the executor over a period of at least two years are excludable from the insured's gross estate.) Except as noted above for life insurance benefits, contributions to a qualified plan are not currently taxed to an employee, and they are allowed to accumulate income tax free until distribution.

The portion of a distribution that is allocable to contributions made in the years before 1974 can receive long-term capital gains treatment (60% exclusion from income tax), whereas contributions allocable after 1974 are taxed as ordinary income. However, a special 10-year forward-averaging tax method is available if a lump-sum distribution is taken and capital gains treatment is not elected on the pre-1974 portion. If payout in annuity form is elected, the receipt of the proceeds is spread over time, and income tax is imposed at ordinary rates on the amounts received each year.

Buy-sell for Business Interest

Professional corporations and partnerships have problems at retirement, death, and disability of the professional since practices are not readily transferable to family members due to the licensing and expertise required.

Sole proprietors, partners, and professional shareholders can plan for these problems by arranging a buy-sell agreement with another colleague or partner. A written buy-sell agreement should provide a formula or fix a price for the sale of an interest. The agreement should require the physician or his or her estate to sell its interest, and the purchasers should be bound to acquire the interest at the stipulated price. The purchase of life insurance can be used to generate the needed liquidity to fund the buy-sell agreement. In case of disability, disability insurance can be purchased to fund a buyout through installments.

If the partners, shareholders, or associates decide to purchase a deceased or retired interest individually, each person will own insurance on each other's life in the amount at least required to cover the interest he or she expects to acquire. The purchase by individual shareholders of stock under a buyout rather than the corporate entity may have income tax advantages to the purchasers.

A properly drafted buy-sell agreement will fix the value of the business as an asset for purposes of federal and state death taxes.

ESTATE PLANNING

A discussion of the various aspects of estate planning will be provided that should enable the reader to appreciate the scope of this subject as well as the necessity for appropriate action in regard to each person's own affairs. One of the primary objectives of estate planning is the retention of the maximum lifetime benefits of property, while making adequate provision for its transfer to the owner's survivors with a minimum reduction for death taxes and other death-related expenses. Although estate planning is necessarily concerned with the reduction of taxes of all descriptions, it is at the same time performed in the context of a particular person's unique desires for both lifetime and testamentary disposition of his or her assets.

Inventory

Before beginning the estate-planning process, the physician should develop a clear and complete inventory of both assets and liabilities. Forms are available at most banks or through life insurance underwriters, which will help the physician with the listing of assets in an orderly fashion in terms of type of property, ownership status, value, and income tax basis, among other considerations. This type of exercise should help the preparer orient his or her thinking concerning the financial needs of various family members and what is or will be available to satisfy them. The process of making an inventory of the physician's financial situation can be done together with or independent of the estate-planning team (i.e., financial advisors, such as an accountant, attorney, life insurance underwriter, or investment counselor). Proper completion of the information requested in such a document will give the physician's advisors the wherewithal to adapt various planning ideas to the particular situation consonant with his or her goals and desires.

Types of Ownership

The various assets shown on an inventory form can be owned in many ways. Some of the more common forms are as follows:

- Outright or sole ownership simply means that one possesses all the rights that it is possible to have with respect to a piece of property.
- Tenancy in common is a form of split ownership in which one possesses all the rights as in sole ownership, except that these rights exist in an undivided interest in property owned together with one or more persons.
- Joint tenancy is an expanded form of split ownership in which there is normally a right of survivorship, meaning that the share of one who predeceases the other co-owners automatically passes pro rata to the survivors. However, such an interest can always be converted to a tenancy in common to preclude this possibility.
- Tenancy by the entireties exists only between husband and wife and is a particular form of joint tenancy. In most states, husband and wife are considered to own such property as an entity, and neither can terminate this situation without the consent of the other. One advantage of such ownership, in addition to the automatic-survivorship feature, is the fact that property owned in this fashion will not be subject to the debts or obligations of either spouse alone, unless that spouse survives. However, this advantage does not hold for any debt for which both spouses are liable.

Community property exists in eight states that have a civil law tradition (Spanish in the West, French in Louisiana). This concept of property ownership maintains that property acquired during marriage while domiciled in a community-property state belongs to both husband and wife equally, much as a tenancy in common. Both spouses may own premarriage property separately as well as postmarriage property, provided that certain legal formalities are followed.

To the concepts above might be added property that is split in ownership in terms of time, such as life estates (the right to income from or use of property for one's life), remainders (the right to property after the death of a life tenant or a term of years), and equitable ownership (the right to the benefits of property held in trust). These various forms of ownership may be created or simply have been transmitted either by lifetime gifts or upon someone's death to a particular person.

Wills

Once the physician has determined the nature of the various property interests that have been accumulated, the need for a will should become apparent. Many couples do not feel that a will is necessary, since they may as husband and wife own property jointly so that upon the death of the first, the property passes automatically by operation of law. However, this assumption does not address all the contingencies that may happen, such as simultaneous death or death shortly after one another. Putting joint property aside, if the person does not exercise his or her right to designate who will enjoy property upon death, the state in which one is domiciled will under its intestate (dying without a will) laws designate how the property will be divided. This law should be carefully examined since there is hardly a situation where this scheme of distribution will adequately meet a family's needs. Other factors that can be important considerations are the provision for guardians of the person and property of a minor and various technical provisions that will provide death tax savings, both federal and state, such as the marital deduction, the orphan's exclusion, tax clauses, and so on. One of the most important aspects of a will is the naming of an executor, someone whom the physician can trust to administer his or her estate properly. Without a will, the state will appoint an administrator, normally a family member. The drafting of a will to negotiate the narrow waters of the tax laws will require an attorney skilled in estate planning.

Federal Estate and Gift Taxes

If the physician requires convincing proof of the necessity for adequate estate planning, he or she should consider the imposition of the federal estate and gift tax. The Tax Reform Act of 1976 created a new tax table that imposes a unified and progressive tax upon the cumulative transfers made by a person during life and the final transfer at death. Exhibit 1 demonstrates the severity of this combined tax on the transfer of one's property. There is some relief, however, in that there is a credit available that offsets the tax once calculated. For the year 1979, the credit offsets $38,000 in tax; for 1980, $42,500; for 1981 and thereaf-

Exhibit 1. Unified Rate Schedule for Estate and Gift Taxes.

If the amount with respect to which the tentative tax to be computed is:	The tentative tax is:
Not over $10,000	18% of such amount
Over $10,000 but not over $20,000	$1,800 plus 20% of the excess of such amount over $10,000
Over $20,000 but not over $40,000	$3,800 plus 22% of the excess of such amount over $20,000
Over $40,000 but not over $60,000	$8,200 plus 24% of the excess of such amount over $40,000
Over $60,000 but not over $80,000	$13,000 plus 26% of the excess of such amount over $60,000
Over $80,000 but not over $100,000	$18,200 plus 28% of the excess of such amount over $80,000
Over $100,000 but not over $150,000	$23,800 plus 30% of the excess of such amount over $100,000
Over $150,000 but not over $250,000	$38,800 plus 32% of the excess of such amount over $150,000
Over $250,000 but not over $500,000	$70,800 plus 34% of the excess of such amount over $250,000
Over $500,000 but not over $750,000	$155,800 plus 37% of the excess of such amount over $500,000
Over $750,000 but not over $1,000,000	$248,300 plus 39% of the excess of such amount over $750,000
Over $1,000,000 but not over $1,250,000	$345,800 plus 41% of the excess of such amount over $1,000,000
Over $1,250,000 but not over $1,500,000	$448,300 plus 43% of the excess of such amount over $1,250,000
Over $1,500,000 but not over $2,000,000	$555,800 plus 45% of the excess of such amount over $1,500,000
Over $2,000,000 but not over $2,500,000	$780,800 plus 49% of the excess of such amount over $2,000,000
Over $2,500,000 but not over $3,000,000	$1,025,800 plus 53% of the excess of such amount over $2,500,000

Exhibit 1. (continued)

Over $3,000,000 but not over $3,500,000	$1,290,800 plus 57% of the excess of such amount over $3,000,000
Over $3,500,000 but not over $4,000,000	$1,575,800 plus 61% of the excess of such amount over $3,500,000
Over $4,000,000 but not over $4,500,000	$1,880,800 plus 65% of the excess of such amount over $4,000,000
Over $4,500,000 but not over $5,000,000	$2,205,800 plus 69% of the excess of such amount over $4,500,000
Over $5,000,000	$2,550,800 plus 70% of the excess over $5,000,000

ter, $47,000. For decedents dying in 1981, for example, the credit translates into the equivalent of $175,625 of property passing tax free. Tax would therefore be imposed at the marginal rate of 32%. Most people are not aware of this large liability, which is imposed without choice at their death and becomes in essence a first lien on their property. Without adequate financial planning, such an imposition will create severe liquidity needs on an estate, and if adequate insurance and other forms of liquid assets are not available, the executor may be forced to sell assets at sacrificial prices, depleting the estate even further for the physician's heirs.

Tax-saving Ideas

The following represent some tax-saving ideas that should be explored with the estate planning team.

$3,000 Annual Exclusion

An amount up to $3,000 may be given free of gift tax each year to any one donee. This amount may be increased to $6,000 per donee if a spouse consents to split another spouse's gift on the gift-tax return (e.g., $3,000 per spouse), or each spouse could give $3,000 to any particular donee.

Gift Tax Marital Deduction

A spouse can give $100,000 to his or her spouse free of gift tax. The second $100,000 transferred to a spouse is treated as a taxable gift. Thereafter, any amounts in excess of this initial $200,000 receive a 50% exclusion, so that only one-half of the gift is subject to tax.

Life Insurance Ownership

The continued ownership until death of a life insurance policy by a deceased insured will subject the proceeds to taxation in his or her estate. It may be advisable for an insured to have ownership of such insurance on his or her spouse or children or an irrevocable trust for their benefit; otherwise, the full face value will not be available when it is needed. (In most states, insurance payable to a named beneficiary other than one's estate or the executor will be free of inheritance tax.)

Estate Tax Marital Deduction

The federal estate tax allows a deduction from a decedent's estate for the value of property passing to the surviving spouse in such a manner that it will be taxable in the survivor's estate at death. This exclusion can be the greater of $250,000 or one-half the adjusted gross estate (the gross estate is the sum of all one's assets less debts and other deductions of administration expenses), provided that such an amount actually passes to the spouse, as noted above.

Marital Deduction Planning

Many people use simple wills that leave all their property outright to the surviving spouse. This disposition, unless desired, will increase tax costs, since the excess over that which qualifies for the marital deduction will be taxed twice, once in the estate of the first to die and then again on the death of the surviving spouse. To alleviate this double-tax burden of passing property to the next generation, many attorneys will recommend a so-called A-B trust plan. This plan simply means that a portion (A) will be set aside for the surviving spouse to qualify for the marital deduction (this portion will normally be reduced by property passing to the spouse outside the will, e.g., joint property). The net balance after taxes and expenses will be placed in trust for the spouse for life with the remainder to the children. The B trust will not be taxed in the surviving spouse's estate if properly drafted, while at the same time the spouse can almost have the full economic benefit of the property, such as income, limited rights of withdrawal, discretionary principal distribution by the trustee, and, perhaps, a limited power of appointment (the right to designate who among a certain class of persons will enjoy the property at her death).

Orphan's Exclusion

An exclusion of $5,000 per year for each year a minor is under 21 years of age will be allowed for property passing to a minor on the death of the last parent to die.

Integration of the Unified Credit

Since by 1981 any person either during life or at death may pass $175,625 of property tax free after expenses and deductions (the property value equivalent of the $47,000 tax credit enacted by the Tax Reform Act of 1976) or the balance if a portion has already been used up by lifetime gifts, it is important to integrate this amount with the marital deduction. It may be advisable in smaller estates (those less than $425,625) to specifically bequeath this equivalent amount first either outright or in trust and then offset the balance of the estate with the maximum marital deduction. If the maximum marital deduction of $250,000 for the smaller estate is bequeathed first to the surviving spouse, the full value of the credit may be lost forever since there may not be enough property left to fully use it, assuming, of course, that there is the desire to reduce taxes in the surviving spouse's estate. This tax credit should be carefully discussed with the physician's advisors.

Trusts

Trusts may be created for many purposes and may take different forms. Depending on how it is structured, a trust may constitute a separate taxpayer for federal income tax purposes, which allows great planning possibilities for family members. A trustee is chosen to hold legal title to certain assets and is given duties for the maintenance and distribution of these assets to the beneficiaries (the equitable owners). Some of the more commonly encountered types of trusts are as follows:

Revocable Trusts
This type of trust, as its name implies, may be changed at will. Such a trust has both life- and death-related uses. During life, the physician may wish to have a trustee administer property and actually see it in operation before death, at which time the trust may then have continued purposes for his or her heirs. A revocable trust can substitute for a will when the person dies. Since it is not subject to probate, the trust goes on without scrutiny. However, it is still subject to federal and state death taxes, since control is maintained until death. Revocable trusts are sometimes used in connection with pour-over wills; that is, the will simply directs the executor to turn over any assets not already in the trust to the trustee. The trust itself, then, has the basic dispositive provisions, including marital deduction clauses. Life insurance may also be placed in such a trust simply to escape state death taxes, since the trustee will be considered a named beneficiary, independent of the estate.

Irrevocable Trusts
An irrevocable trust, as its name implies, cannot be changed once set up. However, most states allow termination if the grantor, trustee, and beneficiaries all concur. Property transferred to such a trust will be subject to federal gift tax to the extent that the grantor does not retain an interest in the trust. To keep such assets out of the estate, the grantor must not retain any beneficial interest or control of the property. Accordingly, such a trust can be a useful planning device for transferring property to benefit the spouse and children, while keeping any appreciation and income thereon out of the estate and, possibly, out of the estate of the surviving spouse. This type of trust is especially useful for the owner and

beneficiary of life insurance policies, since in that case one is making transfers of cash for premiums, which then balloon into the face value at death. To keep insurance out of the estate, the trustee must exercise discretion in both the purchase and the maintenance of insurance policies. These funds may yet be available for estate-liquidity needs if the trustee is empowered to either lend money to the estate or purchase assets therefrom. There are a myriad of possibilities for using an irrevocable trust in one's life- and death-related planning.

Short-term Trusts

Short-term, or Clifford trusts as they are generally called, are created mainly for income tax purposes. Since a trust may be a separate taxpayer if made irrevocable for at least 10 years, income tax savings may be affected by transferring property and having the income therein taxed at the lower tax brackets of the respective beneficiaries. There are quite a few technicalities to observe to ensure that the income is not taxed to the grantor. These rules relate to limiting the grantor's control of, and economic benefits from, the trust. The grantor will, however, be considered to be making a taxable gift to the extent of the present value of the income interest transferred. After the stipulated time, the property reverts to the grantor or the estate. One use of such a trust may be to place property therein that is used in the physician's practice and then rent it back from the trust. The advantage of this approach is that the rental paid is deductible by the physician as a business expense, reducing his or her income at its higher bracket and making the rent taxable at the lower brackets of the beneficiaries, such as children.

In summary, the above are just a few of the many concepts and ideas that can be adapted to help save taxes and yet provide security for present and future needs. There are many intricacies involved in the integration of property law and federal and state tax laws in keeping with the physician's particular needs and desires. Every member of the estate-planning team has a contribution to make in the thinking process involved so that nothing is overlooked. A good attorney is essential to the implementation of the plan through careful and competent drafting of the wills, trusts, or other documents involved. The selection of an attorney is a critical component of the financial planning process. Again, references from colleagues can be helpful, and an attorney reference service is provided by most local bar associations. The physician should be careful to ascertain experience in this particular aspect of legal work and also consider the personal elements of faith and trust.

8
Health Insurance

Robert A. Zelten

Most Americans are protected by some form of health insurance. About 90% of all Americans under the age of 65 are covered by private health insurance, but the vast majority of this coverage is extended to employees and dependents under group health insurance contracts issued to employers, health and welfare funds, and other groups. In addition, an estimated 60% of Americans over age 65 supplement their Medicare coverage with private health policies.

Public third-party payment programs also provide protection against the cost of health care services. In 1977, 26 million people were enrolled in Medicare, and 22 million received benefits under Medicaid.

The widespread existence of health insurance, however, should not be mistaken for complete protection. About 20 million Americans are without any form of health insurance. Moreover, for some who are covered, the layer of protection is thin. Overall, in 1977, 30.3% of all personal health care expenditures were paid directly out of pocket by consumers; that is, they were not paid by insurance (1). The proportion paid out of pocket varied according to type of service (Table 1).

It is the purpose of this chapter to discuss the nature of insurance programs that provide reimbursement for health care services with specific attention focused on coverage for physicians' services. In fiscal 1977, $32.184 billion were expended for physician services exclusive of amounts paid to salaried, hospital-based physicians. Figure 1 summarizes the sources of these payments.

PRIVATE INSURANCE PROGRAMS

Types of Private Insurers

Currently, the private health insurance market in the United States is composed of 69 Blue Cross plans, 69 Blue Shield plans, 800 commercial health insurers, and about 400 other types of organizations, one-half of which are health maintenance organizations (HMOs).

Blue Cross plans pay for hospital services and operate through contracts with hospitals that describe how hospitals will be reimbursed for treating Blue Cross subscribers. Blue Cross plans do not compete with one another; they generally

Table 1. Per Capita and Out-of-Pocket Expenditures for Personal Health Care Services (Fiscal 1977)

Type of Service	Total Per Capita Expenditures	Percent Paid Out-of-Pocket
Hospital care	$297.38	5.9
Physicians' services	145.84	38.8
Dentists' services	45.41	79.5
Other professional services	14.56	43.5
Drugs and drug sundries	56.72	83.1
Eyeglasses and appliances	9.45	91.9
Nursing home care	57.18	41.4
Other health services	19.59	—
Total—all services	$646.11	30.3

Source: U.S. Department of Health, Education, and Welfare: *Social Security Bull.* July 1978.

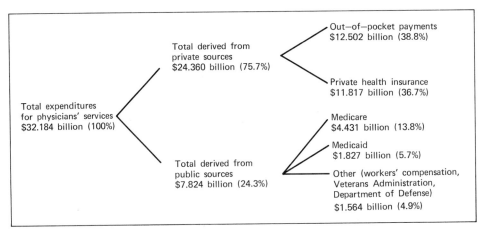

Figure 1. Sources of payment for physicians' services, 1977. (*Source:* U.S. Department H.E.W., *Social Security Bulletin,* July 1978.)

operate in nonoverlapping geographic areas. From a tax standpoint, Blue Cross plans are nonprofit organizations. At the end of 1977, Blue Cross covered 83.5 million people, including 8.6 million with Medicare supplementary coverage (2).* Enrollment in Blue Cross has been stable over the past several years.

Blue Shield pays for physicians' services and generally operates through contracts with individual physicians who are referred to as "Blue Shield participating providers." Even though there are 69 Blue Cross and 69 Blue Shield plans, Blue Cross and Blue Shield plans do not always cover coincident areas. For example, five Blue Cross plans operate in Pennsylvania, whereas there is a single, statewide Blue Shield plan. In recent years, several Blue Shield plans have

*Medicare supplementary coverage refers to a product that provides insurance coverage for many expenses not covered by the federal Medicare program.

merged with Blue Cross plans. In areas where the plans have not merged, however, Blue Cross frequently performs marketing and other services for Blue Shield under joint operating agreements. Joint operating agreements make it easier to combine hospital expense and physician expense coverage in a single insurance contract. Enrollment in Blue Shield has been declining slightly in recent years. At the end of 1977, about 70.9 million people had Blue Shield coverage. An estimated 85% of Blue Cross and Blue Shield subscribers are covered by group contracts.

Commercial health insurers are regulated under the standard state insurance statutes, whereas Blue Cross and Blue Shield are regulated under special enabling laws in most states. There are few commercial insurance companies that have health insurance as their major line of business. The commercial health-insurance field is dominated by life insurance companies. Prudential, Travelers, Aetna, Connecticut General, and Equitable are the five largest, and each has annual health insurance premium income well in excess of $1 billion. Commercial health insurers combine all types of health coverage in a single contract. They do not operate under territorial franchises and compete against each other as well as against Blue Cross and Blue Shield for policyholders. They do not have contracts with participating providers.

About 97 million people have some hospital expense protection through commercial companies. Commercial coverage for physicians' services is held by about 90 million people (3). Some of this protection is limited—primarily that purchased on an individual rather than group basis.

An additional 10 million people have health-expense protection with a variety of other organizations. Most of these people, about seven million, are enrolled in HMOs, a type of organization described in Chapter 1.

Finally, health care providers should be aware of a growing trend among some groups to self-insure and self-administer their employee health-benefits program. These steps are usually taken by employers in an effort to save money by enhancing their cash flow. They may hire their own employees to pay claims or contract with a company that specializes in administering such programs. Increasingly, hospitals and physicians are receiving payment directly from corporations rather than from insurance companies. It is too soon to determine what impact this trend will have on physicians. At a minimum, however, it evidences a growing interest on the part of premium payers to look more closely at the money they spend for health care.

Nature of Private Insurance Coverage

Basic medical expense and major medical expense are the two broad categories of health insurance. Sometimes the basic and major medical benefits are separately identifiable in a benefit program, and sometimes they are combined in a comprehensive medical-expense program.

Basic Medical-expense Insurance
Basic coverage affords protection against three types of medical expenses—hospital, surgical, and regular medical expenses.

Hospital-expense insurance provides coverage for hospital room and board

and nearly all other services provided by a hospital other than personal convenience items. Included are charges for laboratory tests, drugs, x-ray films, use
of operating and recovery rooms, and so on. The room-and-board benefit is
normally stated in one of two ways. Under the service-benefit approach, coverage is provided for the full semiprivate room-and-board charge of the hospital.
This approach is used by nearly all Blue Cross plans and is found in an increasing number of commercial insurance contracts. The second approach provides
coverage for room-and-board charges up to a specified maximum amount per
day. The Health Insurance Association of America indicates that 60% of Americans recently insured by commercial insurers in groups of 25–499 employees are
eligible for hospital room-and-board benefits equal to the hospital's semi-
private-room charge (3). In 1977, group insurance plans reimbursed 91% of
room-and-board charges and 90% of hospital charges for ancillary services for
those covered.

Hospital benefits typically are extended for 120–365 days per admission.
Restrictions are placed on some types of admissions, however. For example,
admissions for nervous and mental disorders and treatment for alcoholism and
drug addiction are often limited to 30 or 60 days. Maternity care may be provided
only if the pregnancy had its inception after the effective date of coverage.

Surgical-expense insurance typically provides coverage regardless of where
the surgical procedure is performed. Coverage is stated on either a fee schedule
or a prevailing-fee basis. Fee schedules specify the maximum an insurer will pay
for each procedure. Prevailing-fee, or usual, customary, and reasonable (UCR),
programs attempt to pay physicians their usual professional fee with some
limitations (physician reimbursement is explained later). An increasing number
of persons have UCR coverage for physicians' services. This coverage applies to
well over one-half of Blue Shield subscribers and to 60% of those covered in new
group health insurance policies issued in 1977 by commercial insurers. Group
health insurance policies provide relatively complete coverage for surgical services (Table 2). Little variation in percentage reimbursement exists according to
age or geographic region, but noticeable differences can be found across procedures.

Table 2. Adequacy of Group Health Insurance Protection for Covered Services

Type of Expense	Percent of Covered Expenses Reimbursed	
	1977	1967
Surgical procedures	83.8	77.0
Private-duty nursing	82.7	72.8
Anesthetist	82.6	84.4
Diagnostic x-ray films and laboratory tests	81.5	75.7
Physician visits, in hospital	74.1	70.4
Prescribed drugs	63.6	60.9
Physician visits, home and office	59.4	59.6

Source: Health Insurance Institute: Source Book of Health Insurance Data 1977–78.

Regular medical-expense insurance was developed after hospital and surgical coverage. It is designed to pay for physicians' nonsurgical services in a hospital, at home, or in the office. Coverage is sometimes provided for diagnostic services. Table 2 indicates the adequacy of regular medical-expense protection for those who have it. Many of the services ordinarily covered under regular medical-expense insurance are covered under major medical-expense coverage.

Major Medical-expense Insurance

Many basic health insurance policies provide extensive coverage, including most Blue Cross-Blue Shield plans and many group contracts issued by commercial insurers. However, in the early 1950s another type of coverage was developed to provide protection against potentially high health care costs. Referred to as major medical coverage, it is sometimes sold as a separate program to supplement existing basic coverage, and in other cases it provides comprehensive coverage by combining basic and extended coverage in a single unit.

With major medical insurance, most health care services prescribed by a physician are covered whether provided in or out of a hospital. In fact, major medical coverage is broader than even most policyholders realize. Maximum benefits of $25,000 per person are common, and limits of much higher amounts (including unlimited benefits) are becoming increasingly common.

One standard feature of major medical insurance is its use of patient cost-sharing. Most contracts contain both deductible and percentage-participation (or coinsurance) provisions. Deductibles are provisions that require the policyholder to pay certain otherwise covered costs out of pocket before major medical benefits begin. Deductibles take a variety of forms. The amount may be stated as an absolute dollar amount or as a percentage of income. They also may be applicable on a per illness, per person, or per family basis. A typical deductible clause would require a policyholder to incur costs of $100 out of pocket over basic benefits before major medical benefits would be payable.

Percentage participation, or coinsurance clauses, require the policyholder to pay a stipulated proportion (commonly 20%) of the cost of all covered services once the deductible has been satisfied. Certain services, such as outpatient psychiatric care, might require a higher level of patient payment (e.g., 50%). Some policies waive the percentage-participation requirement once the patient's out-of-pocket payments reach a stated amount.

Coverage Limitations

Some common limitations and exclusions are found in even the broadest private health insurance contracts. For example, any expenses due to accidental bodily injury or disease arising out of the work environment are excluded because such expenses are covered under workers' compensation. In general, services provided by a Veterans Administration provider, or covered under Medicare or other program, are excluded because the policyholder is not legally obligated to pay for such services.

Cosmetic surgical procedures are excluded from coverage unless necessary as a result of bodily injury. Custodial care and medically unnecessary services are generally excluded. Dental coverage is narrowly defined unless a special dental program is provided. Routine physical examinations or checkups are usually not covered unless a specific disease or injury is revealed or a definite symptomatic condition was present.

Under UCR programs, benefits will not be paid for charges or expenses that exceed the usual and customary charge in the locality.

Other Provisions

Most family health insurance contracts cover the spouse of the policyholder and all unmarried children under 19 years of age. Unmarried, full-time students are often covered up to age 23. Dependents beyond age 19 are also covered if incapable of self-support due to a physical or mental handicap.

Insurance companies attempt to eliminate duplicate payment for a given expense by including "coordination of benefit" provisions in group health-insurance policies. Where more than one group insurance policy is in effect, a priority of coverage is established that is designed to prohibit a patient from recovering more than 100% of the loss. These provisions do not extend to policies purchased on an individual basis.

Provider Reimbursement

Provisions for provider reimbursement vary a great deal. For example, there are major differences between hospital and physician reimbursement. Moreover, commercial insurers reimburse each of these major providers differently than do Blue Cross and Blue Shield. Blue Shield will often treat participating physicians differently than nonparticipating physicians. For convenience, the following discussion is divided into the mechanics and the level of reimbursement.

Mechanics of Reimbursement

Hospitals generally deal directly with insurers. Blue Cross plans establish procedures with their participating hospitals that allow hospitals to bill Blue Cross for services provided to Blue Cross subscribers. Since Blue Cross coverage for inpatient services is quite extensive, Blue Cross assumes responsibility for nearly the entire bill. The Blue Cross subscriber is responsible for the uncovered portion of the bill. This portion includes any deductibles or copayments and the charges for personal convenience items. Since Blue Cross usually accounts for a large portion of a hospital's revenues, arrangements often exist for speeding the flow of dollars to a hospital to minimize any cash-flow problems the hospital might face.

Whereas a hospital typically deals with one Blue Cross plan, it may deal with numerous commercial insurers. Hence, the relationships between hospitals and commercial health insurers are not as formal. Most commercial health insurance, however, permits the covered patient to assign benefits to the hospital. Hospitals nearly always attempt to obtain such an assignment so that they can bill the insurance company directly and thus reduce their bad debts. If the coverage is relatively complete, a commercially insured patient is in the same position as a Blue Cross subscriber. However, a hospital's administrative office will usually estimate how much of the bill will be recovered from the carrier and bill the patient for the estimated balance at the time of discharge.

This description applies to all group health insurance and most individual coverage. However, in recent years there has been substantial growth in the sale of "hospital indemnity" policies by commercial insurers. This coverage generally provides a stated dollar benefit (e.g., $40) for each day a policyholder is hospitalized. Under these policies, which are often sold through the mail, the insurer pays the policyholder directly. Policyholders usually supplement more extensive private or public hospital coverage with hospital indemnity policies.

Physician reimbursement is more complicated than hospital reimbursement. If a patient is covered by Blue Shield and the physician is a "participating" Blue Shield provider, the physician generally will submit the bill directly to Blue Shield on a standard claim form for payment. If not, a variety of procedures may be followed. Some Blue Shield plans do not reimburse nonparticipating physicians directly. Instead, they send payment directly to the subscriber, and the physician must bill the subscriber. Other Blue Shield plans pay participating and nonparticipating physicians on the same basis, whereas others will pay nonparticipating physicians directly if the physician obtains an assignment of benefits from the Blue Shield subscriber. Some Blue Shield plans (e.g., Blue Shield of Massachusetts) cannot, by law, pay nonparticipating physicians, nor may they reimburse subscribers who use them.

The situation is complicated further by the existence of fee-schedule benefit programs and UCR benefit programs. If a patient is covered by a Blue Shield fee-schedule program and uses a participating physician, the physician will bill the usual fee directly to Blue Shield. Blue Shield will pay the physician the fee-schedule allowance; the patient is responsible for the balance between the actual charge and fee-schedule allowance. If the patient has a low income, as described in the fee-schedule program, participating physicians are precluded from billing the patient for any amount in excess of the Blue Shield fee-schedule allowance. Blue Shield's failure to update the definition of "low-income subscriber" and the introduction of Medicaid in the mid-1960s have virtually eliminated the applicability of this full-service protection for low-income subscribers.

If the patient is covered by a Blue Shield UCR benefit program, participating physicians are precluded from billing the patient any amount over the Blue Shield payment. The physician bills Blue Shield directly, and Blue Shield bases its payment upon the "usual, customary, and reasonable" charge for the service in question. (This situation is described more fully below.)

Nonparticipating physicians are not bound by these rules. On the other hand, nonparticipating physicians may have their services covered less extensively than those of participating physicians, and they are generally required to collect their fees directly from the patients rather than from Blue Shield.

Because there are so many of them, commercial insurance companies do not find it feasible to use the concept of participating physicians. Also, because of the lack of standardization in claim forms and benefit programs, most physicians do not deal directly with commercial insurers. Rather, they bill the patient and leave it to the patient to obtain reimbursement from the insurance company. The physician's office staff, however, provides the patient with the information necessary to complete an insurer's claim form. For the most part, commercially insured patients are treated the same as Blue Shield subscribers who use nonparticipating physicians.

Level of Reimbursement

One of the reasons Blue Cross plans are able to provide broad hospital benefits is that their contracts with hospitals give them some control over what they will pay for such services. Commercial insurers do not have such contracts and are often forced to insert some coverage limitations directly into their health insurance agreements to limit their financial exposure. Commercial insurers pay whatever amount the hospital charges for its services up to the limits specified in their contracts with policyholders.

Blue Cross plans employ a variety of reimbursement formulas. A few plans pay charges, some negotiate a discount from charges, and others pay a rate determined by some state rate-setting authority. Many of the large Blue Cross plans, however, reimburse hospitals on the basis of costs.

Under cost-based reimbursement arrangements, a hospital submits its operating budget to Blue Cross just before the beginning of the hospital's fiscal year. Blue Cross personnel review the budget and determine an amount that may be described as the hospital's total allowable costs. Blue Cross essentially agrees to pay its share of allowable costs. A variety of techniques are employed to determine Blue Cross's share of allowable costs. In most cases, however, a fraction is applied to the total allowable budget. The numerator of the fraction may be the anticipated Blue Cross subscriber inpatient days, and the denominator may be the anticipated total inpatient days, that is, the ratio of Blue Cross days to total days. A more common calculation would place in the numerator the estimated charges assessed Blue Cross patients and in the denominator the total charges assessed all patients, that is, the ratio of Blue Cross charges to total charges. The product obtained by multiplying the fraction times the total allowable costs is Blue Cross's estimated share of the hospital's costs.

Once this calculation is made, the total usually is divided by the anticipated number of Blue Cross inpatient days to arrive at a cost per day. This figure is commonly referred to as the "interim per diem payment" and is the amount of money Blue Cross will pay to the hospital throughout the year for each day of inpatient care provided by the hospital to Blue Cross patients. At the end of the fiscal year, an audit is made to determine Blue Cross's share of the budget based on actual data. Any difference between the actual share and the total of interim payments already made is then transferred to the appropriate party to effect a final settlement for the year just ended.

Cost-based hospital reimbursement increasingly has come under attack as inflationary. Administrators of hospitals and hospital medical staffs have little reason to use resources efficiently since virtually any cost incurred is reimbursable. Cost-based reimbursement also provides Blue Cross with some substantial advantages in the group health insurance market. This advantage occurs because "allowable costs" as defined by Blue Cross are often less than "total operating costs" as defined by the hospital administrator. Hence, if a hospital is to recover revenues equal to its total operating costs, it will have to charge other patients enough to recover the costs not allowed by Blue Cross and other cost-based reimbursers. As a result, charges per day of care will exceed costs per day of care, and charge-based payers will be competitively worse off than cost-based payers in regard to patient premiums for insurance. Thus, some patients end up subsidizing others. Some states are attempting to equalize rates to address this problem.

Reimbursement of physicians' services under fee-schedule benefit programs is straightforward. The physician or patient will be paid the fee-schedule allowance unless the actual charge is less. Reimbursement under UCR benefit programs, however, is quite complex. Moreover, there is a good deal of variation in the operation of UCR programs from insurer to insurer.

Under UCR reimbursement arrangements, the insurer pays the physician's usual fee for a particular procedure as long as that fee does not exceed what is considered to be the *customary* fee for that procedure. Generally speaking, the customary fee is the fee that would fully reimburse 90% of the physicians performing that procedure in a designated geographic area. A higher payment could be made if it were reasonable because of unusual features in the particular case.

The typical Blue Shield UCR program creates and maintains "physician profiles." A profile is a collection of the physician's usual fees for the procedures performed by the physician. The usual fee for a procedure is the fee most frequently charged by a physician, as reflected on the claim forms submitted to Blue Shield. The plans update physician profiles with varying frequency. Some plans perform annual updates, whereas others do it quarterly. The less frequent the update, the greater the tendency for physicians to believe that they are being inadequately reimbursed. Some Blue Shield plans have been sued by their participating physicians for failing to update usual fee profiles as often and as liberally as they would like. In any event, the usual fee, as defined by Blue Shield, is what will be paid to participating physicians for procedures performed for Blue Shield subscribers. Moreover, participating physicians may not collect more than this amount by billing the patient.

Physicians whose usual fee for a procedure is above the customary fee for that procedure will not collect their usual fee (Table 3). In general, the maximum that will be paid to any provider for a procedure is the amount that would reimburse in full 90% of the physicians performing that procedure. In other words, physicians in the top 10% would be cut back to the ninetieth percentile fee. According to Table 3, $650 would be the maximum fee paid for Procedure A in 1978.

As noted, there exists a great deal of variation across Blue Shield plans in the actual operation of UCR reimbursement arrangements. Customary-fee levels may be updated at regular intervals of one year or each quarter, or they may be updated at irregular intervals. Some plans subdivide their geographic area of operation for purposes of reimbursement; for example, physicians practicing in urban areas may be separated from those in rural areas when customary-fee limits are calculated. Other plans apply different limits to different specialists performing the same procedure. More than a few Blue Shield plans do not maintain individual physician profiles. They reimburse whatever a physician charges for a covered service as long as the amount billed does not exceed the customary limit. This system permits physicians to get immediate recognition of fee increases, since increases in their individual charges are not limited by their own "usual" fees.

Commercial health insurance companies also offer UCR programs. There is great variety in the administration of these programs as well. It should be noted that commercial insurers have no authority to bind physicians to their payment levels since they do not have contracts with physicians. Some commercial insur-

Table 3. Operation of a UCR Program Calculating the Customary Fee
for Procedure A

Charge for Procedure A	1976 Number of Physicians	1976 Cumulative Percent of Charges	1977 Number of Physicians	1977 Cumulative Percent of Charges	1978 Number of Physicians	1978 Cumulative Percent of Charges
$300 or less	13	3	9	2	2	1
$325	3	4	2	3	0	1
$350	30	10	19	7	9	3
$375	3	11	5	8	2	3
$400	68	26	60	20	22	8
$425	12	29	9	23	5	10
$450	75	45	69	37	36	18
$500	130	77	145	69	119	45
$550	25	84	43	79	44	56
$600	46	94	53	91	112	80
$650	12	97	16	95	28	89*
$650 plus	64	100	60	100	94	100
Total number of physicians with charges	481		490		473	
Highest charge		$950		$1,500		$1,200

*The customary fee or the highest fee allowed in 1978 would be the fee that included 90% of all charges that year.

Source: Support materials furnished in a Blue Shield rate filing in New Jersey. The dates have been changed.

ers contend, however, that physicians often accept the insurer's reimbursement as full payment.

There is growing disenchantment with UCR programs. Much of the concern is that such programs are highly inflationary. Since they are automatically updated, it is easier for physicians to receive increased fees. Also, after UCR programs operate for a period of time, fees "bunch" toward the top of the customary range; that is, the fees for a particular procedure are not evenly dispersed (Table 3). Hence, even though the maximum fee allowed might increase only modestly, total expenditures for a particular procedure may increase dramatically as physicians with fees below the maximum raise their fees to the customary-fee level.

A variety of controls have been discussed or are being introduced into UCR programs to check both fee inflation and total expenditure increases. Some plans have resorted to less frequent updates of both usual fees and customary limits. Others have placed limits on permitted increases for usual fees and for maximum fees. A few plans have applied some sort of index to permitted increases. There is little doubt that UCR programs will come under closer scrutiny as the interest in cost containment grows.

PUBLIC HEALTH INSURANCE PROGRAMS

Medicare and Medicaid are the two principal public programs that provide protection against health care costs (Fig. 1). In the sections that follow, eligibility for benefits, services covered, program administration, financing, and reimbursement will be discussed.

Medicare

Medicare was created when Title XVIII was added to the Social Security Act. It has two parts. Part A of Medicare (Basic Plan of Hospital Insurance) provides benefits to cover the cost of hospital and related care. Part B (Voluntary Supplementary Medical Insurance Plan) provides benefits to cover the cost of physicians' services and certain other medical services not covered by Part A.

Eligibility

Since July 1966, all people entitled to social security benefits or railroad retirement annuities who are 65 or older have been entitled to Medicare benefits whether or not they are retired. In 1973, benefits were extended to certain disability beneficiaries and to any person under age 65 with chronic renal disease. Eligible persons must file an application for benefits. Since participation in Part B requires a financial contribution, eligible persons are given an opportunity to decline Part B coverage, but they rarely do. People over age 65 who are not eligible for Part A benefits can enroll voluntarily by paying the full cost. For such persons, enrollment in Part B is mandatory.

Benefits

Part A provides inpatient hospital care, posthospital skilled nursing services, and posthospital home health care services. Inpatient care is covered for up to 90 days for each episode of illness separated by 60 consecutive days outside of a hospital or skilled nursing facility. Each person also has available a 60-day lifetime reserve to provide added coverage after the 90 days are exhausted. Coverage in psychiatric hospitals has a 190-day lifetime limit. Inpatient benefits are subject to deductible and copayment provisions. A deductible equal to the national average cost of an inpatient day ($160 in 1979) must be paid by the patient, and a payment equal to one-fourth of this average per diem ($40 in 1979) must be paid for each day between the 60th and 90th. Each day of the lifetime reserve is subject to a copayment equal to one-half of the average per diem cost ($80 in 1979). These cost-sharing amounts are recalculated each year.

Posthospital care in a skilled nursing facility is provided for up to 100 days for each episode of illness. To be eligible, a patient must be transferred to the facility within 14 days after a hospital stay of at least three days and with a physician's authorization. A patient copayment ($20 in 1979) is required for every day after the first 20 days of posthospital care.

Posthospital home health care services for up to 100 visits in the year after discharge from a hospital or skilled nursing facility are also covered if the patient had been hospitalized for at least three days and the services are provided by a participating home health care agency.

Part B covers physicians' services no matter where they are furnished. Some services provided by dentists and chiropractors are also covered. Services and supplies incidental to the care provided by physicians are also covered. Other covered services include diagnostic tests and x-ray films, ambulance services, prosthetic devices, radiation therapy, and various other medical services. Part B also covers up to 100 home health care visits in addition to those provided under Part A. The Part B benefit does not require previous hospitalization, however. A limited outpatient psychiatric benefit is also provided.

Part B requires beneficiaries to pay a deductible of $60 per calendar year for covered services and to pay 20% of the remaining covered expenses. Further, Medicare does not reimburse for charges that are considered not to be reasonable based on customary and prevailing charges of physicians. The cost-sharing provisions do not apply to home health care services.

Because of the deductible and copayment provisions of Medicare and the exclusion of certain services from coverage (e.g., prescription drugs, ordinary dental services, and routine physical examinations), Medicare currently covers about one-half of the health care costs of the aged.

Administration

Medicare is administered, for the most part, by private insurers under contract to the federal government. These contractors, known as fiscal intermediaries, administer the program in accordance with rules developed by the Health Care Financing Administration (HCFA). Under Part A, providers select the intermediary through whom they wish to receive payment. Most hospitals, skilled nursing facilities, and home health care agencies have selected Blue Cross. There are currently 77 Part A intermediaries.

In selecting carriers under Part B, the government has the authority to contract with insurance companies and other organizations to handle payment for physicians' services. Such contractors serve specific geographic areas. There are now 46 carriers serving 60 areas.

The job of the intermediaries and carriers is to make payments and to audit payments. They also perform claims adjudication, utilization review, financial accounting, statistical activities, and professional relations.

Financing

Payments to providers of services covered by Part A of Medicare come out of the Hospital Insurance Trust Fund. The deposits to the trust fund are derived from payroll taxes levied on employers, employees, and the self-employed. The trust fund also earns interest income that helps pay for benefits. Persons not eligible for Medicare automatically but who enroll in the program voluntarily are charged a premium intended to cover the cost of services received.

Part B benefits and administrative expenses are paid out of the Federal Supplementary Medical Insurance Trust Fund. Unlike the trust fund for Part A, however, the Part B trust fund derives its money from federal general revenues and from premiums paid by those enrolled in Part B. The premiums are deducted from the monthly retirement-benefit checks of participants. The current monthly contribution for aged beneficiaries is $8.70 (4). The federal government contributes an additional $18.60 per beneficiary per month.

Reimbursement

Because Medicare participation by providers was to be voluntary, liberal reimbursement practices were initially part of the program. Hospitals and other Part A providers are paid the costs incurred by them in rendering care to program beneficiaries. Before Medicare existed, many hospitals had not been fully reimbursed because many members of the aged population were unable to pay their hospital bills.

The cost-based reimbursement method described earlier is employed by Medicare. Hospitals also receive a 2% "nursing cost differential" to recognize that aged patients often require more intensive nursing services than does the average patient.

Until recently, not much attention was paid to the "reasonableness" of a hospital's costs. Now, however, maximum payment levels, or ceilings, have been established for routine hospital costs through peer-group comparisons.

Initially, payments for physicians' services under Part B were based on customary and prevailing fees. Although the terminology is different, this payment method was comparable to the UCR reimbursement method described above. Under Medicare, customary refers to a particular physician's fee profile (the usual fee under UCR), whereas the prevailing fee is the maximum reimbursement allowed (the customary limit under UCR).

After some initial experience, the prevailing-fee limit was set at the 75th percentile rather than the 90th percentile often used in UCR payment programs. The current prevailing fee limit is based on the 75th percentile of prevailing charges in fiscal 1973 adjusted in subsequent years by an index designed to reflect increases in the costs of running a physician's office. If the index method continues to be employed, it is likely that reimbursement for physicians' services will resemble fee-schedule reimbursement since most physicians' customary charges will eventually reach the prevailing limit (4).

Whether Part B reimbursement practices have an impact on a particular provider depends on whether the physician accepts Medicare assignment. Accepting assignment means that the physician must accept the Medicare payment, plus the 20% coinsurance payment required of the patient, as full payment. A physician is permitted to accept assignment on a patient-by-patient basis. The physician may accept or reject assignment for the same patient on a visit-by-visit basis. A physician who accepts assignment under Medicare is in essentially the same position as a physician who participates in Blue Shield. The difference, of course, is that participation in Blue Shield applies to all Blue Shield subscribers, whereas under Medicare it is optional for each patient and each visit.

Physicians who do not accept assignment under Medicare bill their patients directly and may charge whatever they wish. In these cases, the patient is responsible for the bill and must make a claim against the Part B carrier for reimbursement. The carrier will reimburse only the amount eligible for payment under the above rules. Medicare beneficiaries often end up paying more than 20% of the physician's charge when assignment is not accepted by the physician.

Currently, it is estimated that about one-half of physicians' bills paid under Part B involve assignments.

Medicaid

Title XIX was added to the Social Security Act at the same time that Title XVIII was added. Title XIX, or Medicaid, is a public assistance program designed to provide protection against medical expenses for the poor. It is a voluntary program, and no state is required to have such a program.

However, if legislation is not enacted at the state level, federal financial participation is lost. Because the federal support is derived from general tax revenues, there is a strong incentive for states to establish a Medicaid program since federal taxpayers in the state are forced to contribute to federal Medicaid support whether or not they have a program.

The federal legislation establishes standards that a state program must meet to be eligible for federal support. The specific features of Medicaid, however, are left to individual states, which actually administer the program. Hence, wide differences are found among the various state plans, and it is virtually impossible to generalize about Medicaid.

Reference to Figure 1 indicates that Medicaid accounted for 5.7% of national personal health care expenditures for physicians' services in fiscal 1977. This figure is less than half the share paid by Medicare.

Eligibility

Federal financial participation is extended for benefits provided to persons "whose income and resources are insufficient to meet the costs of necessary medical services." Subsequent amendments to the legislation set an upper limit on net income for persons for whom federal support would be available, but states have substantial discretion in establishing specific eligibility standards.

A qualifying state program is required to provide Medicaid benefits to all people receiving public assistance benefits under the state's categorical cash-assistance programs. In addition, matching federal assistance is available for people who are not in financial need, as defined in the cash-assistance programs, but who are placed in financial need because of medical expenses. People in this category are often referred to as the "medically needy." Twenty-eight states extended Medicaid benefits to the medically needy, whereas 21 did not, as of mid-1976. Arizona does not have a Medicaid program.

Benefits

To receive federal support, a state program must provide at least the following services to everyone receiving federally supported financial assistance: inpatient hospital care; outpatient hospital services; other laboratory and x-ray services; skilled nursing facility and home health care services for people 21 and over; early and periodic screening, diagnosis, and treatment for those under 21; family planning; and physician services.

Many states pay for additional services that also are supported partially with federal funds. Some common additional services are:

- Prescribed drugs
- Dental services
- Prosthetic devices
- Optometrists' services
- Eyeglasses
- Podiatrists' services
- Emergency hospital services
- Institutional services in intermediate-care facilities, including institutions for the mentally retarded

States can provide different services for the medically needy as opposed to the categorically needy. Federal financial support will be extended for the medically needy as long as the state program provides a combination of at least seven acceptable benefits.

No qualified state program can require patient cost-sharing for inpatient hospital services used by cash-assistance recipients. Other cost-sharing provisions must be related to the recipients' resources.

Administration
Each state bears the ultimate responsibility for the administration of its Medicaid program. About one-third of the states administer their own programs, whereas the others contract with fiscal agents in the private sector to handle the administration of the program. Contracts vary from state to state. In Texas, for example, the fiscal agent performs an insuring role since he or she is responsible for paying all valid claims in exchange for a predetermined per capita premium. Typically, however, fiscal agents perform only administrative functions and are paid on a cost-reimbursement, fixed-price, or fixed-rate basis (5). Depending on the state, the Medicaid program is operated out of the department of health, department of welfare, or the department of social services.

Financing
As noted above, each state with an approved Medicaid program is eligible for federal financial participation. The federal share of the costs of medical services is based on each state's per capita income. At a minimum, the federal share is 50%. Sixteen states received 50% in 1977; the 78% matching assistance received by Mississippi was the highest. The source of both state and federal funding for Medicaid is general revenues.

The federal government also matches state administrative costs. The proportion matched by federal funds varies according to administrative function.

Reimbursement
Payment for inpatient hospital services under Medicaid is similar to Medicare reimbursement. A great deal of variation exists, however, in the payment for other services. Virtually all states place some limitations on what a physician will be paid. Some are very restrictive and pay physicians on the basis of fee schedules. Others use negotiated charges or pay usual and customary charges

(6). Because Medicaid beneficiaries are poor, the state's Medicaid allowance establishes the maximum payment that a physician is likely to receive for services provided to Medicaid patients.

Other Public Programs

Although Medicare and Medicaid account for most of the public expenditures for physicians' services, several other public programs pay for care provided by physicians. The most important other program is workers' compensation. Workers' compensation programs are state programs that provide income continuation and medical-expense benefits for injured workers. In fiscal 1977, workers' compensation programs paid $1.1 billion for physicians' services. Workers' compensation programs vary across the states as much as Medicaid programs.

CONCLUSION

The characteristics of private and public third-party programs that pay for physicians' services have been described in this chapter. The various programs are complicated. Although these programs rarely place limitations on what a physician may charge for services, they often effectively limit what a physician may be able to collect.

There is growing dissatisfaction with current methods of paying physicians. Fee-for-service payment encourages excessive services. UCR payment programs encourage physicians to inflate fees to reach satisfactory fee profiles. Since profiles are generally updated on an annual basis, physicians often charge today what they hope to be collecting next year.

Experiments with different physician-payment methods likely will continue. Health maintenance organizations will undoubtedly continue to grow. Medicare and Medicaid will also experiment with different payment systems. Whatever emerges in the current cost-containment environment, however, it is not likely to pay physicians more. On the other hand, health services provided by primary care physicians are likely to become more extensively covered by third-party payment programs.

REFERENCES

1. Gibson RM, Fisher CR: National health expenditures, fiscal year 1977. *Social Security Bull.* 41; July 1978, p. 7.

2. Blue Cross Association and Blue Shield Association: *Fact Book 1978*. Chicago, 1978.

3. Health Insurance Institute: *Source Book of Health Insurance Data 1977–78*. Washington, DC, 1978.

4. Myers RJ: *Basic Provisions and Present Principles of the Medicare System, Social Security*. Homewood, Illinois, Richard D Irwin, 1975.

5. Health Care Financing Administration: *Report to the Administrator, Recommendations. Medicare and Medicaid Contracting*. Rockville, Maryland, Department of Health, Education, and Welfare, October, 1978, vol 1.

6. Davidson SM: Variations in state Medicaid programs. *J Health Politics Policy Law* 3:54, 1978.

9
Legal Aspects of Health Care

Arnold J. Rosoff

In recent years, legal regulation has increasingly affected the delivery of health-care services in the United States. This effect is attributable in part to the greatly increased involvement of the federal government in the financing of health care through the Medicare and Medicaid programs begun in the mid-1960s. It is also due to increased demand by the public for legal protection of its interests in a complex and difficult area. To function effectively and with protection of their own interests, physicians and other health care providers must be aware of the requirements placed on them by the legal system.

Regulating health care delivery effectively poses a difficult and somewhat paradoxical challenge. On one hand, the system requires regulation because of intense inflationary pressures and the dangers of poor or inconsistent quality in high-technology medical care. On the other hand, health care regulation is especially difficult because of the complexity of the field and the emphasis on professionalism, which has, as its essence, the notion of self-regulation. If one assumes that the portion of our nation's gross national product available for health care delivery is relatively fixed, the question becomes how many of the available dollars should be spent on the direct provision of care and how many on "watchdogs."

This situation and its inherent complexities underlie the sensitive—but highly interesting—interface between medicine and law, an interface with heavy political overtones. What we are viewing here is the attempted regulation of an area of activity that has until recently not been regulated to any appreciable degree, and one that is highly resistant to regulation. To be effective, the physician must maintain a close, personal and confidential relationship with the patient. Such a relationship can be jeopardized by the intervention of external forces that imply that the physician may not deserve the patient's full trust. Furthermore, the practice of medicine, even in these days of high technologic sophistication, is still very much an art. To adapt to complex clinical situations, the physician must have substantial latitude for personal judgment and decision-making. Regulation that would impose rigid restrictions on professional judgment could be counterproductive to the goal of good patient care.

The objective of this chapter is to give a general overview of the broad range of applicable legal principles—the framework of laws in which the health care practitioner must operate. Given the breadth of the chapter's coverage, many subjects are not fully discussed. Nevertheless, the material should sensitize practitioners to the various legal issues involved in their practices, as well as alert them as to when to secure needed information.

LICENSURE OF MEDICAL PROFESSIONALS

The licensure of health professionals in the United States has a varied and interesting history, with cyclic changes roughly paralleling the political and social development of the emerging nation itself. During the Revolution and the direct post-Revolutionary period, several states attempted the regulation of medical practice by establishing state boards of medical examination and licensure. However, as the country began to expand rapidly in the early 1800s, the need for physicians was so great that many of the states abandoned their attempts to impose restrictions on and requirements for medical practice. During this period, a medical school diploma was accepted as a license to practice, although the schools were highly variable in the quality and content of their teaching.

By the mid-1800s, the number of such schools had grown to about 460, many of questionable academic stature. Promotion of higher standards of medical education was one of the prime objectives of the AMA when it was founded in 1847. As expansion slowed and the country became more settled in the latter part of the nineteenth century, the movement toward reinstatement of medical-licensure laws was slowed by the development of healing cults, each advocating its own particular approach to medical care. Osteopathy was developed in 1872 as a separate and distinct branch of the healing arts; chiropractic made its debut in 1894. Texas, in 1873, was the first state to adopt a modern medical-practice act; numerous other states followed soon after. These laws—still extant in essentially the same form—specified the elements of the medical curriculum, the minimum length of training required, and the acceptable ways of documenting that the requisite training had been received. By 1895, nearly all states had medical-practice acts and licensing examinations, although several states still would accept a diploma from a qualified medical school as proof of the physician's competence to practice.

With the publication in 1910 of the Flexner report on medical education, a movement to standardize the training of medical practitioners began. The number of medical schools had already decreased to approximately 160 by 1900, and after the Flexner report this number fell even lower. In 1912, after the report's issuance, the Federation of State Boards of Medical Examiners was formed. This action was followed in 1915 by the formation of the National Board of Medical Examiners (NBME), the group that today develops and administers the standardized examination accepted in most states and territories as proof of competence to practice. Interestingly enough, in 1915, the first year that the NBME test was given, only eight states were willing to accept the test results as proof of competence. Thirty-two students applied to take the examination; 16

qualified for the test, 10 actually showed up to take it, and only five passed. Today, thousands of medical students around the country take the test each year. Still, although most states now accept the NBME examinations, licensure continues to be handled on a state-by-state basis.

Limitations of the Current System

The limitations of our present state-based medical-licensure system are substantial. Assuming that the system does an adequate job of assuring a baseline level of competence when physicians are initially admitted to practice, there is no guaranty of continuing competence. Disciplinary actions against physicians are few, and the sanctions, in the rare occasions when they are imposed, tend to be extremely weak. Suprising as it may seem, there is no formal link in many states between the judicial determination of liability in a civil action for malpractice and the institution of governmental proceedings to revoke or suspend the practitioner's license. Malpractice reform acts adopted in many states in the mid-1970s have addressed this procedural deficiency.

Even where the current licensing structure performs its function of assuring an acceptable level of competence among practitioners, it still has its negative aspects. The overly rigid specification of the medical curriculum in many states serves as a barrier to innovation in education and to the recognition of new classes of health professionals. Many claim that antiquated and inflexible medical licensure requirements place an undue and anticompetitive restriction on entry into the medical marketplace. Clearly, steps might be taken to improve the contribution of the medical licensure system to the quality of care and access to that care.

Improving the Licensure System

Substantial innovations are being considered and tried. There is a developing trend toward the imposition of continuing-education requirements for the renewal of practitioner's licenses. The requirement for continuing education provides some assurance that practitioners stay current with new developments in their respective medical care fields. There has been talk, but no action to date, of instituting a system of mandatory periodic reexamination, since attendance at continuing-education functions does not, in itself, give adequate assurance that acceptable levels of competence and knowledge are being maintained. As noted above, many states have recently taken steps to tie the medical malpractice litigation system to the process of licensure and professional discipline. Finally, many states are experimenting with the recognition of new categories of health professionals. Physicians' assistants, nurse practitioners, child-health associates, and other forms of "physician extenders" are being tried in many different settings. On the whole, the experience with the use of these new paraprofessionals and with their regulation has been favorable. There is still a long way to go, however, before state licensing systems for health professionals fully meet their responsibility for assuring adequate access and quality in health care services.

THE PHYSICIAN'S DUTY TO TREAT

Does the physician have a legal duty to render medical care in an emergency situation? This question has been raised several times in different contexts, and the answer is quite clear: no. There is, of course, an ethical duty recognized by the medical profession. The "Principles of Medical Ethics," published by the Judicial Council of the American Medical Association, contains the following edict:

> Section 5. A physician may choose whom he will serve. In an emergency, however, he should render service to the best of his ability. Having undertaken the care of a patient, he may not neglect him; and unless he has been discharged, he may discontinue his services only after giving adequate notice.

Thus, the duty to treat is a professionally prescribed, not a legal duty. The 1901 Indiana case of *Hurley vs Eddingfield* (1) remains a definitive precedent on this issue. The defendant, Dr. Eddingfield, had been the decedent's family physician for several years. When the decedent became dangerously ill, a messenger informed the physician of the decedent's violent illness, tendered him the fee for his service, and informed him that no other physician was procurable in time and that the decedent relied on him for attention. Without giving any reason, Dr. Eddingfield refused to answer the call for aid. Apparently, no other patients required the physician's immediate service, and he could have gone to the relief of the decedent if he had been willing. Death ensued, the trial court found, because the physician withheld care. On the basis of the above facts, the Indiana Supreme Court held that the physician had no common law duty to render aid, even in a situation where he had reason to believe that the patient's life was in jeopardy. The plaintiff argued that the physician, by virtue of seeking and accepting a license to practice in the state, assumed a corresponding duty to render care when it was needed. The court held: "In obtaining the state's license (permission) to practice medicine, the state does not require, and the licensee does not engage, that he will practice at all or on other terms than he may choose to accept."

Acknowledging that there is no common law duty to render aid, and that the medical practice act does not compel a licensed physician to do so, the question remains whether there is some other statutory authority that might be invoked on behalf of the duty. In a 1968 Rhode Island case (2), a physician was summoned by state police to render emergency medical aid to a woman who had been injured in an automobile accident. Through his wife, also a doctor, the physician declined, claiming that he was ill. A suit was brought by the police against both husband and wife under an old 1896 statute, apparently never before applied, which read:

> Aid and assistance in execution of office. Every town sergeant and constable, in the due execution of his office, may command all necessary aid and assistance in the execution of his said office; and every person who, when so required, shall refuse or neglect to give such aid and assistance, shall be fined not exceeding $20 (3).

Although the sanction provided in the statute was minimal, the case was nevertheless an important precedent. The trial judge held that the statute did not empower police to order physicians to provide emergency care. The trial judge reasoned that the purpose of the statute was to enlist *unskilled* aid, such as a police officer might want to commandeer to help stop a runaway horse, summon assistance, and so on. It was not intended, the judge reasoned, to authorize police to commandeer the assistance of citizens with particular skills that might be useful in emergency situations. Said the judge:

> Where are you going to limit the use of someone else's brains in an emergency? What if the Mount Hope Bridge starts shaking in the middle? Do the police have the power to summon an engineer from his vacation at the beach? (4).

The court's reasoning raises a paradox: although unskilled persons can be required by the police to render assistance, those who have particular talents or capabilities may not. This ironic result presumably rests on recognition of a property interest that a person acquires in skills or abilities that he or she has invested time, effort, or money in acquiring. Thus, a physician's knowledge and talent are his or her own and can be sold or otherwise disposed of as he or she sees fit, free from any compulsion by private or public authority.

Should There Be a Duty to Treat?

Although the above cases accurately reflect the American jurisprudential position on this question, they run counter to the law of many other countries around the world, especially European countries, which follow a civil law system (i.e., a system based on Roman law). In such countries as France, West Germany, the Scandinavian nations, Poland, the Soviet Union, and Spain, the law requires persons, not just physicians, to render such aid as they can in an emergency situation. The German statutory provision is illustrative:

> Anybody who does not render aid in an accident or common danger or in an emergency situation, although aid is needed and under the circumstances can be expected of him, especially if he would not subject himself thereby to any considerable danger, or if he would not thereby violate other important duties, shall be punished by imprisonment not to exceed one year or a fine (5).

No data are readily available to determine how many prosecutions have been brought under civil-law provisions such as that quoted. One would assume that there have been few successful prosecutions. However, even without aggressive enforcement, such statutory enactments reflect society's expectations about what a person should do to help his fellow man. The American position on compelling aid by physicians is probably based less on principle than on practicality. Obviously, the application of such a mandate would pose important difficulties. For example, if, as in the Rhode Island case above, a physician claimed that he or she was too ill to render useful assistance, on what basis might this claim be challenged? The Rhode Island physician who refused to answer the police call may have indulged to excess in New Year's "cheer" and did not feel sober enough to render aid or assistance. Certainly, a law that robbed him of his right to make such determinations might run counter to the best interests of patients. Or suppose, instead, that a physician is summoned late at night by a telephone call from a distraught mother who insists that her child is deathly ill. How would the courts evaluate the physician's claim that, after listening to a description of the child's symptoms, he determined that the mother's apprehension was groundless? The point of these hypothetical situations is that even if we accept the principle of requiring physicians to render emergency assistance, the application of that principle still may pose substantial difficulties. Is it advisable for legislatures to adopt legal requirements that they know, as a practical matter, cannot be implemented? These are rhetorical questions, but it is worthwhile that they be raised and carefully considered by medical practitioners.

"Good Samaritan" Laws

A discussion of the rendering of care in emergencies must address the laws that most states have enacted to protect "good Samaritans." At last count, all American jurisdictions, with the exception of the state of Washington, had such laws on the books. The following Vermont provision is representative:

> (b) a person who provides reasonable assistance in . . . [an emergency] shall not be liable in civil damages unless his acts constitute gross negligence or unless he will receive or expects to receive remuneration. Nothing contained in this Subsection shall alter existing law with respect to tort liability of a practitioner of the healing arts for acts committed in the ordinary course of his practice (6).

In many states, such grants of statutory immunity are restricted to licensed health care providers. The purpose of the good Samaritan laws is to encourage persons to stop and render assistance in emergency situations. They are a response to fears voiced by practitioners that they might be subject to negligence liability if a bad outcome were to result from the attempt to provide care under difficult conditions. It is interesting to note that there are no important cases recorded of physicians, or other good Samaritans, actually being found liable in such situations. Since the law judges physicians' actions in light of the exigencies of the emergency situation, their fears of being held liable are essentially groundless. It is even more interesting to note that a poll conducted by the AMA in the early 1960s indicated that a smaller percentage of physicians would stop to render emergency assistance in states that had enacted good Samaritan legislation than in those that had not (7). One can speculate that the debates attending the passage of the laws did more to raise physicians' fears than the passage of the laws did to allay them. The results of the AMA study are far from conclusive, and it is mentioned here simply as a point of interest. The fact remains, however, that physicians doing their best to render assistance under emergency conditions would seem to have nothing to fear legally. The good Samaritan statutes merely codify what was already the law.

"Abandonment"

As reflected in the quotation from the AMA's Principles of Medical Ethics, a physician who has undertaken the care of a patient may not discontinue services without the patient's consent unless he or she gives adequate notice. In this context, "adequate notice" means sufficient time, under the circumstances, for the patient to seek care from some other practitioner or source. A physician who discontinues treatment without adequate notice is guilty of "abandonment" and would be legally responsible for any harm that befell the patient as a result of leaving him or her without an alternative source of care.

Cases of abandonment are extremely rare today, given the availability of hospital emergency rooms and other sources to which a patient could turn for care if "abandoned" by his regular physician. Still, every practitioner should understand fully the responsibility assumed when undertaking the care of a patient. If the physician has reason to anticipate that a patient will need his or her services, the physician may not take a vacation or otherwise be unavailable without making arrangements to assure proper referral of the patient to alternative sources of care. Most physicians would make such arrangements anyway as a matter of providing good service to their patients, maintaining goodwill, or professional ethics. It should be recognized, however, that, at bottom, a legal requirement is involved. A physician who causes a patient to rely on him or her and then is not available when the services are needed is in substantial legal jeopardy. A patient who expresses a desire that the physician discontinue providing care thereby consents to that discontinuance and terminates the physician's responsibility. This result assumes, of course, that the physician, if challenged, could prove this fact. It is extremely important that where a physician-patient relationship has existed and is discontinued, the physician adequately document the termination of the relationship and the date—as closely as it can be ascertained—on which that termination took place. As will be seen later in this chapter, the date of termination of a physician-patient relationship may be extremely important for application of the statute of limitations on medical malpractice actions.

RESPONSIBILITIES OF A PHYSICIAN TO A PATIENT

As will be discussed later, the relationship between a physician and a patient is basically contractual, even in the absence of a written document providing evidence of the contract. Beyond this contractual element, however, the relationship is also "fiduciary." In other words, it is a relationship of trust and confidence, in which one party is dependent to an appreciable degree on the other. Other examples of fiduciary relationships include a guardian and his or her ward and a trustee and his or her beneficiary. In such situations, the law places special responsibility on the dominant party for the protection of the dependent party. The essence of this special responsibility is that the dominant party must put the good and welfare of the dependent before his or her own and that the dominant party also treat the dependent person in the same way as if he or she were in the subordinate position. The fiduciary relationship is perhaps best understood by comparison to a standard "arms-length" bargaining transaction, where the parties have more or less equal bargaining power and it is expected that each will act for his own best advantage. The fact that a fiduciary element is involved has important implications for the physician-patient relationship.

The Duty to Preserve Confidentiality

One important aspect of the fiduciary relationship is the obligation of confidentiality, which the physician owes to his or her patient. The duty to keep patient information confidential has long been recognized as a most important aspect of medical practice. The ancient Hippocratic oath included the provision that:

Whatever, in connection with my professional practice, or not in connection with it, I may see or hear in the lives of men which ought not to be spoken abroad I will not divulge, as reckoning that all should be kept secret.

This ethic is reflected in Section 9 of the American Medical Association's *Principles of Medical Ethics,* which states:

A physician may not reveal the confidences entrusted to him in the course of medical attendance, or the deficiencies he may observe in the character of patients, unless he is required to do so by law or unless it becomes necessary in order to protect the welfare of the individual or of the community.

The reasons for this requirement of confidentiality are both sound and obvious. To be effective in his treatment, the physician must know all the facts concerning the patient's situation. In turn, the patient must fully trust the physician and be willing to confide in him or her. That trust would be undermined if the patient could not assume that personal information would be kept in strict confidence. Furthermore, the physician's access to sensitive information places a greater responsibility of silence upon him or her. The physician may be in attendance when the defenses of the patient and the patient's family are let down, such as when the patient is semiconscious or delirious, or in other situations when the physician is privy to information that the average person is not. One further reason for the tradition of confidentiality, not as relevant today as in times past, is the scorn or ostracism that society might place upon a sick person out of its ignorance of the nature of disease.

However, although people are much more understanding about illness today, the reasons for the preservation of confidentiality remain strong. The duty is primarily ethical and professional, although there are legal grounds that could be asserted against a physician who breached a patient's confidence. Cases are extremely rare on this point. To recover damages for a breach of confidence, a patient would have to show either demonstrable harm resulting from the breach or that the breach was motivated by the malice or bad faith of the physician. In the latter case, punitive damages would be assessed. The most important consequence that a physician might fear by breaching confidence is the possibility of the revocation or suspension of his license for "unprofessional conduct." Even disciplinary actions of this sort are rare, however.

Closely related to the doctrine of confidentiality is the so-called physician-patient privilege against testifying in court. To preserve the confidentiality discussed above, the patient has a right to prevent any personal information from being disclosed by the treating physician in court, or otherwise in a legal proceeding, without the patient's express consent. In other words, the physician has a legal right to keep this information secret, a right that only the patient can waive. There are some exceptions to this right, of course, such as where a statute requires health care providers to inform police or other authorities of certain kinds of illnesses or gunshot wounds that they are called to treat. The rationale for recognizing an exception in these cases is the protection of the public welfare, regarded in appropriate circumstances as an objective of higher order than protection of the patient's confidentiality.

It is not the intent of this chapter to delve into the complexities of the law of evidence. For present purposes, it is sufficient that health care providers understand their general obligation to maintain patient information in close confidence.

Theoretically, a question might be raised in a particular case regarding the exchange of information between the patient's attending physician and other health care personnel with whom the physician exchanges information in the course of treating the patient. Cases challenging such exchanges do not arise. If one did, a court would likely find that the patient implicitly agreed to such an exchange as a reasonable adjunct to general authorization of the care being rendered. In a hospital setting, however, many persons with only minimal contact or relationship to a particular patient might have access to information about the patient's condition or activities or those of the family and friends while in the hospital. This information is confidential and should not be treated lightly. Conversations in a crowded hospital elevator between physicians, nursing staff, or other attendants concerning a patient should be scrupulously avoided. Physicians should take care not to discuss confidential aspects of patients' cases while walking in the hall or standing in areas where inappropriate persons might overhear. These prohibitions are meant to be applied intelligently, not with wooden absoluteness, but health care personnel should never lose sight of the obligation that they have to patients in their care.

One other important aspect of the confidentiality obligation, often overlooked in practice, is the need to keep sensitive information from the patient's family members unless the physician knows that the patient has no objection to this information being shared. The health care provider might think, quite naturally, that the spouse, adult offspring, brothers, and sisters of the patient should be kept apprised of the patient's condition and the course of treatment. In general, such a sharing of information will be consistent with the patient's wishes and is advisable, but the health care provider cannot simply make this assumption. It should be an easy matter in almost every case to check with the patient first, tactfully, to ascertain his or her wishes in this regard.

MALPRACTICE AND THE DUTY OF CARE

There are two potential grounds on which a health care provider may be held liable to a patient: tort and contract. A tort is a civil wrong, an injury to one's person, property, or reputation, for which the law will award damages to the aggrieved party. In the context of health care malpractice, tort liability is further subdivided into intentional, or deliberate, torts and negligent torts, that is, those attributable to the practitioner's careless or inadvertent failure to observe the applicable standard of care in treatment. Charges of intentional tort are most often couched as matters of "assault and battery," or lack of consent. The subject of "informed consent" will be dealt with at length in the following section. A physician is seldom held liable on contract law grounds; therefore, this section will deal with the law concerning negligence.

Negligence liability arises when the health care practitioner fails to observe the standard of care required and the patient suffers some harm as a result. The requirements for negligence liability are often referred to as the "four D's": duty, dereliction, damage, and direct causation. The plaintiff must first establish that the defendant owed him a *duty* of care. Stated generally, the duty of physicians and other medical practitioners is to render care of the type and quality that a reasonably prudent practitioner of comparable training would have rendered under the same or similar circumstances. A person purporting to render specialty care is held to the standards of practitioners trained and proficient in that specialty. After establishing what the applicable duty of care is, the plaintiff must prove as a factual matter that the defendant was *derelict;* that is, he or she must show in what way or ways the defendant failed to observe the applicable standard. The plaintiff then must show appreciable *damage* and, finally, prove that the damage was *directly caused* by the negligence of the defendant. It is not enough that the negligence be a contributing factor to the plaintiff's injuries; it must have been the primary, or "proximate" cause.

Need for Expert Testimony

The requirement of proving the four D's is not unique to the medical malpractice area; it applies in tort law generally. The special difficulty in medical malpractice cases stems from the fact that the lay jury—or a judge if the case is not tried to a jury—is not considered competent to make judgments about technical or scientific matters unless the relevant information has been provided to it through expert testimony. Thus, in most cases, the plaintiff in a medical malpractice action must find one or more physicians who are properly qualified and willing to testify as to the nature, extent, and quality of care that should have been rendered in the patient's case. Locating witnesses to satisfy this evidentiary need has often proved difficult for potential plaintiffs, giving rise to the popular belief that there is a "conspiracy of silence" among members of the medical profession. Although it is probably true that many members of the profession are indisposed, as a matter of principle, to testify against their professional colleagues, it is likewise true that many matters relating to proper treatment are so sophisticated and complex that qualified medical witnesses may truly feel incapable of passing judgment upon the way that another professional handled a particular patient. Obviously, there are situations where the treatment is so egregiously wrong that trained medical minds could not reasonably differ as to its propriety. However, a large proportion of cases involve questions of sufficient subtlety that it is difficult for one practitioner to look back, recreate the circumstances under which the defendant was acting, and make a firm judgment that the actions taken were inappropriate. Even in the present ethical climate, when physicians are far less reluctant than formerly to testify against professional colleagues, it may still be extremely difficult for a plaintiff to secure the needed expert testimony to bring a case to court.

Locality Rule

The conspiracy of silence referred to in the preceding paragraph was formerly compounded by a doctrine of evidence known as the "locality rule," which was applied in many states from the late 1800s to the 1960s. The locality rule came to prominence in *Small vs Howard* (8), a case decided by the Massachusetts Supreme Court in 1880. In that case, it was held that a physician practicing in the small town of Bedford (population approximately 2,500) should not be held to the same standards of knowledge and sophistication in treatment as specialists in surgery practicing in the city of Boston. The court recognized the variance in the degree and currency of knowledge of practitioners between rural and urban areas and from one part of the country to another, and it laid down the principle that expert medical witnesses must be drawn from the same professional community, that is, the same geographic area, as where the alleged malpractice occurred. In *Small,* then, the question would be whether the plaintiff received such care as he would have received from a reasonably prudent physician practicing in the town of Bedford.

Although the locality rule may have been an appropriate accommodation to variations among geographic regions existing in the late 1800s, the rule became obsolete as the pace of communications and travel increased and medical education became more standardized in the early 1900s. With the tremendous expansion in the number and quality of professional and scientific journals, the greater mobility of physicians, and the concomitant opportunities for the exchange of information, a legal rule tying standards to a particular community no longer made much sense. Moreover, given the friendships and allegiances likely to exist among professionals practicing in the same area, this stricture on the source of expert testimony probably did serve to magnify the conspiracy of silence in many cases.

Over the years, the strict locality rule of *Small vs Howard* was softened to a more flexible approach that allowed the plaintiff's witnesses to be drawn from the same *or a similar* medical community. The American Bar Association and American Law Institute adopted this modified form of locality rule in 1956, and many states followed suit. Finally, by 1968, the underlying factors that had led to the *Small* ruling had so changed that the Massachusetts Supreme Court overturned its earlier holding and proclaimed, in the case of *Brune vs Belinkoff* (9), that is was no longer appropriate to apply a locality rule. The court reasoned that the standards of appropriate care had become so uniform throughout the nation that a single national standard should be applied to test whether the defendant's actions satisfied his professional responsibility to the patient.

Res Ipsa Loquitur

The doctrine of res ipsa loquitur has long been recognized in tort law, but it reached its prominence in medical malpractice litigation during the period when the locality rule served to heighten the conspiracy of silence problem. Res ipsa loquitur, literally translated, means "the thing speaks for itself." In other words, in some cases, the negligence of a defendant is so clear that it can be adequately assessed by a lay jury without the assistance of expert witnesses. The classic res ipsa loquitur case in the medical malpractice context is that of a sponge or surgical implement being left within the body of the patient during a surgical procedure. This kind of error simply does not happen in the absence of negligence. Since it can effectively be guarded against, it is only reasonable that the law require adequate safeguards to be applied.

For the requirement of expert testimony to be waived under the res ipsa loquitur doctrine, three elements must be present. First of all, the injury to the patient must be of a kind that clearly would not occur in the absence of some-one's negligence. Second, it must have been caused by an instrumentality that was within the exclusive control of the defendant. Finally, there must be no possibility of "contributory negligence," that is, that the plaintiff was partly responsible for the harm sustained. This third element is easily satisfied in most medical malpractice cases, because the patient is commonly a passive participant. There simply is not much opportunity for the patient to be contributorily negligent. This requirement could apply, however, if it could be shown that the patient failed to follow a postoperative regimen prescribed by the physician. A patient who disregarded the physician's orders and played handball within a couple of weeks after having a shoulder fracture set would, of course, forfeit all chance of using res ipsa loquitur in a suit for nonunion of the break.

During the period when the conspiracy of silence was felt to be most acute, many courts responded by relaxing their standards for the application of res ipsa loquitur. The "high-water mark" for the res ipsa loquitur doctrine in medical-malpractice cases is often said to be the case of *Ybarra vs Spangard* (10), decided in California in 1944. In that case, a patient who was put under general anesthesia for an appendectomy awakened after the operation with a sharp pain about halfway between the neck and the point of the right shoulder. The pain spread to the lower part of his arm and, after the patient's release from the hospital, he developed paralysis and atrophy of the muscles around the shoulder. The patient recalled experiencing substantial discomfort in the shoulder area when being positioned on the operating table before losing consciousness. The court allowed application of res ipsa loquitur and found for the plaintiff, reasoning that since he was unconscious at the time of the injury, he could not re-alistically be required to identify the specific negligent action that caused his paralysis. The jury needed to determine only that paralysis of the shoulder does not ordinarily follow an appendectomy and, having made this decision, award a recovery to the plaintiff.

The *Ybarra* case and others of its kind have led numerous commentators to call the res ipsa loquitur doctrine a "rule of sympathy." It is felt that jurors may, when freed from the requirement of identifying specific elements of negligent practice, grant recovery to plaintiffs on what are primarily emotional grounds. More recent cases generally do not go as far as *Ybarra* in allowing the application of res ipsa loquitur. As a general rule, the doctrine is most likely to be applied in cases where the patient was unconscious at the time when the injury allegedly took place, or the injury affected a part of the patient's body other than that which was being treated, or both.

Medical Professional Standards

In *The T. J. Hooper* (11), an admiralty case decided by the federal courts in 1932, the owners of a freighter in coastal service were held negligent for not having equipped the vessel with a radiotelephone, even though relatively few vessels in coastal trade at that time were so equipped. In declaring the court's opinion, Justice Learned Hand stated:

> In most cases reasonable prudence is in fact common prudence; but strictly it is never its measure; a whole calling may have unduly lagged in the adoption of new

and available devices. It never may set its own tests, however persuasive be its usages. Courts must in the end say what is required; there are precautions so imperative that even their universal disregard will not excuse their omission (12).

Although the rationale of *The T. J. Hooper* case has been applied to many industries and situations since 1932, the courts have been reluctant to extend the reasoning of that case to the medical malpractice area. The law, in general, apparently has not felt itself qualified to invade the sanctity of medical professional judgment and impose its own standards in disregard of accepted medical practice.

This reluctance was overcome, however, in the 1974 case *Helling vs Carey* (13), decided by the Supreme Court of the state of Washington. In *Helling,* two ophthalmologists were found negligent for failing to administer a simple pressure (Schiotz) test to check whether a young female patient was suffering from glaucoma. The physicians had claimed, with support by expert witnesses, that it was not usual medical practice to administer such a test to persons under the age of 40, as was the patient-plaintiff, except where there was frank indication of loss of visual field. Despite the court's acceptance that the physicians had accurately described the professional custom in dealing with such cases, it held that:

> . . . the reasonable standard that should have been followed under the undisputed facts of this case was the timely giving of this simple, harmless pressure test to this plaintiff and that, in failing to do so, the defendants were negligent, which proximately resulted in the blindness sustained by the plaintiff for which the defendants are liable (14).

Helling vs Carey has been cited as a landmark decision in medical malpractice law. Its importance lay in its untying of medical negligence determinations from standards regularly observed by the medical profession. The impact of such a change in approach would have been substantial. However, despite early predictions, the *Helling* case has not been widely followed, and, in fact, the legislature of the state of Washington apparently rejected the case's ruling by a statute passed in 1975. That law reads, in relevant part:

> In any civil action for damages based on professional negligence against a hospital . . . or personnel of any such hospital, or against a member of the healing art . . . the plaintiff in order to prevail shall be required to prove by a preponderance of evidence that the defendant or defendants failed to exercise that degree of skill, care, and learning possessed by other persons in the same profession and that, as a proximate result of such failure, the plaintiff suffered damages . . . (15).

It does not appear, however, that the approach of *Helling vs Carey* has been permanently interred. In a 1979 opinion, in *Gates vs Jensen* (16), the Washington Supreme Court overturned a judgment in favor of the defendant, an ophthalmologist, in a case factually similar to *Helling.* The trial jury, applying the above statutory provision, had found for the defendant, apparently believing his performance had been consistent with prevailing medical practice. The Supreme Court reversed, holding that this would not preclude a finding of negligence if the "degree of skill, care and learning *possessed* by other persons in the same profession," as called for by the statute, were found to be higher than that actually *practiced* by the defendant, even though his performance might equal that of his professional peers. The court ordered a new trial, at which the jury was to be instructed that:

> Irrespective of whether you find that any defendant has met or failed to meet the applicable standard of care followed by practicing ophthalmologists . . ., if you find that . . . reasonable prudence under the circumstances required the administration of additional diagnostic tests . . ., failure to perform those tests . . . would constitute negligence (17).

The court's strained construction of the statute, while seemingly counter to the legislative intent, indicates how strongly the court is determined to retain flexibility to apply higher standards where prevailing medical practice seems inadequate to meet patient care needs. The final chapters in this unfolding saga have yet to be written.

Dealing with the Malpractice Crisis

The legislation in Washington State referred to in the preceding paragraph is typical of provisions found in malpractice reform acts adopted by many of the states in the middle 1970s. These laws were a reaction to the perceived "malpractice crisis," a phenomenon characterized by a dramatic increase in the number of malpractice suits brought and the size of judicial awards. Because of the lengthy statute of limitations period allowed for malpractice actions in certain cases—the so-called "long-tail" problem—even relatively minor changes in the incidence and size of malpractice awards can, and do, cause substantial increases in malpractice insurance premiums. Thus, the malpractice crisis was, in fact, a crisis in terms of the availability of affordable liability insurance for practitioners.

In the space of about two years, beginning in 1974, more than half the states adopted legislation designed to improve their malpractice litigation systems. In many of these states, it seems, "improving the system" meant making it more difficult for patients to secure awards against their physicians. Thus, many of the reform statutes passed during this period are "doctors' legislation," drafted and promoted by the medical establishment. Notwithstanding this fact, many of the procedural reforms are commendable, including such points as mandatory arbitration of malpractice claims, the establishment of medicolegal screening panels for malpractice actions, and limitations on the size of attorneys' contingency fees.

Before this spate of new legislation, commentators had noted that as much as 84¢ of each dollar spent for medical malpractice liability insurance was being spent for the functioning of the litigation system rather than for compensation of injured patients. Although this statistic makes a dramatic point about the functioning of the system, it is not altogether fitting that physicians seize upon this fact as evidence of the system's deficiencies. This is because physicians buy liability insurance—or so one would assume—not primarily to compensate injured patients but, rather, to pay the costs of their defense against such suits and, only when that defense is unsuccessful, to pay the actual damage awards rendered. Thus, in one sense, when physicians are successfully defended in court, they are getting their "money's worth," even though little is paid out to injured patients.

Experience under the reform laws of most states is still too limited for proper assessment of their impact. The crisis, however, at least in terms of the availability of malpractice liability insurance, seems to have abated. Although the new legislation may deserve much of the credit for this "leveling off," some of it may also be attributable to increasing awareness on the part of juries that the "deep pocket" of the insurance companies is fed by public resources. Higher damage awards mean higher insurance premiums, which, in turn, mean higher costs for medical care. A growing conservatism on the part of American juries in general may have as much to do with the lessening of the malpractice crisis as does any other factor.

"Crystal-balling" Medical Malpractice Law

Although projecting the future of medical malpractice law is not an easy task, some predictions are possible. Continued movement toward national, rather than local, standards seems assured. Despite the legislative reactions to the *Helling vs Carey* decision (15), it still is likely that the medical profession will no longer be allowed to set its own standards of performance on a totally unilateral basis. Even where the entire profession is slow to adopt new technologies and safeguards, liability still may be assessed against any practitioner who experiences a bad result while using techniques that are outdated. The future will undoubtedly bring much greater use of alternative adjudicative processes, such as screening panels and arbitration, addressing the inadequacy of the traditional tort litigation system to deal with matters of great scientific complexity. Although some commentators have advocated total abandonment of a fault-based malpractice system, the shift to a no-fault system focused more on compensation of injured parties than on the allocation of blame still seems a distant prospect. Physicians and other health care providers will have to maintain their present concern about liability risks, and their need to stay abreast of current legal developments will remain as great as at present.

PATIENT CONSENT TO MEDICAL AND SURGICAL TREATMENT

One of the areas of medical jurisprudence that has undergone the most change in recent years is patient consent to medical and surgical procedures. New standards have been developed to protect more fully the patient's right of self-determination to medical care. This right has long been recognized in American jurisprudence, as reflected in the following quotation from a 1914 opinion written by Judge Cardozo, later to serve on the United States Supreme Court:

> Every human being of adult years and sound mind has a right to determine what shall be done with his own body; and a surgeon who performs an operation without his patient's consent commits an assault for which he is liable in damages (18).

However, despite the longstanding recognition of this right, it has still not been fully defined and put into operation. Nonetheless, as discussed in the following section, dramatic changes in patient-consent rules have taken place over the last 20 years.

Need for Consent

To advance upon and touch a person without his or her consent is an "assault and battery," an intentional tort. A person has a right to be free of all unauthorized touching, and the law recognizes this right in the medical context just as it would in other social situations. The key difference is that patients rarely go to a physician unless they are willing to be treated—and touched, if necessary—by the physician. Essentially, then, the patient gives consent, at least by implication, when he or she goes to the physician for treatment. Although there may not be a formal, written consent document, the physician incurs no liability by touching the patient so long as it appears that this was the patient's intent and the physician so understood it. Since, except in the case of surgical or other substantial invasive procedures, it is not customary for a written consent or contract to be executed, the concept of an "implied consent" is a common accommodation between legal principle and actual practice. For example, a person standing in line with others to receive an injection is presumed to have given consent to that procedure. This presumption holds, however, only if it can be shown that the patient understood, in at least general terms, the care that was about to be given and proceeded of his or her own free will. If there was any duress or coercion, or if the nature of the proposed treatment was not, for some reason, understandable to the patient, the implication of consent is negated.

Emergence of the "Informed Consent" Doctrine

The qualification last stated is the basis of a new subset of consent law known as the doctrine of informed consent. In 1957, a California court held that although a patient may have given formal, written consent to an operative procedure, that consent shall not be deemed legally valid if the patient was unaware of substantial risks or consequences of the treatment (19). Thus, consent, to be legally effective, must be "informed," or knowledgeable. A Kansas court in 1960 attempted to recognize this requirement by enunciating a standard for measuring the information provided by a physician to his patient. Likening the duty of disclosure to other professional duties owed by physicians to their patients, the Kansas court held that disclosure is adequate only if the physician revealed to his or her patient what other practitioners would have revealed under the same or similar circumstances (20).

This approach, herein referred to as the "old rule," links the physician's disclosure obligation to standard practice within the relevant medical community. Using such a professionally based standard leaves open the possibility that even if adequate information were not provided to patients, no liability would ensue as long as this deficiency was common among the medical profession. Moreover, as in medical malpractice cases generally, it exposes the patient to the difficulty of finding expert medical testimony about the "standard disclosure" usually made in cases of this type.

Numerous courts and commentators have speculated that no such standard disclosure exists, since the possible combinations of patient anxiety, physicians' willingness to discuss sensitive information, and other factors are so highly variable. If, in fact, no standard disclosure exists, it is clearly unreasonable to make a patient-plaintiff's informed-consent case depend on the patient's production of expert testimony as to what the standard disclosure is. Thus, since about 1970, numerous courts across the country have abandoned the old-rule standard in favor of a new rule focused upon the informational needs of the patient.

This patient-based standard was articulated most forcibly in *Canterbury vs Spence* (21), a 1972 United States Court of Appeals decision. The *Canterbury* suit involved a young man who became paralyzed after a lumbar laminectomy. The defendant neurosurgeon, Dr. Spence, had told him that the laminectomy procedure was "no more serious than any other operation." No mention was made of the possibility of paralysis, although Dr. Spence testified at trial that he regarded this risk as having a probability of approximately 1%. Attempting to justify his nondisclosure of this risk, Dr. Spence explained:

> I think that I always explain to patients the operations are serious, and I feel that any operation is serious. I think that I would not tell patients that they might be paralyzed because of the small percentage, one percent, that exists. There would be a tremendous percentage of people who would not have surgery and would not, therefore, be benefitted by it, the tremendous percentage that get along very well, 99% (22).

Despite Dr. Spence's unquestioned good intentions, this testimony was precisely the wrong thing for him to say to the court. The physician was attempting to make for his patient the "right" decision and to guard against the patient's veto of that decision by keeping material information from him. The patient, Jerry Canterbury, failed to produce at trial any testimony by medical witnesses in regard to what other practitioners would have revealed under the same circumstances. This lack of expert testimony, the trial court held, was a fatal deficiency. However, on appeal, it was held that the extent of the required disclosure should be measured not by what physicians customarily tell but, rather, by what an average reasonable patient would consider material to his decision. Said the court:

> Nor can we ignore the fact that to bind the disclosure obligation to medical usage is to arrogate the decision on revelation to the physician alone. Respect for the patient's right of self-determination on particular therapy demands a standard set by law for physicians rather than one which physicians may or may not impose upon themselves (23).

As a matter of jurisprudential philosophy, the shift from a physician-based to a patient-based standard is most important. It may be even more important from a practical standpoint, however. By using a patient-based standard, the court allows an informed-consent case to go to the jury without the need for expert medical witnesses. Thus, a substantial impediment to litigation is removed, and many more cases dealing with consent can be expected in the courts as a result. Experience has borne out this expectation, with a substantial increase in informed-consent litigation since the *Canterbury* decision was handed down. Lack of informed consent is not commonly asserted as a freestanding ground but, rather, is appended to a suit brought on other charges of medical negligence. As a cause of action that can be taken to trial without expert testimony, informed consent is a difficult claim to defend against in the pretrial stage.

Seven years after the *Canterbury* decision, the physician community has not yet fully adjusted to the impact of this case and its numerous progeny. Even assuming that a physician reveals to a patient all relevant information about the case and the proposed treatment, liability still is possible if the physician has not adequately documented this disclosure. In other words, it is not enough to actually tell the patient; the physician must be able, if challenged, to prove what was said.

Documentation of the basic fact of consent is not so difficult and has long been handled in an adequate manner. On the other hand, documenting the disclosure of a whole range of informational items—that is, the risks and consequences of the proposed treatment, alternative treatment possibilities, the probability of success of the proposed treatment and its alternatives, and the prognosis if no treatment is given—is another matter entirely. Attorneys have a saying: "To generalize is to omit; to specify is to exclude." Functionally, this saying means that whereas it may be inadequate to simply state in a consent form that "all risks" have been disclosed, there is also potential danger in listing one-by-one the risk items that were disclosed. If a single negative outcome is omitted from the listing and subsequently occurs, the signed consent form then can be used by the patient as "proof positive" that this particular risk was never disclosed. Since risks may vary not only for different treatments but also for different patients, given age, and physical condition, a consent form would have to be specially tailored to each patient's situation to be legally safe. For a physician who treats various kinds of patients for various kinds of ailments, the burden of routinely documenting that an informed consent was obtained may be substantial.

Critics of the informed-consent doctrine claim also that its aggressive application may seriously undermine the physician-patient relationship of trust, which is necessary for effective therapy. In an understandable desire to obtain legal protection, the physician may convey to the patient a sense that their relationship is adversarial rather than cooperative. Although the intent behind the informed-consent requirement is laudable, it is to be hoped that implementation of the doctrine can be achieved in a way that will not have negative side effects.

Consent in Emergencies

Two exceptions to the requirement of informed consent bear special mention. The first applies in the case of emergencies, when it is not feasible to obtain the patient's consent to care that is urgently needed. When the patient is unconscious or otherwise incompetent to consent, the practitioner is obligated to take reasonable steps to secure consent from the patient's next of kin or other person authorized under the circumstances to give a substitute consent. If such consent cannot be obtained within the time available, and if the situation is a true emergency—that is, seriously and immediately threatening to the life or health of the patient—consent will be presumed. In other words, the law will assume that the patient, if he or she had been able, would have given consent to the proposed treatment. It is advisable, of course, for the practitioner to document all the requisite elements outlined above. If possible, the consultation and advice of another health care practitioner should be sought, to confirm the determination that care could not be delayed until a proper consent might be obtained.

"Therapeutic Privilege"

The second major exception to the informed-consent requirement is frequently referred to as the doctrine of therapeutic privilege. As explained in the *Canterbury* opinion, the exception applies

> ... when risk-disclosure poses such a threat of detriment to the patient as to become unfeasible or contraindicated from a medical point of view. It is recognized that patients occasionally become so ill or emotionally distraught on disclosure as to foreclose a rational decision, or complicate or hinder the treatment or perhaps even pose psychological damage to the patient. Where that is so, the cases have generally held that the physician is armed with a privilege to keep the information from the patient, and we think it clear that portents of that type may justify the physician in action he deems medically warranted. The critical inquiry is whether the physician responded to a sound medical judgment that communication of the risk information would present a threat to the patient's well-being.

> The physician's privilege to withhold information for therapeutic reasons must be carefully circumscribed, however, for otherwise it might devour the disclosure rule itself. The privilege does not accept the paternalistic notion that the physician may remain silent simply because divulgence might prompt the patient to forego therapy the physician feels the patient really needs [citations omitted] (24).

The last point made in the above quotation speaks directly to the justification offered by Dr. Spence for his nondisclosure of the risk of paralysis. The vast majority of courts that have dealt with informed consent have recognized some form of therapeutic privilege, although the language used to define the limits of such privilege varies widely according to jurisdiction. Practitioners are urged to become familiar with the law on informed consent in the states in which they practice, giving special attention to the way in which that law defines the scope of therapeutic privilege. As the *Canterbury* opinion suggests, it may be wise for the physician dealing with a therapeutic-privilege situation to make a disclosure to a close relative of the patient (24). Note, however, that such a disclosure could raise confidentiality problems, as discussed earlier in this chapter.

Refusal of Essential Treatment

Another important aspect of the patient's right of self-determination is the question whether a patient should be allowed to refuse treatment that is essential to life. Although some states have repealed or softened their suicide statutes in recent years, it still is against the law in many jurisdictions to attempt to take one's own life. In such a legal context, it can be argued that for a patient to refuse care that is essential to life is tantamount to suicide and, thus, is illegal. Notwithstanding the logic of this argument, many courts and state legislatures are moving toward acceptance of the patient's right to refuse treatment, even when such refusal carries with it a high risk of death.

Consistent with its recognition of the patient's right of self-determination on therapy, the law has recently come to accord greater latitude for patients to refuse therapy, even when such refusal is likely to mean death. In most courts throughout the country, a competent, mature patient will be allowed to choose freely between treatment and nontreatment. Cases to the contrary can generally be explained either by the existence of a minor child or other dependent who relies on the patient for support or by the patient's apparent lack of competence to make rational decisions regarding his or her treatment. The latter point involves something of a "Catch 22," since many would view a patient's refusal of life-saving treatment as an irrational act. The circularity is obvious: only a person who is rational may effectively refuse consent to treatment, but a rational person would not decline treatment. Thus, in the minds of some, the very act of refusing may itself take away the power to refuse effectively. Fortunately, enlightened judicial thought has not been trapped in this "closed loop" of reasoning.

Following the New Jersey Supreme Court's decision of the *Karen Quinlan* case (25), numerous states have enacted so-called right-to-die laws granting terminally ill patients the option to refuse "heroic," life-sustaining care. These statutes contain several important restrictions on the exercise of the right to die, however, most prominent of which is a safeguard against assertion of the right by persons lacking full mental competence. To guard against impulsive action that might be triggered by one's despair upon learning that an illness is terminal, some statutes, such as that of California, impose waiting periods before a direction to suspend life-saving treatment may become effective. Laws of this nature vary significantly from state to state; it is therefore advisable that each practitioner become aware of the laws of the particular state(s) in which his or her practice is located.

Over the last several years, numerous cases involving a patient's desire to refuse life-sustaining treatment have been taken to the courts by medical practitioners unsure of their obligations and potential liabilities. One of the objectives of the right-to-die statutes is to avoid the need for frequent court intervention in matters of great sensitivity. How effective the statutes will be in this regard has yet to be determined.

Consent to Experimental Procedures

Another aspect of patient consent that has raised substantial question is consent to experimental procedures. Despite the law's principle of honoring the right of individual determination, it seems that there are some risks so great that society is not willing to allow a person to undertake them. Thus, in addition to the requirement that the proposed experimental subject be fully informed and make a wholly voluntary choice regarding participation, the law has devised other safeguards against inappropriate medical experimentation.

All research studies involving human subjects that are carried out under federal auspices or by institutions that receive federal funding are subject to the regulations of the Department of Health and Human Services for the protection of human subjects. These regulations require that all biomedical, psychologic, and sociologic studies involving human subjects be approved before their commencement by an "institutional review board" (IRB), which reviews research protocols on the basis of a federally prescribed set of evaluation criteria. These criteria establish a calculus that weighs the benefits of a given experiment against its risks. On the one hand, the probability and severity of the experiment's risks are measured; on the other, the product so derived is measured against the probability that the experimental procedure will be successful and that the benefit can be expected to follow. Experiments that have an expected therapeutic value for the subject are generally viewed more favorably than those that do not. Similarly, the risks of the experiment are accorded less weight if the subject is in critical condition and has a poor prognosis for recovery unless the proposed treatment is administered.

The decision-making in regard to what experiments will or will not be allowed is often quite difficult, and the process defies reduction to a simple mathematical formula. The function of the IRB is to summon the judgment of knowledgeable persons of varied backgrounds—not just scientists and medical personnel but also ethicists, attorneys, philosophers, sociologists, and the clergy. There is no assurance that the decisions reached by such broad-based IRBs will necessarily be humane, but they are more likely to reflect the prevailing values of society than are decisions made by scientists alone.

Assuming that the research in question is methodologically sound and is justifiable under the above criteria, approval still will not be granted unless there is adequate assurance that prospective subjects will be fully informed about the nature of the experiment and its risks and expected benefits and will be given an opportunity to make a free and uncoerced choice regarding participation. In obtaining the subject's consent, the experimenter must make it absolutely clear that the subject is free to decline participation, that he or she may withdraw from the experiment at any time without penalty, and that continued care will not be negatively affected if the subject decides not to participate. The above require-ments are intended to assure that only reasonable and justifiable experiments are conducted and that no one is involved in such experiments unless he or she knowingly and freely chooses to be. There undoubtedly are situations where the progress of scientific knowledge is inhibited by these review procedures, but most agree that a greater good is served thereby.

To a certain extent, much of medical practice is a matter of trial and error. Informal experiments are being conducted all the time in the course of therapy. The practitioner should be fully aware of the constraints placed upon medical experimentation and, even if a formal, federally funded study is not involved, should regard the regulations of the Department of Health and Human Services as a guide to the kind of safeguards that the law would impose. Since consent to experimental treatments is far more sensitive, it follows that the practitioner should document with care the information provided to the pro-spective subject and the fact that the subject consented.

LIABILITY FOR THE ACTS OF OTHERS

The medical practitioner's liability may extend to cover the acts done by others on his or her behalf or subject to his or her control. It is important that both the physician and those who practice in collaboration with the physician be aware of the legal implications of their cooperative relationship.

Employers' Liability for Employees' Acts

The law has long recognized a doctrine known as *respondeat superior,* which means "let the master answer" and holds that an employer is responsible for acts committed by employees in the course of employment. This doctrine is also known as the "master-servant rule." The employer-employee relationship is one defined by law and may exist even in cases where there is no formal contract or understanding of employment. When one engages in work at the request of another, the manner in which the worker is to be compensated and the degree of control that the other party has over the worker are the key determinants of whether an employer-employee relationship exists. It is sometimes difficult to decide whether one performing work for another is doing so as an employee or as an "independent contractor." The respondeat superior doctrine would apply only in the former case, although it is possible for an independent-contractor relationship to rise to liability on the part of the person who commissioned the work to be done.

In the medical care setting, it is obvious that a physician has vicarious liability, under respondeat superior, for any nurses or assistants whom he or she employs. Not so apparent, but true nonetheless, is that the physician may have vicarious responsibility for any person engaged in providing health care services under his or her supervision or control, even one who is not technically employed by the physician. Thus, a nurse who has been hired and is compensated by a hospital may be regarded as the "borrowed servant" of a physician on the hospital's staff while acting under his or her immediate direction and supervision. The law regards the element of control as the key to allocating responsibility for acts done by members of the health care delivery support team.

The distinction between administrative duties (i.e., the provision of regular nursing service) and medical duties (i.e., those relating directly to the physician's care of the patient) is difficult to draw. With the demise of the "charitable immunity" doctrine—which formerly protected nonprofit hospitals and other eleemosynary health care institutions from tort liability—courts have become less disposed to make such a distinction. They tend to hold the hospital responsible for all acts done by its employed staff and look to the institution's insurer for satisfaction of the injured patient's claim. Analytically, however, the distinction is still worth making, since it clarifies the law's attempt to assign responsibility for harm to persons who are in the best position to control the relevant events and guard against harm. In many cases, this person may still be the physician who, as in the operating room, is regarded as "the captain of the ship." It should be understood that vicarious liability of the physician and the hospital may both arise from the same incident and that the person responsible for the harm suffered may be personally liable as well.

This captain-of-the-ship doctrine is closely related to the borrowed-servant rule and, like that rule, is applied more sparingly by today's courts. It is increasingly recognized that although the physician may nominally be in control of all persons assisting in an operation, the physician is, in fact, relying heavily on the knowledge and judgment of each member of the health care team. Thus, if an anesthesia error causes harm to the patient, it is not automatically taken to be the responsibility of the surgeon performing the operation. Rather, the relevant question is whether the surgeon was, or should have been, in control of that particular phase of the patient's care. Even though the surgeon's primary function is not the monitoring of the anesthesia, there are certain indicators of trouble of which he or she is expected to be aware. On the other hand, there are other aspects of anesthesia administration for which it would not be reasonable to hold the surgeon responsible. As the law gains more understanding of the process of patient care generally, it is attempting to make more subtle and equitable distinctions and determinations regarding the physician's scope of control. Over time, as paraprofessionals become more generally regarded as possessing full competence in their particular areas of endeavor, the captain-of-the-ship doctrine should continue to diminish in importance.

Institutional Responsibility for Quality of Care

A related change that is also taking place is the growth of the doctrine of "corporate responsibility," by which health care institutions are held responsible not only for the acts of their employees but also for acts of nonemployed members of their medical staffs. The well-known case of *Darling vs. Charleston Community Memorial Hospital* (26) held that a hospital is responsible for assuring proper consultation among members of its medical staff in difficult cases. Dr. Alexander, the physician treating the patient, Darling, in the hospital for a leg fracture, was considered to be subject to the hospital's control, even though he was an independent practitioner, not a hospital employee. Since the hospital had rules requiring consultation in complex cases, it was responsible for seeing that those rules were observed. Harm caused to the patient by the failure to follow these rules was held to be as much the hospital's fault as that of the attending physician. It is this concept of corporate responsibility, articulated in the *Darling* case and subsequent decisions, that has contributed heavily to the decline of the distinction between administrative and medical services. All aspects of the patient's care are considered to be, to some extent at least, the responsibility of the institution wherein that care is provided.

Of course, recognition of the hospital's responsibility for malpractice committed by a nonemployed member of its medical staff raises substantial dilemmas. Facing potential liability for malpractice, the hospital must assure itself that only competent and qualified people are allowed to practice within its facility. Moreover, it must take reasonable steps to assure that rules relating to that practice are scrupulously observed. The medical staff of the hospital is no longer regarded as an independent and autonomous unit. The structure of its bylaws and the routine adherence to their provisions are as much the responsibility of the hospital as of the staff members themselves. Thus, the obtaining of patient consent for procedures, the proper maintenance of treatment records, and the conduct of consultation in appropriate cases have been added to the hospital's responsibility for preserving the quality of the care that its patients receive.

Limitations Upon Control of the Medical Staff

The hospital's job of assuring standards of care is made more difficult by legal developments in recent years restricting the institution's ability to exclude practitioners from staff membership. It has been held that a physician's staff privileges are a form of property and cannot be removed without due process of law. If a hospital proposes to revoke, suspend, or restrict the staff privileges of an affiliated physician, it must give the physician advance notice of such action and provide an opportunity to be heard on the action's appropriateness. A formal hearing with witnesses and counsel for the physician is not required in all cases, but the hospital must see that the subject practitioner is given a full and fair chance to present facts and arguments on his or her side of the issue. Valid reasons must exist for the hospital's action, and the hospital may not discriminate against particular physicians or act in an arbitrary and capricious manner. Nor may the hospital, in reaching its decision, rely upon information that is kept secret from the affected party. The physician must be apprised of all information considered and be given an opportunity to refute it or present opposing arguments.

The frustration of hospitals over the growth of these due-process requirements has been considerable. On one hand, they are required to accept more and more responsibility for care rendered in their facilities by medical staff members. On the other, they are—as they see it—being left with less and less ability to exclude or restrict practitioners whom they regard as posing an excessive risk. The paradox is genuine, and the law has yet to achieve a successful reconciliation of the two interests. The only advice that can be given for the present is that hospitals should choose carefully physicians whom they admit to staff privileges and if they have any suspicions regarding the mental, physical, or professional competence of a staff member, they should monitor that member carefully and take all reasonable steps to guard against patient harm. Although this advice places a responsibility upon health care institutions that they have not traditionally borne, it is a responsibility that they are uniquely suited to discharge. Moreover, there is currently no other practical way to protect patients from poor quality in medical care.

New approaches are being developed, however. In recent years, several states have enacted statutory provisions dealing with "impaired" practitioners and providing for measures short of license revocation or suspension to safeguard against the harm that these more severe sanctions can cause to the physician. A physician calling proper attention to the error or incompetence of a professional colleague is, in many states, protected against charges of defamation, provided that he or she acted in good faith. In Arizona, physicians are charged with a statutory duty to inform appropriate officials of deficiencies that they observe in other practitioners (27). Other states, such as Florida, have "sick doctor" statutes that make special provision for the identification, monitoring, and rehabilitation of problem practitioners (28). It is likely that statutes of this nature will become widespread in the near future.

DRUG REGULATION

A medicolegal issue that has provoked substantial controversy in recent years is the nation's mechanism for controlling the introduction of new therapeutic drugs. Jurisdiction over this area is vested in the Food and Drug Administration (FDA) of the Department of Health and Human Services. The FDA has as its main function the supervision of testing of new drugs before their introduction to the market and the routine monitoring of drug manufacture to assure production quality.

The first step toward the present system of drug regulation was taken in 1906 with the passage of the Federal Food and Drug Act (29). This act did not address safety or efficacy as such but simply prohibited the "misbranding" of drugs and the use of false or misleading claims in their sale. Not particularly strong in its basic concept, the law was weakened even further by unfavorable judicial interpretations. Since there was no requirement for prior approval of drugs before their introduction in the market, all enforcement was after the fact. When, in 1937, 107 persons died from the use of sulfanilamide, the resultant hue and cry forced Congress to pass the Food, Drug, and Cosmetic Act of 1938 (30). This law, the foundation of our present regulatory system, required premarketing approval of all new drugs and specified that no drugs could be approved unless first proved safe for use under the conditions prescribed, recommended, or suggested in their labeling. Note that only the drug's *safety* was addressed by the premarketing approval process; efficacy continued to be dealt with by treating false therapeutic claims as a form of misbranding. The 1962 Kefauver amendments to the Food and Drug Act (31), the law currently applicable, provide that new drugs can be approved only if they are shown to be both safe and efficacious when used as prescribed in their labeling. Specific research steps are mandated for the premarketing review, and the FDA applies a "benefit-risk ratio" by which it weighs the benefits from the drug's use against its risks. On the benefit side of the equation, account is taken of both the drug's effectiveness and the seriousness of the illness or illnesses that it is designed to treat.

Two-stage Review Process

Under the prior approval structure, as modified in 1962, a drug must pass through two separate stages of review before being generally marketed. The first stage is necessary for the drug to be granted "investigational new drug" (IND) status. To be approved as an investigational new drug, the drug must first have been tested in the laboratory and by controlled studies on animal subjects. If the drug has been in use in human beings in other countries, properly documented evidence of the results of such use may be submitted in lieu of animal tests. Given the stringency of United States testing requirements and the long lead time required before the introduction of any new drug onto the American market, it is not uncommon for a drug to be in widespread use overseas before undergoing the FDA approval process. This fact has given rise to the claim that American drug laws consciously allow people in other nations to be the human guinea pigs for testing of drugs before they are offered for sale to American consumers.

In applying for IND status for a new drug, a manufacturer must submit a carefully prescribed plan for research and monitoring of that drug's effects on human subjects. If the FDA is unsatisfied with the research methodology proposed, a lengthy process of negotiation may be required before the agency and the manufacturer agree on a mutually acceptable testing program. Although time limitations are placed upon the FDA's review of IND applications, in practice these limits are not firm, and considerable time may elapse before actual testing in human beings begins. Vigorous restrictions are imposed on the testing and monitoring, including procedures for informing human subjects that they are going to be exposed to an investigational drug. No judicial review is provided for either the denial of IND status or its withdrawal by the FDA once granted.

After testing under the IND phase has taken place, the manufacturer petitions the FDA to allow sale of the drug. This petition is known as a "new drug application" (NDA). The law specifies that the FDA is to act on NDAs within six months of their filing; however, there are numerous ways in which the six-month period can be extended. Once an NDA has been granted, the drug can be sold on the market, but experience with it continues to be carefully monitored. If at any time the FDA decides that the drug is either unsafe or ineffective, it may withdraw its approval and block further sale of the drug.

Delay in Approving New Drugs

With these two levels of review, the time that elapses from a drug's discovery to its general marketing may be as long as seven to 10 years. Many have criticized this delay, arguing that the lengthy and cumbersome process keeps valuable new drugs from being made available to American consumers as expeditiously as they should be. These objections do have validity, as the gestational period for a new drug is substantially longer in the United States than in many other countries. However, the cautious and conservative approach incorporated in the FDA's approval process has its positive aspects as well. For example, the FDA's delay in approving sale in the United States of the drug thalidomide prevented children in this country from suffering the congenital deformities that afflicted hundreds of babies born in Great Britain, Canada, Portugal, West Germany, and other countries. Dr. Frances Kelsey, the FDA physician who processed the application of an American drug company to market the drug under the brand name Kevadon, was presented with a special award for distinguished civilian service by President John F. Kennedy. Clearly, the thalidomide disaster is a classic example of the kind of harm that the FDA approval process is intended to prevent. However, lives can also be lost or harmed by preventing the timely introduction of new and useful drug technology. Obviously, a balance must be struck between caution and progress. Many claim that the latter is not being properly served by our current system for approval of new drugs.

Quality Control Review by the Food and Drug Administration

The other main aspect of the FDA's operation is the assurance of manufacturing quality on a continuing basis. A relatively small number of FDA inspectors tour drug-manufacturing plants across the country, observing quality-control techniques, collecting samples, and generally attempting to assure that drugs are safely made and packaged. One common problem that these inspectors encounter is the cross contamination of one drug by another in factories where the same equipment is used sequentially for manufacture of different substances. Penicillin, for example, is light and fluffy and easily carried by air currents. Poor control of dust and poor cleaning of equipment can lead to problems with impure and adulterated drugs. In addition to its direct inspections, the FDA supervises the process by which companies keep records of drugs produced and distributed. Thus, when a problem arises in regard to a particular drug, it is possible to track down the various bulk units of that drug originating in the same production run. Preserving the integrity of manufacturers' record-keeping is another important aspect of the FDA's job.

Drug Prescription According to Generic Name

A final drug-regulation issue bearing mention is the current trend toward encouragement of generic prescription, that is, prescribing drugs by chemical classification rather than by use of specific brand names. As health care costs have risen dramatically in recent years, new approaches to cost containment have been sought. It has long been recognized that there are substantial price differences between drugs that are essentially the same but are produced and marketed by different manufacturers. The so-called antisubstitution laws enforced in several states make it illegal for a pharmacist to dispense any drug other than the one specifically named in the physician's prescription. If the physician, for convenience or other reason, chooses to prescribe by brand name, these laws prevent the pharmacist from substituting a cheaper brand of the drug, even though both have precisely the same chemical composition. Substantial pressure now exists for repeal or modification of those antisubstitution laws, to allow pharmacists, subject to certain constraints, to dispense less expensive drugs and pass the savings back to consumers. It is argued, however, that differences in manufacturing quality and bioavailability do exist from one manufacturer's product to another and that removal of all restrictions on pharmacist substitution would be going too far.

The Department of Health and Human Services has placed itself squarely behind generic prescription by implementation of its maximum allowable cost (MAC) reimbursement regulations under the Medicare and Medicaid programs (32). Under MAC, the Department of Health and Human Services will reimburse suppliers for covered prescription drugs only up to the cost of the least expensive generic equivalent. MAC regulations apply only to drugs specifically listed by the Department as being chemically and functionally equivalent.

NEW HORIZONS IN HEALTH CARE REGULATION

In concluding this chapter on health care law, it is worthwhile to note briefly some other developments that may affect the course of health care delivery in the near future.

Antitrust Laws and the Health Care Industry

One potentially far-reaching development is the increased interest in applying federal antitrust laws to the health care system. It had long been believed that the Sherman Antitrust Act of 1890 did not apply to the "learned professions," that is, law, medicine, and so on. This belief came to an abrupt end in 1975 when the United States Supreme Court decided the case of *Goldfarb vs Virginia State Bar Association* (33). The court held that there is no exemption for professional activity. Since the *Goldfarb* ruling, several other judicial decisions have further narrowed exemptions and immunities that previously had been thought to apply to the health care field (34). The Department of Justice and the Federal Trade Commission have shown great interest in the possible application of antitrust laws and principles to the health care industry. The basic belief underlying their intervention is that this industry can be made to function more or less like a conventional economic market.

To accomplish the objective of making the health care marketplace more competitive, many existing structures and relations will have to be revised. In the name of professionalism and preservation of quality, many traditional forms of competition—such as the advertising of services and prices—have been virtually outlawed by the medical establishment. In times past, when cost was not as important a consideration as currently, no one seriously challenged the complex system of interdependencies and protective relationships that were being formed in the health care field. Thus, there are many well-established traditions in health care that would clearly be regarded as illegal, anticompetitive restraints in other contexts. It is these relationships that are now being questioned.

The Federal Trade Commission has, for example, challenged the power that the AMA holds over medical education in this country. The system of specialty board certification has also been questioned as a means of limiting competition and restricting the entry of new professionals into a given market. Physicians' advertising of their qualifications, services, and fees is being encouraged, as is the abandonment of "relative value scales" as a basis for fee setting. Even the federal health-planning program established under Public Law 93-641 (35) and the Professional Standards Review Organization program (PSRO), developed for the monitoring of quality and usage of services under the Medicare and Medicaid programs (36), have been called into question. All these features of the health care system, long accepted and, in some cases, even encouraged by the government, are now being subjected to searching inquiry.

Dealing with the Endpoints of Life

Another major area that inevitably will experience dramatic change in the near future involves life itself—its origin, nature, and limits. During the 1970s, there have been dramatic changes in the law governing the endpoints of life. The Supreme Court's *Roe vs Wade* decision in 1973 (37), recognizing a woman's constitutional right to have an abortion during the first two trimesters of pregnancy, has brought much change and controversy to the health care system. Even in 1980, seven years after that momentous decision, many related legal issues remain to be adjudicated. Moreover, the ramifications of the rationale underlying *Roe vs Wade* extend deep into other areas of the law of health care. As medical science and technology push back the frontiers of knowledge, the law has increasingly come to recognize areas of individual privacy where one can choose his or her own course in matters of great personal sensitivity.

One of these areas involves genetic counseling and, potentially, genetic engineering. As it becomes possible to predict with greater accuracy the characteristics of offspring before they are born, the law will have to face questions of how far parents may go in choosing the type of children that they wish to bring into the world. The use of amniocentesis to test for Down's syndrome is now relatively common, with abortion available as a matter of right if the test is positive. Presumably, under the rationale of *Roe vs Wade,* the same latitude for individual choice would apply if a mother chose to abort because the fetus was of the "wrong" sex. The development of fetoscopy and other techniques for in utero examination of fetuses could extend much farther the possible reasons for choosing to abort.

Another related medical development that will inevitably call forth new legal guidelines is the extrauterine fertilization of a human ovum and the subsequent implantation of the resulting embryo in the womb of either the donor of the ovum or of a "surrogate mother" who volunteers to carry the baby to birth. The legal questions that can arise from such a procedure are many and complex; the only certainty is that they will, in fact, arise and require settlement. A fair amount of jurisprudential thought is already being applied to anticipating the possibilities and providing for them by statute law.

At the other end of the spectrum of life, questions of the transition from life to death are equally troublesome. The decision of the New Jersey Supreme Court in the case of *Karen Quinlan* (25) is illustrative of the type of issue that lies ahead. As noted above, courts in several states have held that a person has the right to refuse life-prolonging treatment, subject to limitations that, as yet, have not been fully defined. Further, many state legislatures have enacted laws recognizing a person's so-called right to die or to seek "death with dignity." Finally, in recent years, the health care system has come far toward accepting the "hospice" movement, which seeks not to postpone the death of the terminally ill but, rather, to lessen the physical and psychologic suffering that attends the inevitable event. All the above instances reflect attempts by medical science, and society as a whole, to accommodate to the changing limits of its ability to deal with the forces of life and death.

Preventive Medicine and Protection of the Environment

Recent developments in health law have not been confined to the narrow field of medical care. Many have focused as well on safeguarding the physical environment and promoting more rational approaches to personal health maintenance. Examples of the former are state and federal laws governing water and air pollution and those setting occupational safety and health standards. Traffic rules (such as the 55 mile per hour national speed limit) and automobile safety standards (i.e., head restraints, seat belts, and structural roll-over protection) also fall into this category. The encouragement of personal health maintenance, to date less well developed as a legal matter, is an area in which substantial future change can be expected. An example is the Surgeon General's caveat on cigarette packs and the current cautionary legend on items containing artificial sweeteners.

CONCLUSION

These and other public health initiatives are implemented by means of the legal system, and all such developments belong to the fast-growing field known as "health law." The scope of this chapter does not permit full exploration of all these subjects, but they are worth mentioning, if only briefly, to raise the level of health practitioners' awareness of the many ways in which the law impacts on their field. The objective is not to stir feelings of unease in health care personnel as they witness the approach of new actors into their traditional domain. Rather, it is to help them understand the various forces that they will encounter, so that they may deal with them more comfortably. Despite its occasional pretensions of being something more, the law is simply the formal embodiment of society's public policy determinations. People who understand changing societal values and mores can predict more accurately the turns that the law will take; conversely, those who follow developments in the law will have an additional and important clue to trends and countertrends in popular thought.

REFERENCES

1. 156 Ind 416, 59 NE 1058 (1901).
2. Williamson C: Physicians' legal liability for refusing emergency aid. *R I Med J* 51:261, 1968.
3. General Laws of Rhode Island, §45-16-6, as amended (G L 1896, Ch 232).
4. *Providence Journal* February 6, 1968, p 16, col 3-4.
5. Criminal Code of Germany, Art 330c (1953). Note: Emergency care: Physicians should be placed under an affirmative duty to render essential medical care in emergency circumstances. *Univ Calif Davis Law Rev* 7:246, 1974.
6. Vermont Statutes Annotated, Tit 12, §519b (1972).
7. Chayet N: *Legal Implications of Emergency Care,* New York, Appleton-Century-Crofts, 1967.
8. 35 AmR 363, 128 Mass 131 (1880).
9. 354 Mass 102, 235 NE 2d 793 (1968).
10. 25 Cal 2d 486, 154 P 2d 687 (1944).
11. 60 F 2d 737 (2d Cir 1932).
12. *Id* at 740.
13. 83 Wash 2d 514, 519 P 2d 981 (1974).
14. 519 P 2d at 983.
15. Revised Code of Washington §4.24.290 (1975).
16. 92 Wash. 2d 246, 595 P 2d 919 (1979), rev'ing 20 Wash App 81, 579 P 2d 374 (1978).
17. 595 P 2d at 923, n.3.
18. 211 NY 125, 129, 105 NE 92, 93 (NY 1914)
19. *Salgo vs Leland Stanford, Jr University Board of Trustees,* 154 Cal App 2d 560, 317 P 2d 170 (1957).
20. *Natanson vs Kline,* 186 Kan 393, 350 P 2d 1093, modified 187 Kan 186, 354 P 2d 670 (1960).
21. 464 F 2d 772 (DC Cir 1972).
22. *Id* at 794, n 138.
23. *Id* at 784.
24. *Id* at 789.
25. *In the Matter of Karen Quinlan, an Alleged Incompetent,* 70 NJ 10, 355 A 2d 647 (1976).
26. 33 Ill 2d 326, 211 NE 2d 253 (1965), *cert denied* 383 US 946.
27. *Arizona Revised Statutes Annotated* §32-1451A, as amended 1971.
28. *Florida Statutes Annotated* §458.1201, as amended 1975.
29. Act of June 30, 1906, Ch 3915, 34 Stat 768.
30. Act of June 25, 1938, Ch 675, 52 Stat 1040.
31. 21 USC §321(p) (1) (1976).

32. 45 Code of Federal Regulations, Part 19; 40 *Fed Reg* 32284 (July 31, 1975).

33. 421 US 773 (1975).

34. Rosoff A: Antitrust laws and the health care industry: New warriors into an old battle. *St Louis Univ Law J* 23:429, 1979.

35. 42 USC §300k to 300t (Supp V 1975).

36. 42 USC §1320c (1976).

37. 410 US 113 (1973).

10
Regulation and Health Planning

Denis J. Lucey, III
Ellen S. Smith

Government's increasing financial involvement in health care, particularly through Medicare and Medicaid, has led to expanded attempts to regulate and plan medical care in this country. As medical care expenditures have skyrocketed, the government has sought ways to control costs. Emphasis has been placed both on planning to determine the need for various resources and on the control of expenditures through definitions of appropriate amounts and types of service. At present, planning and regulation of health care have been combined in the National Health Planning and Resources Development Act of 1974—Public Law 93-641—which is best known for establishing the health systems agencies.

In this chapter, we shall focus on the aspects of P.L. 93-641 that have relevance to the practicing physician. The history of health care regulation and planning will be reviewed, as will the successes and failures of the various efforts at planning and regulation of facilities and services.

Planning can be defined as the ". . . specification of means necessary to achieve a prescribed end, before action takes place" (1). Regulation, on the other hand, refers to ". . . principles, rules or laws imposed by external authority for controlling or governing behavior" (2). It is important to recognize these two complementary and, at the same time, competing functions that the law has recently assigned to planning agencies. Regulation in health care has been enacted in a piecemeal fashion in this country. This has hindered the evaluation of its effectiveness and frustrated many physicians who have dealt with the regulatory agencies. It is understandable that some would ask whether the primary care physician should be involved in the health-planning process at all. Indeed, some physicians would say that they should not. However, since the major indirect and direct effects of regulation on practitioners are related to their use of services within the hospitals with which they have affiliations, resources approved through the planning process may determine the amount and types of services that practitioners can obtain for hospitalized patients.

THEORIES OF PLANNING

The hierarchic nature of planning is described by Webber in Chapter 14. In general, there are two broad distinctions of planning theory: positive and normative theory. The positivists plan for future changes on the basis of new ideas, whereas those espousing normative theory tend to plan on the basis of the accepted norms and values of their particular situation. Most health planning has been done in a normative fashion.

Four strategies of planning have also been described. The *rational* strategy attempts to maximize the preferred alternative. This strategy often results in a long lead time for plan development, and implementation is rare since the plans may be outdated by the time that they are developed. *Incremental* strategy, as its name implies, occurs in a stepwise manner, often in reaction to a problem. Rarely is there a well identified plan. With the *mixed scanning* approach, changes are made in a somewhat incremental fashion; however, the changes occur within the context of a larger defined plan. *Radical* strategy would make major changes in all areas of health care delivery.

HEALTH CARE REGULATION

Rosoff has outlined the multiple areas of regulation in health care in Chapter 9 and has reviewed their impact on the physician. Health care planning, as defined by Hyman (3), is "long range and forward looking and uses a systematic process for developing what is needed to improve the health care system of a community." Thus, health care planning specifies the means to reach a desired end—improved health care. On the other hand, "regulation is a means oriented function, used to implement the goals of an area-wide health plan" (3). The National Health Planning and Resources Development Act of 1974 combines both functions of planning and regulation.

The diversity of health care services and entities makes health care regulation difficult and piecemeal (4). In turn, America's ambivalent attitude toward regulation in general increases the difficulty of designing appropriate regulatory strategies and methods. The ambivalence stems from a desire, on the one hand, to protect the free-market system and, on the other, to protect the general welfare of society. Another reason that regulation in health care has been difficult is the conflict between the public's need for safe and effective health care and the professional's demand for autonomy (5).

HISTORY OF PLANNING

In this section, the history surrounding the federal government's involvement in planning, regulating, and delivering services will be described. Specifically, concentration will be placed on the Hill-Burton program, Regional Medical Programs, the Comprehensive Health Planning Act, Section 1122 of the Social Security Act, and the National Health Planning and Resources Development Act. Successes and failures of these programs will be described.

Early Planning Legislation

The Hill-Burton program is generally considered to represent the first generation of federal health planning legislation. This program was designed in response to a perceived national shortage of modern acute-care hospital facilities, particularly in rural areas. World War II helped spur the passage of the Federal Hospital Survey and Construction Act of 1946, which established the Hill-Burton program and provided federal aid to states for hospital construction if the states created hospital planning councils and developed plans describing how bed needs would be satisfied. The federal government made available one-third of the loan money, and two-thirds had to be provided by state governments. The act was amended in 1954 and extended to cover nursing homes, rehabilitation facilities, and diagnostic or treatment centers. Ten years later, the hospital and medical facilities amendments (Hill-Harris amendments) set aside funds for modernization or replacement construction and required a component of free care by the hospitals. The strengths of the Hill-Burton program and subsequent additions to the act were an improved federal and state working relationship, an increased number of hospital beds, and a modicum of standardization of physical facilities. The major weaknesses of the act included fixed and narrow goals, inability of the poorer states to obtain matching grants because their own funds were limited, and the use of a method of planning that was based on demand, was hospital oriented, and was based largely on past population and utilization trends.

The Regional Medical Program (RMP) Act (P.L. 89-239) refocused health planning away from hospitals and toward categoric medical programs. By use of the cooperative activities of local health care providers organized into regional units, the act focused on solving the problems of heart disease, cancer, and stroke. In 1970, the Regional Medical Program Act was extended to include kidney disease. Management and operational difficulties resulted in the impoundment of funds by President Richard Nixon. The regional medical programs were provider oriented and therefore concentrated on helping develop technology and high-quality staff. A lack of interstate cooperation contributed to the program's downfall.

The Comprehensive Health Planning (CHP) Act of 1966 (P.L. 89-749), also known as the Partnership for Health Act, followed the enactment of Medicare legislation and increased governmental expenditure for health care. The act provided funds to single state agencies for health planning, including the development of an official state health plan. Each state developed an "A" CHP agency that was advised by a state health planning council. The act also provided for organization of local and regional or areawide "B" CHP agencies. This act and its amendments provided additional federal grants for education in health planning, for provision of public health and mental health services, and for health-services development projects. The B agencies were given little power but were charged with comment and review. They had no review authority over the use of private dollars for capital expansion. The act introduced and emphasized the concept of consumer participation in health planning.

Section 1122 (enacted in 1972) of the Social Security Act was an early attempt by the federal government to find ways of controlling medical care costs; the act stipulated that the Department of Health, Education, and Welfare could deny Medicare and Medicaid reimbursement unless state approval was obtained for hospital capital expenditures resulting from hospital expansion exceeding $100,000, or any expenditure involved in increasing the number of beds or introducing new services that changed the facility's mission. The recent movement toward tax-exempt revenue bonds for large capital-expansion projects of hospitals has strengthened the Section 1122 review process.

Since 1964, 37 states have enacted "certificate of need" statutes. These statutes expressly prohibit an increase in facility capacity, equipment, or services without prior state approval. As of fiscal year 1977, all states except Missouri had enacted some program comparable to certificate of need, but there were 8 states in which the legislation was being challenged. Since 1974, the National Health Planning and Resources Development Act has required the enactment of state certificate-of-need laws.

Certificate-of-need and Section 1122 review were enacted as the government's financial involvement in health care increased. A major flaw of Section 1122 legislation as carried out was the lack of allowance and mechanism for regular appropriateness review or decertification of need. There is minimal evidence that these processes save money, however, and some states have enacted rate-setting commissions to help control costs from another vantage point.

Public Law 93-641

Public Law 93-641 was signed into law by President Gerald Ford in the first week of January 1975. The act attempts to correct earlier problems with health planning by partly dismantling one system (CHP, Regional Medical Program, Hill-Burton) and supplementing it with another. The law mandates an official health-planning system. It is likely to exert future influence on health care, and we shall, therefore, present a detailed consideration of its provisions.

The law itself is complex, specific, and, highly detailed, in part, because it was developed in a period of congressional distrust of the executive branch of government and in part because it passed only after struggle and compromise among strong interest groups, including physicians, other health care providers and consumers, hospitals, and government. Nevertheless, the purpose of the act is explicit, even if, in the short run, its goals are difficult to achieve.

In developing the new planning law, Congress based the legislation on the following conclusions:

1. The achievement of equal access to quality health care at reasonable cost is a priority of the federal government.
2. The massive infusion of federal funds into the existing health care system has contributed to inflationary increases in the cost of health care, has failed to produce an adequate supply or distribution of health resources, and, consequently, has not provided equal access for everyone to such resources.
3. The many responses to these problems by the public sector (federal, state, and local) and the private sector have not resulted in a comprehensive, rational approach to the problems of
   a. the lack of uniformly effective methods of delivering health care

b. the maldistribution of health care facilities and manpower

c. the increasing cost of health care

4. Increases in the cost of health care, particularly of hospital stays, have been uncontrollable and inflationary, and there are presently inadequate incentives for the use of appropriate alternative levels of health care and for the substitution of ambulatory intermediate care for inpatient hospital care.

5. Since the health care provider is one of the most important participants in any health-care delivery system, health policy must address the legitimate needs and concerns of the provider if it is to achieve meaningful results; thus, it is imperative that the provider be encouraged to have an active role in developing health policy at all levels.

6. Large segments of the public are lacking in basic knowledge regarding personal health care and effective use of available health services (6).

Congress identified 10 priority areas in fomulating national health-planning goals and in developing and operating state and areawide health-planning and resource-development programs:

1. The provision of primary care services for medically underserved populations, especially those that are located in rural or economically depressed areas

2. The development of multi-institutional systems for coordination or consolidation of institutional health services (including obstetric, pediatric, emergency medical, intensive- and coronary-care, and radiation therapy services)

3. The development of medical group practices (especially those whose services are appropriate and are coordinated or integrated with institutional health services), health maintenance organizations, and other organized systems for the provision of health care

4. The training and increased usage of physicians' assistants and especially nurse clinicians

5. The development of multi-institutional arrangements for the sharing of support services necessary to all health-service institutions

6. The promotion of improvements in the quality of health services, including needs identified by the review activities of Professional Standards Review Organizations under Part B of Title XI of the Social Security Act

7. The development of health service institutions able to provide care (including intensive care, acute general care, and extended care) on a geographically integrated basis

8. The promotion of disease prevention, including the study of nutritional and environmental factors affecting health and the provision of prevention health care services

9. The adoption of uniform cost-accounting, simplified reimbursement, uniform reporting systems, and improved management procedures for health-service institutions

10. The education of the general public concerning personal (including preventive) health care and effective use of available health services (6)

The act is administered through an elaborate governmental and quasi-governmental structure. A central National Advisory Council on health planning was created. Its establishment was delayed, however, and there has been minimal staff support. The National Advisory Council has not exerted much influence; for example, in 1977–1978, the Department of Health, Education, and Welfare (DHEW) promulgated controversial health-planning standards without the opinion of the National Advisory Council. In the beginning, activity was decentralized into the 10 DHEW regional offices. More recently, the making of policy has reverted back to Washington.

The act established a State Health Planning and Development Agency (SHPDA) in each state. In some states, this agency is the department of health; in others, a department of human resources; and in still others, a part of the governor's office. Each agency is funded through a combination of state and federal monies. Agencies are responsible for performing final reviews according to Section 1122 or certificate-of-need legislation, for aggregating the plans of areawide agencies into a preliminary state health plan, and for developing a state medical-facilities plan (to supercede the Hill-Burton Plan).

Over 50 state health-coordinating councils have also been established. These councils are analogous to the A agency councils under P.L. 89-749. Each council is appointed by the governor from a pool of areawide agency representatives and other interest groups. A majority of the appointees must be health care consumers, and at least 60% of the membership must represent the areawide agencies. Thirty percent of the health care providers must be direct providers (e.g., physicians, nurses, and dentists).

The functions of the state health-coordinating councils are as follows: to advise the state agency (SHPDA), to review and approve the state health plan, to review and comment on areawide health-systems agency budgets and federal designation agreements, and to review and comment on the official state plans of other health-related state programs (e.g., maternal and child health, mental health). State health-coordinating councils vary substantially in size from state to state. Common problems have included both inadequate representation of health professionals because of the multiplicity of new health professions and the exclusion of consumers because of narrow definitions. Consumers are excluded if they have a 10% fiduciary interest or a policy-making role in a health-care institution or if they are close relatives of such persons.

Governors, some interest groups, and legislators have been threatened by the state health coordinating councils. Legislators resent the roles that the councils have with their constituents; governors view the development of policy by the councils as usurpation of executive authority; and special interest groups dislike the umbrella role assigned to the councils for program review and plan development.

The most important administrative subdivision created by this legislation is the Health Systems Agency (HSA). The nation was divided into over 200 health service areas, and each Health Systems Agency is responsible for its own health services area. Health-service areas were intended to be "natural" health care service areas, and each area was to contain a population of between 200,000 and 3,000,000. Each area was to coincide with boundaries for Professional Standards Review Organizations, existing planning areas, and state planning and administrative areas. Areas were established by the Secretary of DHEW upon the recommendation of the governor. Special provisions established interstate areas. In many cases, the areas were the same as those of the old CHP B agencies; however, some metropolitan areas were split, and political considerations influenced some decisions. Redesignation of areas has occurred but is discouraged by DHEW.

A Health Systems Agency can be a nonprofit private corporation, a public regional planning body, or a single unit of local government (Chicago has the only Health Systems Agency that is a unit of local government). Private, nonprofit corporations dominate in the northeastern states. The staff of the agency must demonstrate expertise in administration, data collection and analysis, health planning, and health-resource development and use.

The governing body of the Health Systems Agency must be composed of residents from the area, the majority of whom must be consumers. The remainder must be providers (those who deliver health-care service directly), institutional administrators, health care insurers, and health-professions educators. The consumers must be broadly representative of the social, economic, linguistic, and racial populations; the geographic parts of the health-service area; and the major purchasers of health care (6). The mandate thus provides for membership in the Health Systems Agency for minority groups and for business and labor interests. Areas smaller than the entire health-services area may be represented through a subarea advisory council. Persons may be elected board members by the board, by an outside constituency through a general election, or by holding a political office. Health Systems Agencies may provide opportunities for additional consumers and providers to serve on task forces, project review or plan implementation committees, and administrative committees. Public Law 93-641 maintains that Health Systems Agencies exist for the purposes of:

1. Improving the health of residents of a health-service area
2. Increasing the accessibility, acceptability, continuity, and quality of health services provided to them
3. Restraining increases in the cost of providing health services
4. Preventing unnecessary duplication of health resources (6)

The two principal operations of a Health Systems Agency are plan development and project review, two roles that can produce conflicting goals. Health Systems Agencies are charged with developing health-systems plans and annual implementation plans. Health-systems plans and annual implementation plans are concerned with the health status of people within the health care system serving them. Health-systems plans cover three to five years; annual implementation plans cover one year. Both plans must be updated annually. The DHEW has promulgated elaborate rules for the format, content, development, and approval of health-systems plans. There is considerable evidence of the increasing insistence of the DHEW on specifics, such as quantifiable objectives. Because of this insistence on specifics, there are complaints that the Health Systems Agency is not a local enterprise or even a federal-state-areawide collaboration but, instead, a federal intrusion.

The other chief function of the Health Systems Agency is initial review of projects under Section 1122 or certification-of-need legislation before review by the state review body. In theory, such review should follow development and acceptance of the health systems plan; in fact, the reverse has largely occurred because of delays in plan development. The content of some plans, therefore, is the consequence, and not the cause, of project-review decisions. The process then becomes a normative planning process.

Section 1122 and certificate-of-need processes occur in reaction to proposals that are initiated by health care facilities. Larger hospitals and health care facilities have their own long-range planning committees that review intrahospital proposals generally in the context of a long-range plan and determine which proposed capital expenditures the facility will present to the Health Systems Agency. Members of the committee usually include physicians, administrators, and other personnel involved in the planning process. The staff of the Health Systems Agency review a project and recommend approval or disapproval to the board of the agency. These decisions are made on the basis of local, state, and federal guidelines that consider community needs, potential for cost containment, and financial feasibility.

In addition to substantive reviews required for expenditures of $100,000 or more, changes or expansion in service or facility, changes in bed complement, or substantial cost increases, there are nonsubstantive reviews. Nonsubstantive reviews are performed when capital expenditures are under $100,000, when local institutions apply for federal grants (called a proposed use of federal funds [PUFF] review), and when federally funded projects identified by the Office of Management and Budget are undertaken (called A-95 reviews, because the projects are identified in circular A-95). These review activities tend to be less important.

If the local Health Systems Agency has a subarea council, review proceeds first through that council, then to a project review committee, and, finally, to the board. Final authority rests with the state agency, but relative financial weakness and the needed political alliances with the Health Systems Agencies make the recommendations of the agencies influential. Applicants denied approval may take objections to an administrative hearing for resolution.

A major handicap to a good working relationship between provider applicants and the regulators of the Health Systems Agency and within an agency between plan-development advocates and plan-implementation (i.e., project-review) supporters is that the agency is able to review a project and thus promote changes in the system only when an applicant initiates a project application. This handicap shields from review institutions that should make changes but fail to submit applications. The law originally provided for periodic review by the Health Systems Agency of all institutional health services, but this provision has been effectively discontinued since adequate funding was not available for the extensive staff work required.

Finally, P.L. 93-641 established planning and technical-assistance centers to consult with Health Systems Agencies, SHPDAs, and state health coordinating councils and to study health-planning issues. One such center was funded for each of the 10 federal regions. The results have been uneven; at this writing, several centers are expected to be consolidated.

According to a survey conducted by the American Health Planning Association covering the 24 months ending in July 1978, 44% of the Health Systems Agencies were new organizations, and 56% grew out of the CHP agencies. The Health Systems Agencies in this period reviewed a total of $12 billion in capital expenditures and disallowed $3.4 billion.

The Health Planning and Resources Development Amendments (P.L. 96-79) signed into law in October 1979 expanded national health priorities from 10 to 16. Some of these new priorities emphasized cost containment, identification and discontinuance of unneeded services and outpatient care. Other major areas included in the amendments were recommendations concerning Health Systems Agencies, SHPDA's, SHCC's and appropriateness review. The amendments have clarified regulatory procedures under the act. Health Systems Agencies are allowed to review only those services which are brought to them for review. They cannot bargain about other services.

THE PHYSICIAN AND PUBLIC LAW 93-641

What is the effect of the National Health Planning and Resources Development Act of 1974 (P.L. 93-641) on the health care practitioner? It is useful to consider the practitioner in three settings: the private office, the publicly funded program, and the hospital.

In the office, the effect is minimal and generally positive or promotional. Health-system plans, annual implementation plans, and state health plans can encourage physician recruitment, suggest an improved distribution of physicians, and recommend economic incentives for physicians providing primary care—all in response to the priorities of P.L. 93-641. Other activities are possible; for example, there is intermittent interest in review of capital expenditures in private offices. However, such review was not authorized by P.L. 93-641.

In publicly funded programs (e.g., the Appalachian Regional Commission centers or the Urban and Rural Health Initiative Projects), there is a greater probability of review by the Health Systems Agency and SHPDA. The record shows, however, that reviews are usually positive for these organized group practices, probably because of support from consumers, who dominate the public agencies.

The greatest effect of these reviews is on the hospital and thus indirectly on the physician who practices in the hospital. Unfavorable reviews of hospital projects can decrease cash flow, restrict access to expensive equipment, or limit the number of beds available for admissions.

Given the potential benefits, the possible hazards, and the great uncertainty associated with current planning programs, how should the primary care practitioner respond? The practitioner should become involved with the health-planning process at every level. As a start, the practitioner should become familiar with the current law (P.L. 93-641), its successor act, the provisions of Section 1122 of the Social Security Act, health-planning regulations and guidelines, and the state's certificate-of-need legislation. The practitioner should become active in establishing health-planning positions with the local hospital association and medical society. The practitioner can become a member of a Health Systems Agency, serve on a technical advisory committee, or become appointed or elected to a Health Systems Agency board.

Through rational planning, it is possible that improvements in quality, effectiveness, and efficiency can be made. On the other hand, bureaucratic planning may level the system in favor of arbitrarily imposed constraints and mediocrity. The practitioner can best determine the outcome by participating in the process of planning.

REFERENCES

1. Foley AC, House RJ, Stern K: *Managerial Process and Organizational Behavior.* Glenville, Illinois, Scott, Foreman and Company, 1976.

2. American Hospital Association: *Hospital Regulation: Report of the Special Committee on the Regulatory Process.* Chicago, Illinois, 1977, p 1.

3. Hyman HH: *Health Planning: A Systematic Approach.* Germantown, Maryland, Aspen Systems Corporation, 1975.

4. Ball RM: Background of regulation in health care, in Institute of Medicine: *Controls on Health Care.* Washington, DC, National Academy of Sciences, 1975, p 3.

5. Yerby AS: Regulation of health manpower, in Institute of Medicine: *Controls on Health Care.* Washington, DC, National Academy of Sciences, 1975, p 84.

6. Public Law 93-641, 93rd Congress S. 2994, January 4, 1975. National Health Planning and Resources Development Act of 1974.

7. American Health Planning Association: *Second Report, 1978 Health Planning Agencies.* 1979.

11

Professional Standards Review Organization: Utilization Review and Quality of Care

Veronica C. Oestreicher

Helen L. Smits

The physician who enters medical practice in the United States in the early 1980s will be faced with a bewildering array of rules, regulations, and advice regarding the "appropriate" use of medical services, particularly for patients who are hospitalized. These rules have many sources. Blue Cross, private insurers, and the local Professional Standards Review Organization (PSRO) each has authority over a separate group of patients. Although the basic principles of utilization review are similar, the details applicable to the various types of patients may differ: what is covered under a Blue Cross plan may not be covered by Medicare, and services considered necessary and appropriate under Medicare may not be included under Medicaid, despite the fact that both are government programs managed by the same agency within the Department of Health and Human Services.

There are two basic reasons why every practicing physician needs at least a working knowledge of the intricacies of utilization review and quality assurance. First, one must understand and follow the basic rules to protect patients from unexpected denial of insurance coverage, denial that can be devastating when applied to all or a substantial portion of a hospital stay. Second, physicians do have an opportunity to participate in, and influence, decisions that are having an increasing influence on practice patterns in this country. Although not every physician will wish to be an active member of the local PSRO or sit on the utilization review committee in his local hospital, all should at least understand the opportunities that exist to influence the judgments made for each patient and to alter standards or criteria that appear to be unreasonable.

The main focus of this chapter will be the PSRO program, a series of independent, government-funded organizations that are responsible for the amount and quality of services provided to federally funded patients under Medicare and

Medicaid. This network of organizations is now nationwide; its size and consistency contrasts with the more variable individual review programs sponsored by Blue Cross plans and private insurers. We will indicate where PSRO activity overlaps with other required utilization review as well as the best ways of learning more about non-PSRO aspects of utilization review in any local situation.

The PSRO program was created by Congress as part of the 1972 Amendments to the Social Security Act. The law was developed in response to profound congressional concern about the rapid rise in the costs of medical care funded under federal programs and was designed to assure that health care services provided under Medicare, Medicaid, maternal and child health, and crippled children's programs are necessary, of good quality, and performed at the most economical level consistent with quality care. The program is designed around four fundamental concepts: that physicians are the most appropriate persons to assess the quality of medical care that they deliver; that local, community-based peer review and local standard setting is the most effective means for ensuring that health care resources and facilities are appropriately utilized; that effective quality assurance should eventually include all facets of the health care delivery system; and that peer review organizations must have a broad base of practicing physicians in the community to avoid the bias inherent in a system that is primarily hospital based (1).

Professional Standards Review Organizations are organized and administered by physicians in the PSRO area. These organizations are supported by grants from the Health Care Financing Administration and receive considerable direction from the federal government. Many PSROs also contract with private insurance agencies to carry out review of nonfederal patients. Currently, the country is divided into 195 PSRO areas, each within state boundaries. The law requires that PSROs review the services provided in hospitals and long-term-care facilities; review of ambulatory care may eventually be required. At present, however, review of hospitalized patients is by far the most important responsibility of PSROs. In addition to case-by-case review, PSROs conduct audits of the quality of care and analyze the practice profiles of physicians and institutions within their area. The review process is based on locally determined criteria for acceptable practice.

DEVELOPMENT OF PSRO LEGISLATION

The medical profession in the United States has traditionally taken an interest in assuring the quality of medical practice. In 1918, the American College of Surgeons began a process of voluntary accreditation of hospitals in response to evidence that many institutions were delivering substandard care. In 1952, the voluntary accreditation of hospitals became the responsibility of the new Joint Commission on Accreditation of Hospitals (JCAH), an organization formed by the College of Surgeons, the American College of Physicians, the American Medical Association, and the American Hospital Association. Standards developed by the JCAH encouraged institutions to deliver high-quality care with medical staff overseeing one another's work by such means as "tissue committees" to review the pathologic findings on tissue removed at surgery.

In 1954, the Commission on Financing Hospital Care, organized by the American Hospital Association, evaluated methods for hospital cost controls. Promotion of effective utilization by medical-staff review of other staff members' patients was proposed as one way to decrease overuse of services. Interest in this idea grew in many areas in the 1950s; in 1957, the Pennsylvania commissioner of insurance ordered that hospitals develop a utilization review plan before Blue Cross contracts could be approved. Utilization review committees were formally sponsored in the late 1950s by the Tenth Council or District of the Pennsylvania Medical Society. Soon Blue Cross plans all over the country encouraged or required the formation of these committees, which had the dual function of limiting excess use of services, while improving the quality of patient care. In 1963, the JCAH added a requirement that hospitals evaluate the quality of their medical care on the basis of documented evidence. This requirement meant that utilization review committees had to at least oversee the quality of care if an institution was to meet conditions for accreditation.

With the enactment of Medicare in 1965, when the federal government became a major health care financer, utilization review became a legal requirement for all hospitals and nursing homes accepting Medicare patients; the goal of review, however, was expected to be the control of excess use of services rather than quality assurance. This goal grew out of Congressional concern that Medicare and Medicaid would lead to increased health care costs through over-utilization. In 1967, utilization review requirements were extended to include Medicaid patients. The utilization review committees were responsible for evaluating the medical necessity of services. Final decision-making did not, however, rest with the committee; payment could be denied retrospectively by the Medicare intermediary, by the state for Medicaid patients, and by Blue Cross or other insurers for their own patients. Even though rare, these denials could be costly and distressing to the patient and were frustrating to utilization review committee members, who found themselves held responsible for a task without adequate authority to carry it out.

During the late 1960s, experiments with innovative utilization review systems were undertaken in several parts of the country. Many of these experiments were conducted by groups organized through local medical societies in cooperation with insurance companies. Some of the most successful experiments involved sharing of risk by physicians; savings were passed on to the participating physician group, whereas uncontrolled increases in services decreased the groups' practice income. Prototype PSROs appeared as federally funded experimental medical care review organizations (EMCROs). The primary goal of all these programs was to develop and test mechanisms for reviewing medical care. The apparent success of the best systems greatly influenced the design of the PSRO program and contributed to the success of PSRO legislation.

By 1970, estimates of the future costs of the Medicare hospital insurance program for the next 25-year period overran the original estimates made in 1967 by about $240 billion. One of the major reasons for this precipitous rise was increased utilization of services provided to beneficiaries; the increasing per diem cost of hospital care as well as the rising costs of medical and surgical procedures compounded the problem. Existing utilization review committees in hospitals appeared, in the aggregate, to have little or no effect, largely because there were wide variations between institutions in the standards set for necessary and appropriate care.

Cost control and quality were the overriding concerns of Congress as it searched for a more effective substitute for utilization review. In 1972, Senator Wallace Bennett (R, Utah) introduced the PSRO program for the second time as an amendment to the Social Security Act and in his September 27 speech to the Senate he stated:

> The PSRO amendment represents the best, and perhaps the last, opportunity to fully safeguard the public concern with respect to the cost and quality of medical care while, at the same time, leaving the actual control of the medical practice in the hands of those best qualified—America's physicians (2).

PSROs became part of Public Law 92-603, the 1972 Amendments to the Social Security Act.

PROVISIONS OF PSRO LEGISLATION

Organization

Each PSRO is required to be a nonprofit organization with membership limited to licensed doctors of medicine or osteopathy engaged in the practice of medicine or surgery in the PSRO's area. Other practitioners, such as dentists, may become members if they have independent hospital admitting privileges. To qualify as a PSRO, an organization must include at least 25% of the physicians in the area as members. PSRO membership is voluntary and open to all active physicians in the area and is unrestricted by membership or payment of dues to any organized medical society or association.

Delegation

If a hospital is found by the PSRO to be capable of performing the review functions required by law, the PSRO is required to delegate review to the hospital; otherwise, the PSRO itself carries out review in the hospital. When a hospital is "delegated," the PSRO monitors the hospital to assure its performance remains adequate. Delegation essentially means that the hospital's utilization review committee has final authority to certify the necessity of all federal admissions. Delegation has the great advantage of allowing the utilization review committee to coordinate federal and nonfederal review activities. From the PSRO's perspective, however, delegation may preserve local practice idiosyncracies, such as long stays after a given surgical procedure, so that delegated institutions must remain responsive to the standards of the wider practicing community if they are to retain their delegated status. Delegated hospitals are paid for their review activity as a part of their overall payment for the care given to Medicare patients. These payments are made directly to the hospital by the fiscal intermediary.

Binding Review and Appeal Rights

Once a PSRO or delegated hospital determines the necessity, or lack of it, for a given admission or set of services, the PSRO's determination is binding and cannot be reversed by the state or the Medicare intermediary. When services are considered unnecessary, the determination is usually made before the care has been given; both the patient and the practitioner are notified by letter of the decision. Of particular importance to the practicing physician is the fact that a disputed decision may be appealed to the PSRO either by the physician or the patient. If the PSRO reaffirms its decision, the practitioner or beneficiary has further appeal rights.

Data Collection and Confidentiality

To assess regional patterns of care, PSROs must collect and analyze a great deal of information. Much PSRO data is based on an abstract made of each hospital discharge. These abstracts can be analyzed for various patterns, such as the length of stay for a given diagnosis at each hospital in an area or the length of stay by each practitioner who cares for a given type of patient. Estimates of quality of care can be made on the basis of death rates from specific surgical procedures or the frequency with which practitioners and institutions perform technically difficult procedures. In addition, PSROs collect information related to the quality of care when they conduct audits. There has been a profound and legitimate concern among physicians that the close link between PSROs and the federal government will lead to disclosure of information that could endanger patient confidentiality and adversely affect physician practice. Even apparently straightforward information, such as how often a physician performed a given procedure, could be damaging. One example involves a western state where antiabortion advocates were able to obtain the names of all surgeons who had billed for Medicaid abortions in the previous year; some of the involved physicians then received anonymous threats of physical violence against themselves and their families.

The PSRO law requires the disclosure of some kinds of information. Data must be disclosed to appropriate agencies in the form of aggregate statistics on a geographic, institutional, or other basis reflecting the volume and frequency of services furnished or the demographic characteristics of the population subject to review. A major purpose for releasing such aggregate utilization information is to assist health-planning agencies in determining the need for appropriate and adequate health care services in their communities. Federal regulations describe in much more detail what information may and may not be released. The local PSRO is the best source of information for anyone concerned by this complex and delicate issue.

PSRO HOSPITAL-REVIEW SYSTEM

The hospital, with its high costs, was the first setting in which PSRO review was implemented and is still, by far, the most important area for PSRO review. The

Table 1. Criteria for Performing Cataract Removal*

Reasons for Procedure (one of the following)
1. Lens opacity, proved by slit-lamp and ophthalmologic examination, that accompanies either of the following:
   a. a decrease in visual acuity to 20/70 or less
   b. diminished visual acuity substantially interfering with the patient's mode of living or ability to function
2. Lens opacity that prevents visualization of the interior of the eye for other intraocular surgical procedures
3. Phacogenic glaucoma
4. Phacogenic uveitis

Contraindication
Presence of other visual disorder resulting in such visual loss that no appreciable improvement in vision could be expected after removal of cataract

Comment
Verification of visual acuity at time of hospital admission is suggested to local PSROs

---

*Developed by the American Association of Professional Standards Review Organizations (AAPSRO) for the Department of Health, Education, and Welfare. These sample criteria are for screening patient care for subsequent physician review only and do not constitute standards of care.

three basic methods of review are: concurrent review, medical care evaluation studies, and profile analysis. Ideally, each review mechanism modifies and changes the focus of the others.

The system places heavy emphasis on the use of explicitly stated standards, which are established by the PSRO itself. The technical terminology that has evolved is used to distinguish various areas of review. *Norms* are local patterns of length of hospital stay for specific diagnoses. Since these figures are averages, some patients can be expected to have shorter stays, some longer. A knowledge of local norms for common diagnoses will allow the physician to anticipate when a stay is likely to be questioned. *Criteria* are used to evaluate the reason for an admission or the reason for a procedure; an understanding of these criteria will help to ensure adequate documentation in the record so that unnecessary questioning by reviewers can be avoided. A typical set of criteria for a surgical procedure is shown in Table 1. *Standards* are simply the local professional's expressions of the range of acceptable variation from a norm or criterion—standards are, understandably, much harder to quantify (3).

Local PSROs perform concurrent review, medical care evaluation studies, and profile analysis with considerable flexibility, although the fundamental aspects are generally the same.

Concurrent Review

Concurrent review is the process by which the PSRO certifies the necessity, appropriateness, and quality of services provided during a hospital stay. The basic concurrent review process is shown in Figure 1.

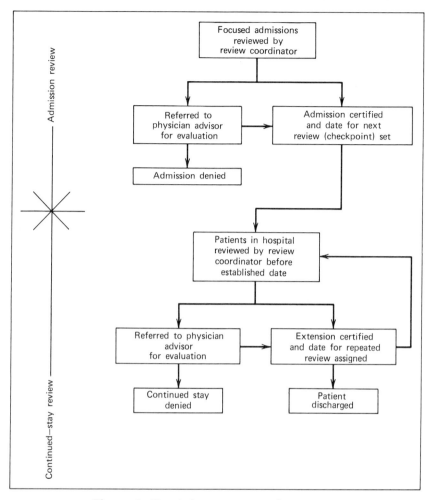

Figure 1. Hospital concurrent review process.

Review is conducted by nonphysician coordinators with physicians serving in an advisory capacity. Review coordinators are registered nurses or other health professionals who have received additional training in the review process. The review coordinator begins by checking the chart on admission, using the PSRO's criteria, to see if hospitalization is necessary.

The admission purely for diagnosis, for example, will be questioned unless the diagnostic tests themselves require hospital services, as in cardiac catheterization. Therapeutic admissions for problems that could be handled on an outpatient basis, such as the stabilization of a person with diabetes who is minimally out of control, will also be questioned. Once the admission is certified as necessary, a standard initial length of stay, or "checkpoint," is assigned on the basis of local norms for the specific diagnosis. This system assures payment for the given number of days; it should also remind the physician when he will be expected to discharge the uncomplicated patient. Standard checkpoints might be 15 days for uncomplicated myocardial infarction and four days for cataract surgery. Many patients are, of course, ready for discharge before the checkpoint.

When the checkpoint assigned on admission is reached, the review coordinators examine the chart to see if further hospital days are needed. The coordinator is looking for evidence that there is a need for additional hospital services. Careful documentation of complications or medical problems unforeseen at admission will avoid unnecessary questioning of the physician's judgment at this point. When this review indicates that further stay is necessary, a second length of stay checkpoint is assigned, certifying payment up to that point. The entire stay is reviewed in this fashion until discharge. If, at any point in the review process, the review coordinator discovers a problem, the case is referred to a physician advisor, who may either decide to approve the case or to deny payment. In many instances, the physician advisor, who is usually a member of the same hospital staff as the attending physician, will discuss the case in detail with the private physician before making a decision. If the case is denied, the usual reason is that hospital care is no longer needed; the patient will then be allowed one to three "grace days" after which time federal payments will cease. Patients may, of course, elect to pay out of pocket for a continued stay if they and the physician wish, but such arrangements are rare.

During the grace period, either the physician or the patient may appeal the decision to the PSRO. Denial may also be of a specific procedure; denial of procedures in the case of a patient who is approved for continued hospital stay is unusual, but can happen.

Medical Care Evaluation Studies

Medical care evaluation studies are currently the most important aspect of the quality-assurance efforts of PSROs. These studies are similar to the patient-care audits required by the JCAH. To develop a comprehensive analysis of care, medical care evaluation studies include all patients, or a sample of all patients, in a given category, rather than only those who are paid for under federal programs.

A medical care evaluation study is an in-depth investigation of a specific area of medical care. Topics may be the care rendered to patients with one diagnosis, such as myocardial infarction, or one presenting complaint, such as chest pain. Topics may also focus on specific treatments, such as the use of blood, or specific techniques, such as the care of urinary catheters. A medical care evaluation study may cover all the relevant patients on a single service, all the patients in a hospital, or patients in all hospitals in a geographic area. The latter method, known as an "areawide" study, has the great advantage of allowing institutions to compare their performance with that of others in the same area.

Medical care evaluation studies may use a wide variety of procedures and methods, but eight basic steps are considered essential for a valid study (4):

1. *Determine the objective of the study.*   The topic chosen should be one that occurs with reasonable frequency, one in which medical care makes a difference and one in which some problem is at least suspected.
2. *Establish criteria.* One of the utilization review committee's most interesting

and challenging jobs is to set the criteria for "standard" medical care. These criteria may be elaborate, complex, and involve branching logic, as in the case of criteria for treatment of myocardial infarction. They may also be extremely simple; one PSRO conducted an audit of the use of blood in which the only criterion for identifying charts for physician review was transfusion of a single unit of blood.

3. *Design the study.* The utilization review committee must decide on the conduct of the study: will all charts be examined or only a sample; how long will the work take; is any extra training of review coordinators needed?

4. *Collection of data.* Information is usually collected from patients' charts by review coordinators or medical records personnel by means of a form designed by the utilization review committee.

5. *Develop reports.* The results of data collection are aggregated and displayed for committee consideration.

6. *Analyze results and identify deficiencies.* The committee must determine if variances from the criteria are justified; they must decide how serious any deficiencies are and how best to correct them.

7. *Develop a corrective plan.* Development of such a plan usually involves work with specialty departments as well as with physicians who appear at fault. Seminars, grand rounds, and special hospital bulletins may all be used to notify staff of problems.

8. *Restudy.* After the corrective plans have been implemented, restudy after a reasonable period of time should ensure that the problems have been corrected.

An Example of a Medical Care Evaluation Study

General Hospital found an unusually high incidence of admissions for pneumococcal pneumonia compared with that of the other hospitals in its area. The hospital's medical audit committee decided to conduct a study to determine the cause. The committee decided that to establish the diagnosis of pneumococcal pneumonia, it was necessary to have a positive sputum culture or characteristic Gram staining, coupled with evidence of pulmonary parenchymal involvement by a chest x-ray film or physical examination. The records of the last 50 patients discharged with the diagnosis of pneumococcal pneumonia were reviewed by two review coordinators. In 20 of the records, the review coordinators could not find evidence that the criteria had been met. These charts were referred to the full medical audit committee for review and interpretation. After discussion with the responsible physicians, the committee decided that in five of the cases, there was evidence to establish the diagnosis, which had not been recorded in the record. In 15 cases, the committee decided that the diagnosis was incorrect, that respiratory conditions other than pneumococcal pneumonia were present, and, since all 15 had received unnecessary therapy with penicillin, that a change in practice was needed. As a result of the study, the committee made the following recommendations to the medical staff:

1. That the physicians responsible for the five poorly documented charts be informed of the findings

2. That the physicians responsible for the incorrect diagnoses participate in a local continuing medical-education program on the diagnosis and treatment of respiratory conditions

3. That the diagnosis of pneumococcal pneumonia be routinely checked against the committee's criteria during the concurrent review process

4. That the topic be restudied in six months

The recommendations were adopted, and faculty from the nearby medical center were invited to give a postgraduate course in the diagnosis of respiratory diseases.

A reaudit six months later, performed by means of the same procedures and criteria as in the original study, revealed no instances of incorrect diagnosis. As a result, the medical staff decided to discontinue the current review requirement for validation of the diagnosis of pneumococcal pneumonia (5).

Profile Analysis

Profile analysis is a relatively new form of review that has not been used by utilization review committees but that is required by law of PSROs. The model can be found in some Western European countries, as well as in this country, in some independent review programs, such as those developed by health maintenance organizations (HMOs). The technique analyzes patterns in aggregated patient-care data (4). Data may be aggregated according to practitioner, such as how many times in a year a surgeon did a given procedure; according to patient, such as all narcotic drugs prescribed for a patient over a set period of time; or according to institution, such as death rates or infection rates for a common surgical procedure at one hospital. Profiles are used chiefly for purposes of comparison and can provide the practitioner with fascinating insights into his or her performance. A profile might, for example, show a change over time in the physician's prescribing habits or reveal that a series of worrisome postoperative complications were actually statistically similar to the experience of other surgeons in the area. Professional Standards Review Organizations will increasingly be using profiles to identify problems deserving emphasis in concurrent review or medical care evaluation studies. A profile is not, in and of itself, a final answer—a disturbing postoperative death rate may be the result of referral patterns of critically ill patients, thus reflecting great surgical skill rather than incompetence. Nevertheless, profiles provide physicians with a unique opportunity to compare their performance with that of others.

Regardless of delegation status, the PSRO is responsible for conducting profile analysis. However, delegated hospitals are expected to participate in the analysis of their own profiles. The PSRO is required to provide continual feedback to both delegated and nondelegated hospitals on the results of profile analysis.

Review of Nonfederal Patients

Review of nonfederal patients usually follows much the same pattern as PSRO review, with a check on the appropriateness of the original admission and subsequent checks on the length of stay. Whether approval by a hospital utilization review committee will mean payment of a given claim for a privately insured patient depends on the agreement between the hospital and the insurance company. In some instances, the insurer's staff may reverse the committee's decision, or an apparently insured patient may not actually be covered for a given illness. For example, chronic or recurring conditions are often not covered until a policy has been in effect for a year or more; transfer of coverage from a private insurer to a Blue Cross plan may be treated like a new policy. The hospital's financial counselors are usually the patient's best guides to complex insurance rules.

ISSUES IN THE PSRO PROGRAM

The evolution of the PSRO program has been difficult and plagued by controversy. The technical and political problems have included implementation difficulties, both locally and in Washington; budget pressures; continued skepticism that physicians could oversee themselves; and limitations in the state of the art.

Although the PSRO legislation makes it clear that the program is to address both cost and quality, the first major controversy was whether the program was oriented to cost or to quality. Many critics insisted that the roles were incompatible. Supporters argued that they go hand in hand. Over time, the latter argument has gained more acceptance, especially with the evergrowing concerns over cost containment. Donabedian supports the compatibility of cost and quality as follows:

> Quality is the appropriate application of medical knowledge, with due regard to the balance between the hazards inherent in every medical intervention and the benefits expected from it. As to cost, I take the position that unnecessary services and the use of more costly procedures or sites of care without distinct gains, in effect represent a lesser level of quality because they signify poor medical judgment and social waste (6).

Although the PSRO review system is more advanced than previous review systems, there remain serious limitations in review methodology. One of the most commonly cited limitations is the difficulty of measuring good care. The PSRO system is based primarily on measurement of the process of care rather than the outcome of care. Some critics argue that measurement should use outcomes to avoid enforcing medical "styles," which may be of little direct benefit to the patient. Although studies of outcome are obviously essential for scholarly evaluations of the quality of care, these studies pose many practical problems for a review system. Even clear-cut outcomes, such as death after a surgical procedure, can be affected by factors beyond the physician's control, for example, the patient's overall condition. Although a few fields, such as obstetrics and certain kinds of acute care, do lend themselves to measurement of outcome, much of the impact of medical care can be evaluated only over long periods of time. Although there are limitations in the process-oriented approach, limitations in the use of the outcome-oriented approach make it impractical for evaluating care in the short run. Combinations of process criteria with short-term outcomes (such as postoperative infections) can maximize the benefits derived from quality evaluations.

Difficulties in implementation created another set of problems for the PSRO program. These difficulties ranged from the initial lack of physician enthusiasm in many parts of the country to early funding problems that reflected both bureaucratic and congressional skepticism about a physician-run review system. One of the major difficulties in implementation arose because there were insufficient data to focus review on problem areas. As a result, almost 100% of federal hospital patients were reviewed in detail, an extremely inefficient and costly process. More recently, budget pressures have led to an emphasis on "focusing," in which most cases receive only statistical evaluation, while nurse coordinators and physician reviewers concentrate on particular cases, and often on particular practitioners, where problems can be expected.

With review resources targeted on problem areas and away from areas of good performance, the PSRO will have proportionately more dollars and energy available for review of priority problems. As local PSROs correct unnecessary admissions and excessive lengths of stay, resources will increasingly be directed toward other hospital activities. Some of these activities include review of ancillary services and physician services, as well as hospital emergency room and outpatient services.

Perhaps the most serious problem that the program faces at present, however, is the continued skepticism of legislators and bureaucrats, both at the state and the federal levels, that physicians can properly oversee one another. The old adage of the fox watching the chicken coop appears regularly in discussions by opponents of the program, a fact that may surprise many physicians, who have difficulty believing that colleagues could prey on their patients. The real issue here seems to be the great difficulty that some laymen have in understanding why there are no "national standards" for medical decisions. It is hard for the nonphysician, for example, to understand that the decision to replace a severely arthritic hip in an elderly patient is influenced not only by the patient's overall medical status, but also by such subtle social issues as whether the person's life revolves around playing chess or hiking. Similarly, laymen and insurance companies are baffled by the fact that such factors as weather and geography can legitimately affect medical decisions, even though early discharge after myocardial infarction is clearly a different matter in Florida and northern Minnesota, at least in the winter.

REVIEW OF LONG-TERM AND AMBULATORY CARE

Current law requires eventual PSRO review in all long-term-care institutions and allows the Department of Health and Human Services to require review in ambulatory settings. Neither area has received much funding, and there is a real possibility that the program will eventually be limited chiefly to review of hospital services. Some understanding of the possible impact of review in both settings may prove useful, however, to the physician who practices in them. This impact is particularly applicable to long-term-care institutions, where review by states of Medicaid patients can be expected in the absence of PSRO review.

Review of Long-term Care

Although long-term care is so different from hospital care that it may not seem reasonable to carry out similar review systems in nursing homes, several factors argue for a strong role in this field. First, the enormous federal investment in long-term care requires the government to be accountable to both the recipients of care and the taxpayers. In 1978, for example, the costs of long-term care constituted 40% of Medicaid expenditures. Second, the persons served (the elderly, the lonely, the confused, and the sick) are highly vulnerable and often unable to voice complaints or make simple inquiries for themselves. Nursing home patients, especially under Medicaid, have little or no real choice of services. Quality care must be assured for them. Last, the demographic characteristics of the population are shifting—the proportion of the population over age 65 has grown from 7% in 1940, to 11% at present, to a predicted 20% by the year 2030. Thus, review of the care given to the elderly will become increasingly more important.

The PSRO requirement for review of long-term-care facilities refers to services provided only in the more sophisticated and well-staffed skilled nursing facilities. Other institutions providing long-term care, referred to as intermediate-care facilities, are reviewed by Medicaid state agencies unless they wish the PSRO to take over the job.

The PSRO review system for long-term care is conceptually like the hospital review system; however, it is operated with some flexibility and imagination. It differs in emphasis in the following important areas (7):

1. Review of the hospitalized patient to be admitted to a long-term-care facility is integrated with the hospital's continued-stay review; the patient and physician can be assured before transfer that Medicare or Medicaid will pay at least for the patient's initial stay in a skilled nursing facility.
2. Concurrent quality assurance is emphasized during continued long-term care. The concurrent quality-assurance process seeks to identify and correct problems while the patient is in the institution and while care can still be modified.
3. Interdisciplinary involvement in review is stressed to reflect the greater role of professionals, such as nurses, social workers, and physical therapists, in the care of patients in long-term-care facilities. The goals of the review are, of course, the same as in the hospital—to assure that admission and services are necessary and that the services meet professionally recognized standards of care.

There are complex problems in the review of long-term care. The number and variety of institutions make review difficult. In addition, the distinction between "skilled" and "intermediate" care is arbitrary at best and is frequently made by Medicaid state agencies in a fashion that is quite different from that of Medicare. In addition, the patient who does not "need" nursing home care is unlike the one who does not "need" a hospital—no alternative may exist. The PSRO physicians who have been involved in the review of long-term care believe that the real impact of the program is on the improved quality of services, with the intangible benefits that come from increased physician involvement in a long-neglected aspect of medical care.

Review of Ambulatory Care

Although ambulatory services, which represent somewhat less than 20% of the costs of medical care (8), are not associated with the same high costs as hospital care, they accounted for close to one billion visits annually during the early 1970s, as compared with fewer than 30 million annual short-stay hospital discharges (9). In addition, much of ambulatory care is practiced without the important informal controls over behavior that are present in the hospital. It is no surprise that some of the worst abuses of the Medicaid program, including the famous "Medicaid mills" and the excessive prescribing of narcotics, have taken place in offices where no organized medical staff could comment on the behavior of the physicians involved. Decreasing hospital use will also transfer more care into the ambulatory setting, making some kind of quality assurance in the office more important.

Professional Standards Review Organizations have conducted a few demonstration projects in ambulatory care; review of ambulatory services is also mandated for federally qualified HMOs. In addition, many group practices, both prepaid and fee-for-service, have a well-established tradition of peer review. Major PSRO intrusion into office practice does not seem likely in the foreseeable future, although review of problem practices, such as the Medicaid mills, will continue and expand. What physicians can expect, however, is expansion of techniques that are based on claims submitted for services. Bills for services rendered can be subjected to "screens," which are statistical methods for spotting possible trouble, with detailed review of records undertaken before any conclusion is reached regarding whether a problem exists. Screens used in existing review systems have looked at such factors as high rates of injections in offices, high rates of prescribed sedatives, and high rates of certain ancillary services. Matching of diagnostic codes to tests ordered is also common, which means that careful attention must be given to coding by office staff if the diabetic patient with hepatitis is not to have payment rejected for tests of liver function.

Although ambulatory review is never likely to be as pervasive as hospital review, the office-based physician can eventually expect to see profiles of his or her office practice and to experience continued claims review, at least on a statistical basis, of the care given in the office.

THE PHYSICIAN'S ROLE

The PSRO program is based on the concept that practicing physicians are best qualified to assure that the health care services delivered by their peers are necessary, appropriate, and of professionally recognized quality. Physician support and involvement are obviously crucial for the success of this concept.

Physicians can have three different roles in the PSRO process: as a member of the PSRO, as a physician in the review system being reviewed, and as a physician who is actually participating in review, that is, a physician advisor.

Active Member

Any physician is eligible to join the local PSRO. Active involvement may mean joining the medical audit or utilization review committee of a delegated hospital, or serving on a PSRO committee, such as one that develops areawide audits or is responsible for overseeing the performance of delegated hospitals. Many physicians find that the intellectual challenge of establishing standards for care is a particularly interesting form of continuing education. The interaction of the PSRO with local health agencies and with the federal funding system is a challenging, educational—and sometimes frustrating—task for someone interested in the political problems of medical practice.

Physician Under Review

Any physician who provides treatment to federally reimbursed patients has been or will be under PSRO review. Therefore, the physician needs to be prepared to explain to the patient what PSRO review means, what a denial is, and what can be done in response to a denial that appears unreasonable. PSRO review, as well as nonfederal review, makes it mandatory that decisions about patient care be well documented to avoid misunderstandings by reviewers.

Physician Advisor

The physician advisor acts for the medical-staff review committee or the PSRO, whichever is responsible for review activity in the hospital. The physician advisor is expected to review problem cases with the exception of those in which he or she was directly or indirectly responsible. Since no one physician advisor can be completely knowledgeable in every aspect of medicine, it is expected that he or she will call upon other professionals for assistance. Serving as a physician advisor is not easy or always pleasant. The decisions are often difficult, and resistance can be expected from the members of the medical staff who are most frequently subject to denials. The job is central, however, to genuine peer review and is necessary if the basic program is to survive. Most PSROs and hospitals rotate this responsibility to avoid turning one staff member into a permanent "bad guy."

CONCLUSION

The PSRO legislation represents the most recent and dramatic trend toward the increased interest in quality assurance. It differs from previous attempts in a number of ways:

1. There has been a change in emphasis from assessment of the structure of medical care to assessment of the actual process of giving care and, where possible, of the outcome of care.
2. Review has moved from a system based in single institutions to a community-based system.
3. Physicians rather than claims-payment agencies are responsible for deter-

mining whether a service is necessary or appropriate, and this determination is made before a service is rendered, not retrospectively.

4. The nature of quality assurance has shifted from looking at an isolated segment of care to a total profile of care, and this profile is gradually being extended from the hospital setting to the long-term-care and ambulatory settings.

The PSRO program is a unique experiment in professional self-regulation. It is an experiment with many built-in tensions: between bureaucrats who expect standardization and physicians who are accustomed to the infinite variety of medical practice; between a Congress that varies from year to year in its willingness to fund the program and PSRO management that needs financial stability; and between insurance companies that think they should set the rules and physicians who see the importance of local, professional control.

No one expects PSROs, in and of themselves, to hold down the costs of health care. Clearly, many other measures, such as the closing of unneeded beds, must be undertaken if overall costs are to be kept under control. But utilization review, when it works, is an important link in the process: an unneeded bed cannot be closed unless it has been kept empty; purchase of an unneeded x-ray machine cannot be avoided unless excess demand for the service has been curbed. Where PSROs and other peer mechanisms do offer unique benefit is in the area of oversight of medical quality, a task that nonphysicians cannot be expected to undertake. Despite the innate frustrations of the interaction between the bureaucracy and a fiercely independent profession, the PSRO program remains the physician's best chance to continue to manage the standards of practice.

REFERENCES

1. Goran MJ, Roberts JS, Kellogg MA, et al: The PSRO hospital review system. *Med Care* 13(Suppl):1, 1975.

2. Gosfield ATD: *PSRO's: The Law and the Health Consumer.* Cambridge, Massachusetts, Ballinger Publishing Company, 1975, p 109.

3. Office of Professional Standards Review Organizations: *PSRO Program Manual.* Rockville, Maryland, Department of Health, Education, and Welfare, 1974.

4. Goran MJ, Roberts JS, Kellogg MA, et al: The PSRO hospital review system. *Med Care* 13(Suppl):1, 1975.

5. Office of Professional Standards Review Organizations: *Technical Assistance Document—Medicare Care Evaluation Studies.* Rockville, Maryland, Department of Health, Education and Welfare, 1978.

6. Donabedian A: Effects of Medicare and Medicaid on access to and quality of health care. *Publ Health Rep* 91:322, 1976.

7. Office of Professional Standards Review Organizations: PSRO Transmittal No. 62: *Guidelines for PSRO Long Term Care Review.* Rockville, Maryland, Department of Health, Education, and Welfare, 1978.

8. Cambridge Research Institute: *Trends Affecting the U.S. Health Care System.* DHEW Publication No. (HRA) 76-14503, 1975.

9. United States National Committee on Vital and Health Statistics: Ambulatory Medical Care Records: *Uniform Minimum Basic Data Set: Final Report.* Vital and Health Statistics. Documents and Committee Reports, Series 4, No. 16, DHEW Publication No. (HRA) 75-1453, 1974.

12

The Nurse Practitioner and the Physician's Assistant

Kathryn J. Bowman

Andrea Zubick

In the 1960s, nonphysician health care providers were recognized as one way of alleviating the perceived shortage of physicians in the United States. Even though the number of physicians has increased, physicians' assistants and nurse practitioners continue to serve as valuable health-manpower resources. In addition, the public's concerns about excessive costs and impersonal technology and nurses' concerns about self-esteem and personal autonomy have led to an expansion of the nurse's role in both traditional and nontraditional settings. The return of many medical corpsmen from the Vietnam conflict coincided with this redefinition of the role of nursing and gave impetus to the development of the physician's assistant (1,2). Consequently, two career paths emerged—one as a direct assistant to the physician and another as a practitioner who provides basic health and medical care, often independently.

The literature of the past decade is filled with information on the advent, role, cost effectiveness, performance, and evaluation of the "new health professionals," who have been variously referred to as "midlevel practitioners," "physician extenders," "health associates," "nurse clinicians," and a host of other terms often connoting special areas of practice (1–7). For purposes of clarity, only the terms "nurse practitioner" and "physician's assistant" will be used in this chapter.

DEFINITIONS

The Council of Primary Health Care Nurse Practitioners of the American Nurses' Association (ANA) provides the following role definition (8):

> The nurse practitioner/clinician is a registered nurse who is a diversified primary care provider prepared to assist in giving comprehensive, continuous personalized care. . . . Although a major contribution of (these providers) is in the area of health

181

promotion, they assume responsibility for selected components of health care conventionally in the realm of medical practice. Family health care is a team effort. The composition of this team may include nurses, social workers, physicians, therapists, and others; (thus the) imperative that there be mutual recognition of each provider's . . . expertise. Where there is overlap, a mutually agreed upon framework must be developed for the provision of joint care.

The American Medical Association's Council on Medical Education, in collaboration with, among others, the American Academy of Physicians' Assistants, has established the following description of the role of the physician's assistant (9):

> The assistant to the primary care physician is a skilled person, qualified by academic and clinical training to provide patient services under the supervision and responsibility of a doctor of medicine or osteopathy who is, in turn, responsible for the performance of that assistant. The assistant may be involved with the patients of the physician in any medical setting for which the physician is responsible. The function of the assistant to the primary care physician is to perform, under the responsibility and supervision of the physician, diagnostic and therapeutic tasks in order to allow the physician to extend his services through the more effective use of his knowledge, skills, and abilities.

By official definition, then, nurse practitioners and physicians' assistants could have similar roles, and in some instances, they undoubtedly do. However, also implied in the definition of the nurse practitioner is a broader, more autonomous role beyond providing collection of medical data and performing diagnostic and therapeutic services. Such a role may include involvement in group and community health education or the development of health care services in less traditional areas, such as school or industrial-health programs.

EDUCATIONAL CRITERIA

Nurse practitioners may train in an organized program of continuing education that meets the "Guidelines for Short-Term Continuing Education Programs Preparing Adult and Family Nurse Practitioners" of the ANA (8). Federal guidelines in the Nurse Training Act of 1975 specify that "the (nurse practitioner) training program shall be a minimum of one academic year (nine months) in length and shall include at least four months (in the aggregate) of classroom instruction" (10). Nurses in continuing-education programs are first required to have basic preparation in a two-year associate-degree program, a three-year diploma program, or a bachelor's- or master's-degree program in nursing. Some continuing-education programs accept candidates with degrees other than in nursing. Graduates of all these programs receive a certificate and are then eligible to apply for certification in states where certification exists (only about 10 states as of this writing) (11). The guidelines of the ANA and the federal government also specify that such programs shall be conducted in collegiate schools of nursing, medicine, or public health or shall be carried out in close collaboration with such schools (8,10). Curriculums must include both didactic material and clinical experience. The majority of nurse-practitioner programs are continuing-education programs, but other types of nurse-practitioner programs are also important (13). First, several bachelor's-degree programs prepare nurse practitioners for certification. Second, master's-degree programs prepare family nurse clinicians. The programs vary in length from one and one-half to two academic years. Still other programs qualify persons who enter with a nursing degree for a master's degree, a registered nurse's license, and a nurse practitioner's certificate, all in three years. Many continuing-education programs are being offered that teach basic physical examination, but neither these short courses nor informal on-the-job training qualifies a person as a nurse practitioner.

Educational programs for physicians' assistants vary as well. The guidelines of the AMA's Council on Medical Education specify a minimum requirement of a high-school diploma for entrance. However, some programs require as much as two years of college plus direct experience in patient care. Definition of this experience generally is not clear (9,12).

Sadler and Bliss have divided programs into those that train assistants to primary care physicians, those that train assistants to specialists, and federal programs that serve prisons and the Indian health care programs administered by the Public Health Service (12). Programs vary in length and outcome. They may be 12 months long and grant a certificate of completion, two years long and grant an associate degree, or 30 months to three or four academic years in length and grant a baccalaureate degree on completion.

The variability of educational experience required to become a "new health professional" poses a perplexing problem to any prospective employer: how to evaluate the quality, preparation, and competence of the employee. Beyond careful interviewing and references as well as a period of evaluation at the beginning of the job, the answer eventually lies in state and national certification procedures.

LEGAL CONSIDERATIONS

Bullough states that because the medical profession took the lead in writing regulatory practice acts, the statutes governing all other health professions (e.g., pharmacy, dentistry) are technically amendments to the medical practice acts in the various states (3,13). Since the advent of mandatory licensure in 1938, nurses have been independently licensed providers of health care. Because of vague and broad statutory language, however, the legal definition of the scope of nursing practice is unclear in many states. In 1955, the ANA attempted to clarify the scope of practice by providing a model practice act, which was not adopted by all states. This model either excluded or specifically restricted acts of medical diagnosis and treatment by nurses (13,14). Statutory change to delineate an expanded role for nurse practitioners has thus proven to be cumbersome.

Some states, such as California, have now modified their definition of nursing to make it easier to specify an expanded-practice role. Others, such as Pennsylvania, have amended their nursing statute in collaboration with the state medical board. These amendments authorize rules and regulations, promulgated by the joint professional boards, that define the circumstances under which nurse practitioners may perform acts of medical diagnosis and treatment. Still other states, such as Tennessee, have amended their medical-practice acts to authorize physicians to delegate medical tasks to nurses, provided that the tasks are performed under the supervision of physicians. Supervision has been defined in different ways by different states. Nurse practitioners have not been expressly recognized in several other states. These states may assume that the expanded role of the nurse practitioner is not appreciably different enough to place the nurse in a new professional category requiring new legal definition beyond what already legitimizes nursing practice.

New legislation has been required in every instance to permit physicians' assistants to practice since they were not covered previously in any existing provider statute. Most states have now amended their medical-practice acts to allow for practice by physicians' assistants (14). The authority for the definition and regulation of physicians' assistants clearly lies with the medical profession.

Adoption of Educational and Examination Requirements

States vary in their use of examinations for licensing and certifying nurse practitioners. (Nurse midwives and nurse anesthetists are included in this definition of nurse practitioners.) Only six states (Alabama, Arizona, Kentucky, Mississippi, New Mexico, and South Carolina) specifically require nurse practitioners to pass a nationally recognized examination before they receive their license to practice. The ANA sponsors national certification examinations for special areas of practice (4,7). Some states require other examinations, and in lieu of examinations, some states (e.g., Pennsylvania) require approval of educational programs (10). Application costs and renewal standards vary from state to state. Reciprocity for certification has not yet clearly evolved (11). The controversy over national as opposed to state certification will probably continue until educational programs become more uniform.

States also differ in their use of examinations for licensing and certifying physicians' assistants. The development of a national examination has caused a high proportion of states to require national examinations; currently, 22 states require an examination for the certification of a physician's assistant. In almost all states that recognize physicians' assistants, the educational program must be approved before certification (14).

Requirements for Physician Supervision

Many states require direct physician supervision of nurse practitioners, although supervision may be described as collaborative working arrangements or "via telecommunications." The number of nurse practitioners that a physician may supervise is not restricted, thus allowing the physican considerable freedom (10). By contrast, the requirements for physician supervision of physicians' assistants may be more explicit, with many states specifying the number of physicians' assistants that a physician may supervise (14). However, both Illinois and Iowa have liberal regulations allowing the physician's assistant to practice away from the physician as long as there is some form of periodic supervision.

Prohibited and Permitted Activities

In states that have statutes and regulations for nurse practitioners, considerable attention has been paid to the activities that they are permitted to perform. For example, in Arizona, New Hampshire, and New Mexico, the procedures have been carefully identified according to specialty. The procedures are especially well defined for nurse midwives (10). Again, because of the great variability from state to state, the prospective employer and employee should understand the statute of their state.

Most states have spent only limited efforts in circumscribing the activities of physicians' assistants because of the degree of physician supervision required in the statutes (14). The potential range of services of the physician's assistant is thus very broad and quite responsive to the needs of the physician.

Drug-prescribing and Dispensing Requirements

There is some similarity in the statutes regulating the authority of both nurse practitioners and physician assistants to prescribe and dispense legend drugs (neither are allowed authority to prescribe controlled drugs). In only a few states (e.g., Arizona, California, Maine, North Carolina, and Washington) can they actually write and sign prescriptions. In other states, there may be authorization to prescribe in the practice statute, but prohibitions in the pharmacy statutes may override the practice regulations. In other states (e.g., New Hampshire), the nurse practitioner or physician's assistant may have to practice in an isolated setting to be able to prescribe a limited type and number of drugs. Only in North Carolina, where all three statutes (nursing, medicine, and pharmacy) were changed, does there appear to be allowance for comprehensive drug prescription by either nurse practitioner or physician's assistant (14).

THIRD-PARTY REIMBURSEMENT

Third-party reimbursement for the services of nurse practitioners and physicians' assistants varies throughout the United States. Many states have not coordinated their reimbursement policies with the legislation and regulations governing practice. The states that do have explicit policies have not provided adequate definitions to guide either their agencies or the providers who wish to be reimbursed. A similar problem prevails with the Rural Health Clinic Services Bill, passed in November 1977. This bill was designed to provide reimbursement to clinics in rural areas and also in some undeserved urban areas; however, in many cases, the legal status of these clinics is unclear because requirements for physician supervision are so poorly defined in the state laws. For example, direct reimbursement to clinics may be denied, except when physicians are on site, thus partially defeating the purpose of increased accessibility to health care services. At this point, nurse practitioners in rural and underserved urban areas are the only ones eligible for Medicare reimbursement (14).

In the private sector, the policy of Blue Shield and the Health Insurance

Association of America allows for reimbursement of physicians' assistants and nurse practitioners only when their services are provided under the direct supervision of a licensed physician. The physician must bill for the service, and payment is made to the physician. The lack of reimbursement to nurse practitioners and physicians' assistants by the private sector is due not only to the policies of each company but also to the state laws that regulate insurance practices (14). Mississippi and Maryland have recently changed their insurance laws to allow for direct reimbursement of nursing services (14a).

FINANCIAL CONSIDERATIONS

Cost Effectiveness

Many copractices involving physicians with nurse practitioners or physicians' assistants report financial success, with increases in productivity ranging from 10% to 400% (15–19). This result is important for the physician, whose income and working hours are affected. It is also important for patients, whose access to medical care is improved. It is not clear how long it takes a new copractice to become financially viable, but one would suspect that just as it takes time to build a relationship between copractitioners, it also takes a comparable period of time to increase the number of patients and develop an efficient practice. Most nurse practitioners can see an average of 9 or 10 patients in an eight-hour day (14,20,21,22). They spend approximately 30 minutes per patient (20,23).

A nurse practitioner's productivity will increase as experience and independence increase, and it will vary directly in proportion to the willingness of the physician to delegate duties (16,24). This willingness will naturally develop over time, as the physician and nurse practitioner learn and become comfortable with each other's skills. With this increase in the productivity of the nurse practitioner, there tends to be a concurrent increase in the productivity and efficiency of the physician (7,16,25).

Fees

Nurse practitioners and physicians' assistants are encouraged to charge the same fees for a visit as the physician since any decrease might be interpreted by the patient to mean a lower standard of care (16).

Salaries

When setting salaries, one must consider several variables: the section of the country in which the practice is located, whether it is rural or urban, the extent of training of the physician's assistant or nurse practitioner, whether the practice consists of a group or a solo practitioner, and the amount of responsibility the employee will be assuming.

Salaries vary across the country. They tend to be higher in rural areas, higher for a nurse practitioner with a master's degree, and higher in group practices

(24). The overall range of salaries in 1978 for nurse practitioners was $10,000–25,000 (26).

The negotiated salary should be clearly stated in a job contract along with the plan for salary review, the criteria for salary increases, the amount of paid vacation and sick time, malpractice insurance coverage, and educational allowances.

If either the new nurse practitioner, physician's assistant, or physician needs help in collecting relevant information to negotiate salaries, the Small Business Administration can be a valuable resource. Their SCORE (Service Corps of Retired Executives) chapters provide free counseling about accounting, legal issues, advertising, and tax problems (22).

Trial Period

Some physicians may consider hiring nurse practitioners or physicians' assistants but may be reluctant because they have no previous experience working with them. One way to gain experience is to become a preceptor for a student by signing up with an educational program for nurse practitioners or physicians' assistants and offering this service. Such offers are generally welcomed by the school, even if considerable travel time is involved. The physician must remember that the primary goal of this arrangement is education rather than service and that it requires substantial instruction and supervision. In some cases, this student-preceptor relationship can serve as an evaluation period ending in full-time employment.

DEVELOPING THE PRACTICE

Expanding the Practice

Most patients' health problems seen in an office practice are minor (20,26,27). Patients may be divided into the well, the worried well, the asymptomatic sick, and the sick (11). The treatment of choice for the well and worried well is often patient education and counseling: teaching patients what they can do for themselves, what requires a visit and how to use the health care system, explaining normal body function throughout the life cycle, reassuring, explaining reasons for medications, providing an unbiased ear, making agency referrals, and intervening in many other ways that require knowledge, patience, and time. The nurse practitioner and the physician's assistant may be especially effective in these situations.

The care a nurse practitioner delivers is of high quality (7,15,31), patients are very accepting (15,29,30,32,33), and the nurse adds emphasis to the health-maintenance aspects of care (15,30,34). With this knowledge, the physician can be reasonably sure that hiring a nurse practitioner will be advantageous for the practice.

However, providing more and better services may not be the primary reason for adding a nurse practitioner or physician's assistant to the staff. Glenn and

Hofmeister give 10 potential incentives that might influence a physician to employ a nurse practitioner (35). They are listed below, in order from most to least probable:

1. Increase net income.
2. Provide more control over working hours.
3. Continue a concept that worked well in medical school or residency.
4. Reward a trusted employee by additional training.
5. Provide expanded care.
6. Be more innovative in delivering care.
7. Compete with local colleagues who already employ a nurse practitioner.
8. Decrease charges to patients.
9. Try a new idea that has been reported favorably in the literature.
10. Make practice optimal.

One can see that business-related incentives are ranked at the top of the list.

Nurse Practitioner-Physician Relationship

Developing the nurse practitioner-physician relationship (copractice) may seem quite natural since physicians and nurses have been working together in private practice for years. This notion, however, is not generally true. Conflicts occur primarily because of changes that must take place in both professional self-images as well as in the relationship itself.

The beginning nurse practitioner must develop a new professional identity. In this process, he or she must answer some difficult questions. Should the nurse practitioner become an independent provider, continue to follow orders, or combine the two roles? How assertive should the nurse practitioner be in defining the new role and setting limits? These questions are even more difficult to answer for the office nurse who has become a nurse practitioner and returned to the same office (36).

Most physicians are accustomed to making all decisions alone. Delegation of even a small portion of traditional responsibility may be a problem, and the physician's perceptions of the appropriate role may not coincide with those of the nurse practitioner or physician's assistant. The physician frequently is concerned about patient acceptance, the needs of the practice, and the medicolegal risks of employing a new health professional (14). The physician may also be reluctant to share relationships with patients (36). It is clear that this working relationship does not come easily. Physicians need training to work effectively with the new health practitioners.

The role of the nurse practitioner is negotiated between employer and employee. It will be shaped by the type of practice; the nurse practitioner's philosophy, abilities, and wishes; the philosophy and preferences of the employing physician; and the patients' needs (14).

To develop a cooperative practice of outstanding quality, the nurse practitioner and physician must combine their knowledge and skills so that both gain satisfaction and accomplish their individual and joint goals for delivering patient care. These goals can be accomplished only through continual discussions of problems and expectations. Schenger et al. have described the "essential elements" of a copractice (37). The most important are:

1. Both the physician and nurse practitioner accept the philosophy of sharing patient-care responsibilities.
2. Both agree to maintain open lines of communication concerning all aspects of the practice. Communication includes regular meetings, reviews, and evaluation of roles.
3. Both are professional colleagues. The physician maintains a general supervisory role over medical care.
4. Each, by mutual agreement, may choose to specialize in the care of certain problems of patients.
5. Patients will have the option to express preference for either provider.
6. They may see the patient alone or together at their discretion.
7. When one is absent, the other will assume primary responsibility for patient care.

As in any close relationship, minor differences will occur from time to time in the copractice. If basic agreement cannot be reached about the essential elements of the copractice, these minor differences can disrupt the overall relationship.

Staff Relationships

The relationship with the physician is not the only one that needs to be thoughtfully developed. Nurses without additional training can feel threatened by a nurse practitioner or physician's assistant, possibly leading to situations that disrupt the operation of the practice (38). All employees in the office need to understand why the nurse practitioner or physician's assistant has been added to the staff and how the new employee's role differs from the traditional roles of the other employees. Periodic staff meetings, both before and after the physician's assistant or nurse practitioner's arrival, will help clarify and correct any problems that arise.

Patient Relationships

Most patients need an explanation of the role of the physician's assistant or nurse practitioner. Distributing brief printed descriptions of the new employee's role and how he or she will function in the practice is most helpful and most likely to increase acceptance. Appointment cards printed with the names of both the physician and the nurse practitioner will also help. One copractice displayed a sign in the waiting room stating: "This office has both a physician and nurse practitioner. You may see one or both on your visits here. If you have a preference, please let us know" (39). The physician should make an effort to increase familiarity and instruct patients in how to use and benefit from the services of the physician's assistant or nurse practitioner.

An efficient copractice takes about one year to develop (28,36). Once developed, the relationship tends to last. A study of 99 nurse practitioners and 78 associated physicians in Canada showed that over 80% of the nurse practitioners were still in their original employment after a five-year period (21). Physicians who have worked with nurse practitioners usually want to keep them. A high percentage would hire another nurse practitioner if their present one left (40).

Sharing Responsibility

One of the first decisions that must be made is how the work will be shared. Glenn and Goldman have identified the following three strategies for patient flow in practices employing nurse practitioners (19):

1. *Series strategy.* All patients are seen initially by the nurse practitioner, who talks with the physician about all patients. A decision is made as to whether the physician will see the patient alone or whether the physician and the nurse practitioner will see the patient together. The nurse practitioner does not have the option to see the patient alone.

2. *Parallel strategy.* The patient may be seen by either the nurse practitioner or the physician. The nurse practitioner may see the patient either with or without physician consultation.

3. *Consultative strategy.* All patients initially see the nurse practitioner, who sees the patient either alone or with physician consultation. The physician has a consultative role in the strategy. No patients are scheduled specifically to see the physician. This strategy is used primarily when more than one nurse practitioner is employed.

These strategies have four variables: the manner of making appointments for patients, the manner of delegating management of patients, the number of nurse practitioners working with one physician, and the communication that occurs between them. The greatest productivity gains can be made with the parallel strategy since it provides the maximal delegation of duties and the greatest degree of independence for the nurse practitioner—factors that have the greatest effect on productivity.

Glenn and Goldman also point out that one could begin by using the series strategy and progress to the parallel and consultative strategies as mutual trust, confidence, and experience grow (19,21). This approach will provide support to both the physician and the nurse practitioner.

Selecting Appropriate Patients

Nurse practitioners and physicians' assistants care for almost all types of patients, but those with the following problems are mentioned most frequently in the literature (15,21,34,40,41): obesity, contraception, counseling, diabetes, hypertension, stable chronic problems, acute episodic problems, and patient education. The physician assistant's or nurse practitioner's scope of practice will gradually expand with experience; therefore, scheduling guidelines may need frequent revision. These guidelines should be clearly communicated to the appointment secretary to eliminate confusion. The guidelines should include new patient assignment, follow-up patient assignment, appointment-time intervals, provider preferences, times to be left unscheduled, and time of the last appointment of the day. A sample set of guidelines follows:

1. Patients who are new to the practice, are over 40 years of age, and have a defined problem should be assigned to the physician for the first visit.
2. All patients with chest pain will be seen by the physician.
3. Patients who are new to the practice and request a routine checkup should be assigned to the nurse practitioner or physician's assistant.
4. Patients who have been seen previously in the practice and are returning for a routine follow-up examination may be assigned to either provider.
5. The appointment times of the nurse practitioner or physician's assistant will be left unassigned each day
   a. from 3:00 to 4:30 p.m. to accommodate emergency or walk-in visits
   b. from 11:30 a.m. to noon and from 4:30 to 5:00 p.m. to return patients' telephone calls.

Taking Telephone Calls

Studies have shown that with the support of physicians, nurse practitioners can safely and effectively share the responsibilities of night and weekend coverage of telephone calls. One study has shown that nurse practitioners handle patients' problems over the telephone more thoroughly than do house officers and private practitioners (40). The after-hours telephone responsibilities should be shared, although sharing may not work in all practices (39). Nurse practitioners may be able to handle most pediatric calls alone since they often relate to well-child care or minor problems but may not be able to handle calls in a consultative-cardiology practice.

Protocols

A protocol explicitly directs the step-by-step collection of subjective and objective data, directs the analysis of the data, and recommends the appropriate action (44). Some states require that nurse practitioners work with such protocols. The advantages of such protocols are that they provide guidance, help ensure a defined standard of care, and make it easier to audit care (44–46). Some believe that protocols stifle clinical judgment and do not recognize patients' individualities (39,44), and a nurse practitioner should be allowed to make independent judgments that go beyond the protocols. Many protocols have been written for physicians' assistants and nurse practitioners in the past few years, and most can be adapted to a variety of settings. They can also serve as helpful references, especially for the beginning nurse practitioner (47–49).

Once a copractice has been established, it can be expanded. For example, nurse practitioners or physicians' assistants can develop group teaching sessions for patients with common problems. With additional training, they can counsel patients about sexual problems (26). A nurse practitioner with a master's degree can conduct clinical research related to common health problems. Some nurse practitioners see nursing-home patients (44), and some make house calls. Although some make hospital rounds (15,26,39), this practice is presently controversial.

Continuing Education

Just as the physician in practice regularly updates his or her professional training, the physician's assistant or nurse practitioner should also carry out a plan for continuing professional education. The copractice should provide the physician's assistant or nurse practitioner as well as the physician with protected time and resources for books, journals, audiovisual materials, and travel. The physician employer should ensure that a plan has been designed; the physician's assistant or nurse practitioner should determine its content.

REFERENCES

1. Edmunds MW: Evaluation of nurse practitioner effectiveness: An overview of the literature. *Evaluation Health Profess* 1:69, 1978.
2. Fisher DW, Horowitz SM: The physician's assistant: Profile of a new health profession, in Bliss A, Cohen E (eds): *The New Health Professionals.* Germantown, Maryland, Aspen Systems Corporation, 1977, p 40.
3. Bullough B: Influence on role expansion. *Am J Nurs* 76:1476, 1976.
4. Bliss A, Cohen E (eds): *The New Health Professionals.* Germantown, Maryland, Aspen Systems Corporation, 1977.
5. Health Care Financing Administration: Executive summary: Survey and evaluation of the physician extender reimbursement program. Rockville, Maryland, DHEW Contract SSA 600-76-0667, Systems Science, 1978, p 17.
6. Runyan J: The Memphis chronic disease program: Comparisons in outcome and the nurses' expanded role. *J Am Med Ass* 213:264, 1975.
7. Spector R: Burlington randomized trial of the nurse practitioner. *Ann Intern Med* 90:137, 1974.
8. American Nurses' Association: *Scope of Primary Nursing Practice for Adults and Families.* Kansas City, 1976.
9. American Medical Association Council on Medical Education, et al: Essentials of an approved educational program for the assistant to the primary care physician, in Bliss A, Cohen E (eds): *The New Health Professionals.* Germantown, Maryland, Aspen Systems Corporation, 1977, p 385.
10. U.S. Department of Health, Education, and Welfare: Federal Nurse Training Act of 1975. *Fed Regist* 4:16, 1976.
11. Mayers J: Personal communication, January 29, 1979.
12. Sadler AM, Bliss A: *Physician's Assistant, Today and Tomorrow.* New Haven, Connecticut, Yale University Press, 1972.
13. Bullough B: The law and the expanding nursing role. *Am J Publ Health* 66:249, 1976.
14. National Center for Health Services Research: *Review and Analysis of State Legislation and Reimbursement Practices of Physicians Assistants and Nurse Practitioners: Final Report.* Rockville, Maryland, U.S. Department of Health, Education, and Welfare, 1978.
14a. Smith FH: Personal communication, 1979.
15. Holmes G, Bassett R: Nurse clinician. *J Kans Med Soc* 77:553, 1976.
16. Nelson E, Jacobs A, Cordner K, et al: Financial impact of physician assistants on medical practice. *N Engl J Med* 293:527, 1975.
17. Voltman J: Jamestown medical clinic system. *J Am Med Ass* 234:303, 1975.
18. Seigal B, Jensen D, Coffee E: Cost effectiveness of FNP versus physician staffed rural practice, in Bliss A, Cohen E (eds): *The New Health Professionals.* Germantown, Maryland, Aspen Systems Corporation, 1977, p 180.
19. Glenn J, Goldman J: Strategies for productivity with physician extenders. *West Med J* 124:249, 1976.

20. Feldman R, Taller S, Garfield S, et al: Nurse practitioner multiphasic health check-ups. *Prev Med* 6:391, 1977.

21. Scherer K, Fortin F, Spitzer W, et al: Nurse practitioners in primary care. *Can Med Ass J* 116:956, 1977.

22. Edmunds M: Rectifying salary problems. *Nurse Practitioner J* 4:36, 1979.

23. Subin L: The business aspects of private nursing practice. *J Nurs Administ* 7:13, 1977.

24. Scheffler R: The employment utilization and earnings of physician extenders. *Soc Sci Med* 11:785, 1977.

25. Schultz P, McGlone F: Primary health care provided to the elderly by a nurse practitioner-physician team: Analysis of cost effectiveness. *J Am Geriatr Soc* 25:443, 1977.

26. AMA Council on Medical Service: Functions and reimbursement of nurse practitioners. *Conn Med* 42:183, 1978.

27. Andreoli K: Ambulatory health care and the nurse practitioner. *Ala J Med Sci* 14:57, 1977.

28. National Joint Practice Commission: Joint practice: A new dimension in nurse-physician collaboration. *Am J Nurs* 77:1467, 1977.

29. Kahn L, Wirth P: Perceptions and expectations of physician supervisors. *Nurse Practitioner J* 3:27, 1978.

30. Cohen E, Crootuf L, Keenan K, et al: An evaluation of policy related research on new and expanded roles of health workers. New Haven, Connecticut, Yale University School of Medicine, 1974.

31. Levine D, Morlock L, Mushlin A, et al: The role of new health practitioners in preparing group practice. *Med Care* 14:326, 1976.

32. Lewis C, Resnik B: Nurse clinics and progressive ambulatory care. *N Engl J Med* 277:1236, 1967.

33. Kushner J: A benefit-cost analysis of nurse practitioner training. *Can J Publ Health* 67:405, 1976.

34. Branman G, Walker W, Reisinger C: A nurse practitioner role in ambulatory care and emergency service. *Nurs Clin North Am* 12:553, 1977.

35. Glenn J, Hofmeister R: Will physicians rush out and get physician extenders? *Health Serv Rep* 11:78, 1976.

36. Bates B: Physician and nurse practitioner: Conflict and reward. *Ann Intern Med* 82:702, 1975.

37. Schenger J, Baton M, Flaherty S: A nurse practitioner in a family practice residency program—Role description and impact on continuity of the practitioner-patient relationship. *J Family Pract* 5:791, 1977.

38. Gibson K: One nurse said we weren't fit to work. *R.N.* 40:38, 1977.

39. O'Shaughnessy C: Diary of an angry nurse. *Am J Nurs* 76:1165, 1976.

40. Levine J, Orr S, Sheatsley D, et al: The nurse practitioner role, physician utilization, patient acceptance. *Nurs Res* 27:245, 1978.

41. Reedy B, Phillips D, Newell D: Making better use of our nurses. *Br Med J* 1:1360, 1977.

42. Perrin E, Goodman H: Telephone management of acute pediatric illnesses. *N Engl J Med* 298:130, 1978.

43. Goodman H, Perrin E: Evening telephone call management by nurse practitioners and physicians. *Nurs Res* 27:233, 1978.

44. Pearson L: Protocols: How to develop and implement within the nurse practitioner setting. *Nurse Practitioner J* 2:9, 1976.

45. Greenfield S, Komaroff A, Pass T, et al: Efficiency and cost of primary care by nurses and physicians assistants. *N Engl J Med* 298:305, 1978.

46. Sor H: The training of physician assistants. *N Engl J Med* 288:818, 1973.

47. Hoole A, Greenburg R, Pickard C: *Patient Care Guidelines for Family Nurse Practitioners.* Boston, Little, Brown and Company, 1976.

48. Hudak C, Redstone P, Hokanson N, et al: *Clinical Protocols: A Guide for Nurses and Physicians.* Philadelphia, JB Lippincott Company, 1976.

49. Capell P, Case D: *Ambulatory Care Manual for Nurse Practitioners.* Philadelphia, JB Lippincott Company, 1976.

13
Social Workers
and Primary Care

Joan Bonner Conway

Judith Frank Hirschwald

This chapter addresses the role of social workers in the delivery of primary health care. First, social work is defined in its historical perspective with special emphasis on health care. Next, the rationale for the social worker's involvement in primary care is described. A glossary of available resources is then presented to help the physician identify community resources for patients' social needs. The role of social workers in solo and group practices, in health maintenance organizations, in emergency services, and in hospitals are reviewed, and, finally, guidelines are provided for selecting a social worker.

WHAT IS SOCIAL WORK?

Social work is a profession that helps people to help themselves. It helps "individuals, families, groups and communities to prevent or to resolve problems caused by social or emotional problems" (1). Social work finds its focus and its object in helping people who face in their social relationships inadequacies, frictions, and limitations that frustrate the full realization or their own capacities and wants as individuals (2). Social work respects man's right to self-determination and choice; social workers have a profound respect for the dignity of individual human beings and their right to find and fulfill themselves within the society of which they are a part (2).

Social workers in health care settings assist patients and their families with social and emotional problems that cause illness, interfere with treatment, or prevent recovery. They assist physicians and other health care personnel to understand the social implications of disease and the effect of the social situation on the patient's medical care (3).

To develop a cadre of qualified social workers to carry out these tasks, standards and educational requirements for social workers have been developed. In an informal sense, the first brief training course for social workers was initiated in 1898 by the Charity Organization Society of New York (1). Most training in this early period was conducted by agencies. By 1917, when the country became involved in World War I, 13 schools of applied philanthropy, social administration, social economy, and social work had been organized. Social agencies no longer housed nor sponsored educational facilities (4). Funding from the government became available for training of personnel to meet the emotional needs of soldiers and veterans. An important advance was the Army's new classification of psychiatric social workers.

In the years that followed, several professional social work organizations were formed, representing various aspects of practice. In 1955, seven of these organizations merged to form the National Association of Social Workers. At the same time that the practice of social work was moving toward a single organization to represent all members, social work education was also moving toward a single voice. In 1952, the Council on Social Work Education was created to reduce conflicts that existed between the two previous organizations, which focused on educational standards for social work (5). The Council on Social Work Education's Commission on Accreditation has "responsibility at the national level for establishing criteria for and accrediting graduate social work education" (5). It also offers accreditation to undergraduate educational institutions for social work. In September 1976, there were 85 member graduate schools of social work, including those working toward membership, and 185 undergraduate programs in social work (5).

SOCIAL WORKERS AS PARTNERS IN PRIMARY CARE

The social worker can act as a consultant for some patients who go to the physician's office. Some patients who do not feel well are there because of conditions that are better treated by a social worker. Other patients need the services of both the physician and the social worker.

Social workers in primary health care settings are concerned with a wide spectrum of problems, which can be divided into two categories. The first is composed of "tangible" problems. Social workers have an intimate knowledge of community resources and the expertise to help the patient to accept and use resources, such as county welfare agencies, social security agencies, the Veterans Administration, and transportation systems. It is often not sufficient to give the patient the name of a resource and suggest that he or she use it. Some patients feel that the use of these resources is a sign of charity. Others avoid using a resource because they do not understand the eligibility requirements. The second class of problems that social workers manage include "intangible" social and emotional problems that require counseling or referral to still another resource. Examples of such problems are depression and anxiety that might be caused by marital or family problems, parent-child conflict, loss of employment, alcoholism, drug dependence, and the reaction of the patient to a family member's illness or death or to the patient's own medical problems.

If one understands the patient as an individual, a family member, and a member of a community and society, and if one sees medical diagnosis and treatment as part of a broader health care system, one understands why it is necessary for the primary care physician and the social worker to care for patients together. Consumers, as patients and prospective patients, increasingly view the health care system as the largest organized provider of services and ask it to meet the entire spectrum of human need. Although the system can never satisfy all human needs, it is increasingly sought out by consumers with acute and chronic feelings of illness and the inability to function.

Indeed, there is a relation between emotional or social stress and physical illness. Our experience shows that there is an increased need for professionals who can support patients troubled by anxieties and the problems of daily living. Part of this support should be provided to people before they interpret their problems as medical illnesses (6). For example, the primary care physician cannot cure the severe headaches of the suburban wife and mother without treating the increasing tensions of a deteriorating marriage and the resultant behavior of the children. The physician may wonder why an elderly diabetic patient is not responding to insulin therapy when the patient cannot afford the medication or regular, well-balanced meals. The primary care physician who assumes responsibility for the whole range of patients' needs will often need to ask the social worker to participate in patient care.

Many professionals and much of the lay public erroneously believe that "social workers only work with the poor" or, conversely, that "only the poor need the services of social workers." Illness is, in fact, a great equalizer. The basic difference between the executive and the janitor is that the executive probably will have more power to purchase service. However, neither the executive nor the janitor will know what service is needed, what the alternatives are, or where to go for service. The executive and the janitor may have identical anxieties caused by a personal or family illness. Marital discord, disturbances in parent-child relationships, alcoholism, drug abuse, cancer, and stroke do not necessarily choose income levels. The patient and the physician unfortunately often share the same bias for referrals to social workers, with the result that the middle- and upper-income patient and family do not gain access to the services of social workers. Some programs may be different, and entry into the system may vary, but the same needs for service exist. If the physician involved in the referral procedure is sensitive to the potential bias of the patient and family toward the services of social workers, the referral will generally be accepted.

GLOSSARY OF HUMAN RESOURCES

The first frustrating lesson one learns when seeking a resource to meet a person's need is that the system is generally not comprehensive. It is often available only to people who meet specific criteria. For instance, an elderly woman living alone in an urban area after an operation for her fractured hip may need temporary assistance with household chores, meal preparation, and some aspects of personal care. The services of a homemaker or home health aide with Meals on Wheels should meet her needs for this short-term convalescence. However, there are many potential problems. First, in most urban areas, the waiting lists for both services are long (perhaps four to six weeks), and this waiting period may eliminate the resource immediately. Second, she will probably also have to meet income requirements and age requirements and live in a specified geographic area to qualify for service. Once all the requirements are met and she qualifies for service, limitations on services may prevent adequate care. The homemaker or home health aide often is able to offer service only four hours a day, five days a week. Therefore, patient's personal-care needs are met only part of the day. What is she to do on Saturday and Sunday? Meals on Wheels will deliver a hot meal once a day, usually at noon, and leave a sandwich or similar food in the refrigerator for the evening meal. However, some agencies do not deliver meals over weekends and holidays, so the patient may be forced to fend for herself during these times. In short, the person who made the referral and the patient need to be aware of these gaps in service so that supplemental resources, such as family, friends, or neighbors, can be called.

Funding sources, agency charters, and regulations, as well as supply and demand in the marketplace, will govern which categories of service can be offered, to whom, and for what period of time. Resources vary tremendously from state to state, from urban to rural area, and, sometimes, from month to month for the same service in the same area. However, in developing a file of available resources, there are some helpful sources.

Health and Welfare Council

The majority of urban areas and rural counties have an "umbrella agency" for human services. The agency probably has a directory that is periodically updated, listing resources and including a brief description of the services provided and the eligibility criteria. A copy of this directory will provide the nucleus of the resource file.

Department of Public Welfare

The nearest state, county, or local department of public welfare can provide a description of services available within the community. In many areas, the department of public welfare will provide some services directly and will contract with existing agencies for other services.

County Board of Assistance

This agency exists in every county. Its complexity and size are dependent on the population and service needs of the county. In general, the smaller the county, the more available and productive it is. Although this statement may seem paradoxical, experience in urban areas reveals that a highly complex bureaucratic structure frequently responds to individual and family needs less effectively. For any person without a source of income, temporarily or permanently, the county board of assistance is the referral source for basic human needs. In most states, the food-stamp program, medical assistance, and other welfare programs are administered through this office. However, most people without prior knowledge of the system overestimate the income levels required for public assistance, which vary from state to state.

Telephone Book Yellow Pages

The Yellow Pages of the telephone book list many resources. For example, under "Social Service Organizations" in one urban telephone book, there is a comprehensive list of resources in all areas. Other examples of headings for general categories of need are: "Alcoholism," "Drug Abuse," "Handicapped," "Counseling," and "Child Care." Usually a telephone call to one agency will identify all agencies within the community that provide the needed services.

Self-help Groups

In almost every community, there exist groups of people with similar experiences, problems, and concerns who have organized themselves to share these experiences and provide support to each other. For some people, a referral to such a group provides the support needed to assist in a life crisis. New organizations are developing all the time, but some of the possibilities are listed below:

· Self-help groups are available for the alcoholic person, for his or her family, and for the children of alcoholic parents.
· "Easy Breathers" and other groups are available to assist patients with emphysema and other chronic pulmonary disorders.
· "Reach for Recovery" helps mastectomy patients, and "One Day at a Time" assists patients with all types of cancer.
· "Parents Without Partners" helps single parents.
· Self-help groups are available to help widows, widowers, and parents who have lost children from sudden infant death syndrome.
· Many organizations provide social and support services to patients with specific diseases, for example, cancer societies, heart associations, multiple sclerosis societies, arthritis foundations, spinal cord injury foundations, stroke clubs, and cerebral palsy societies.

Family-service Agencies

Most communities will have at least one agency, if not many, that advertises itself as a family-service agency. Such agencies are good initial points of contact for learning about resources and may serve as a starting point for the patient or family with many problems. In some areas, the county board of assistance may provide this service.

Social Work Department of the Local Hospital

Within the community, one or more of the hospitals will have either an organized social work department or a service called "discharge planning." The director of the social work department or the person in discharge planning can be a valuable resource for services available in health-related areas and will probably also have a working knowledge of community resources for needs not related to health. If a university-affiliated teaching hospital exists in the community or region, this hospital is probably a good place to start.

Community Nursing Services or the Public Health Agency

This agency can also serve as a referral point for needed services in the home, especially those requiring medical or nursing skills. Visiting nurses are available to provide medically prescribed treatment in the home. In some areas, home-health aides, physical therapists, occupational therapists, and speech therapists are also available for home treatment.

National Association of Social Workers and the Society for Hospital Social Work Directors

These two organizations can serve alone or in combination as valuable consultants in identifying community resources. They will also be aware of unmet needs within the community and will probably be working actively to develop programs to meet these needs. Working closely with them will help offer comprehensive care to patients. If one has difficulty locating local offices of these organizations, the national offices can be reached by writing to the addresses or calling the telephone numbers at the bottom of this page.*

The National Association of Social Workers (NASW) also provides a publication entitled *NASW Register of Clinical Social Workers*. Degrees, licensing, and other service qualifications are listed in this directory. The directory provides a compendium of social workers available for consultation or for direct patient referral. Many social workers are in private practice and can work on a collaborative basis with physicians in managing patients' needs. An additional publication, entitled *National Registry of Health Care Providers in Clinical Social Work*, provides a listing of social workers in private practice. This directory can be obtained by writing to the National Registry at 1025 Dove Run Road, Lexington, Kentucky 40502.

THE SOCIAL WORKER AND THE PRIMARY CARE TEAM

The health care system has been making increased use of social workers as an integral part of the primary care team. One-half or more of the patients seen for outpatient medical services present with exacerbated symptoms and functional illness caused by social and emotional problems (7). If the goal of health care is either simply the cure of illness or "social, mental, and physical well-being," as defined by the World Health Organization, social work services

---

*National Association of Social Workers, 1425 H Street N.W., Washington, D.C. 20005 (202) 628–6800; Society for Hospital Social Work Directors, 840 North Lake Shore Drive, Chicago, Illinois 60611 (312) 645–9400.

should be included as part of the services provided by the primary care team to reach that goal.

Primary Care Physician in Solo or Group Practice

Physicians in solo and group practices are hiring more and more social workers or referring patients to social workers in private practice (8). In many ways, other countries (e.g., Canada, England, Australia, New Zealand, and Israel) have pioneered in the integration of social work into their primary care system (8). One can speculate that the most important reason for fewer innovative models in the United States is its peculiar funding mechanism for health care, with the predominance of fee-for-service payment. Twersky and Cole report that questionnaires returned by 30 social workers practicing in family medicine settings showed that 18 charged a fee for their service, and an additional four planned to charge; the remaining eight did not plan to charge fees (8).

The primary care physician can view the hiring of a social worker, either as a direct employee or on a contractual basis, as an additional expense. Certainly, the social worker's salary is an additional cost that must somehow be borne by the medical practice and that may contribute to increased patient fees. Since reimbursement for the services of a social worker is primarily on a fee-for-service basis, usually with a sliding scale for low-income patients, the revenues generated usually will not meet the cost. The current salary recommendation by the NASW for a person who has just received a master's degree is $16,805; for a person with certification by the Academy of Certified Social Workers (two years of supervised experience beyond a master's degree and successful completion of a qualifying examination), the recommended salary is $19,452. Fringe benefits would add to the cost. Even at full reimbursement by each patient or family of $25 per hour, the practice would need to generate well over 600 fully reimbursed interviews yearly, which is probably unrealistic. Obviously, employing a social worker part-time or contracting for service would reduce the cost.

Despite these financial difficulties, the services of social workers are increasingly being considered by primary care physicians, who are hiring full-time or part-time social workers and contracting with individual social workers or groups of them.

In addition to the trend toward increased usage of social work in primary care settings, some strides are being made toward obtaining direct third-party reimbursement for the services of social workers. As of June 1979, six states (California, Colorado, Maryland, New York, Utah, and Virginia) had passed such legislation. However, the laws are not uniform from state to state, either in the mechanisms to provide reimbursement or in the enforcement of the existing legislation. Some private insurance companies offer social work coverage as an option in certain policies. In some policies and in some states, the supervision of a physician is required for reimbursement. In some states, social work is recognized as a reimbursable provider of psychiatric outpatient services under Medicare. However, the demonstrated supervision of a physician is often required.

In short, reimbursement mechanisms for social work services are currently inconsistent, generally inadequate, and vary widely from state to state. However, strong lobbying efforts are continuing on national and state levels by the social workers to attain adequate reimbursement from all third parties for service. The national office of the NASW or the local NASW chapter would be an appropriate resource to define reimbursement mechanisms in a given geographic area and to identify changes in legislation as they occur.

At this point, the effect of a national health insurance program in providing increased reimbursement for social work services is difficult to predict. The outlines, however, of all currently proposed programs emphasize the areas of prevention, of health maintenance in the broadest definition, and of adequate provision for catastrophic illness. In all three areas, economic and social factors are unquestionably interwoven with the accomplishment of these goals. Therefore, one could speculate that if a national health insurance program is enacted with strong emphasis in the above areas, professionals with demonstrated skills in the prevention of emotional, social, and economic deterioration and breakdown will be reimbursed for their services. In addition, the strong component of cost containment, certain to be a part of any new health legislation, may also help to create specialized health care teams, including physicians, social workers, nurse practitioners, physicians' assistants, and other specialized health care personnel not yet defined.

Primary Care Physician in a Health Maintenance Organization

With the signing into law of Public Law 91-222 in December 1973, health maintenance organizations (HMOs) received legislative sanction and federal support. Among basic services provided by an approved HMO are short-term, outpatient evaluation services, crisis-intervention services, referral services for drug and alcohol abuse, and home-health services. The social and emotional aspects of patient care have emerged as important priorities in HMOs, which emphasize comprehensive care, continuity of care, and preventive care.

Health maintenance organizations also are required to have one-third consumer representation on their policy-making boards and to develop a meaningful grievance procedure for consumer concerns. Recognizing the expertise, both demonstrated and potential, of social service in these areas, social workers have been integrated into the staffs of many developing HMOs.

Traditional family and patient services continue to have important roles in HMOs, but social workers have also demonstrated knowledge of communities, especially in identifying cultural and social patterns of health care usage. Therefore, they have helped to market services to the community and to plan services for the HMO. In conjunction with the nurse practitioner, they have assumed roles in community-health education. In some HMOs social workers have served as the liaison between consumer and health care provider by assisting communities and consumer groups to provide meaningful and representative consumer board members. Finally, the social worker may serve as a consultant to the consumer advocate or ombudsman (9,10).

Primary Care Physician Providing Emergency Service

Two recent changes in the character of emergency services have become evident. First of all, emergency services no longer treat only medical emergencies. They have become the primary care provider for two groups—people who are unable to contact their personal physicians and those who have no personal physician. The second change that has occurred is that emergency services are more frequently staffed and administered by groups of full-time practicing physicians. These physicians must organize a system of care to deal not only with medical emergencies but with 24-hour nonemergency health care.

Particularly in urban areas, the people who use emergency services as their primary source of medical care suffer from chronic medical conditions, have many social problems, and may be afflicted by severe emotional disturbances. Many are elderly, lonely people living a marginal existence within the community. A typical emergency service is equipped with highly specialized medical personnel and equipment to deal with the acutely ill patient. Frequently, it is not equipped to deal with the chronically ill, depressed patient or the family that has many social and emotional problems.

The social worker routinely manages the many different social and emotional problems encountered in the emergency service. By having a social worker manage this aspect of emergency care, not only will the quality of care improve, but the physician may concentrate on managing medical problems. In addition, a social worker can sometimes work with a patient and family and help them find more appropriate care for their medical needs in the future—a service both to the patient and the emergency room staff.

The trend is toward increasing hours of social work coverage in the emergency service. In many hospitals, social workers rotate according to an on-call system and thus are available during the evenings, nights, and weekends. Many emergency services have found that needs are more effectively met by providing social work staff through the evening hours (11).

Primary Care Physician in a Hospital

The social worker who deals with hospitalized patients or those followed by the hospital's outpatient services is an excellent resource to primary care physicians and their patients. The 1979 standards of the Joint Commission on Accreditation of Hospitals now require that social work services be available to patients and their families to help in the "adjustment to the impact of illness and to promote maximum benefits from the health care provided" (12).

The standards further state that the method of providing social work services shall depend on the size and scope of services offered by the hospital (12). The physician can in all likelihood be assured that if the hospital is large or treats certain types of patients, a department with qualified social workers of sufficient size will exist. No matter what the size or purpose of the hospital, there now should be a social work department within the institution, or there must be some arrangement made for providing patients with the necessary services of social workers. Information regarding the types of services and kinds of persons available for delivering these services may be obtained directly from the social work department or from the office of the hospital administrator.

Various methods exist in hospitals to deliver the services of social workers. In some institutions, there is a central intake, with assignment of patients and their families to social workers in rotation. In many others, staff are assigned to specific clinical services, such as surgery, medicine, and obstetrics and gynecology. Sometimes social workers are assigned according to the inpatient or outpatient status of the patient as well as according to specific disease or diseases. Hospitals with hemodialysis services, maternal- and infant-care programs, and rehabilitation centers are required to have social workers with master's degrees who supervise or deliver services to these special groups of patients.

Ideally, social work services should begin when the patient enters the hospital, particularly the patient who will need social planning for aftercare (more popularly described as discharge planning). Obviously, each patient comes from some place and must return to some place. This place may be the patient's home, the home of a relative, a chronic-care facility, a nursing home that provides skilled nursing or intermediate care, a boarding home, a rehabilitation center, a hospice, or some other kind of setting that is concerned with the patient's specific needs (13).

It is often difficult for physicians and others to differentiate between and to decide which of the various aftercare facilities are best for a particular patient. To make such a decision, one must be aware of the type of health and personal care that the patient needs. One also needs to know what kind of personnel are needed to render the care as well as the patient's current and future potential for self-care. Only then can one match the patient to available community resources. Local, state, federal, and other accrediting agencies regulate the kind of care these facilities may or may not provide. Some facilities are licensed to provide more than one level of care. They may, however, impose their own restrictions for the entry level of care in their institution.

A *skilled nursing facility* provides inpatient services that are directed by a licensed physician and that are rendered directly by or under the supervision of licensed professional nursing personnel (14).

An *intermediate-care facility* renders service under the direction of a licensed physician. These services are administered by nonprofessional health personnel under the direction of a licensed nurse (14).

A *boarding home* is a facility where room and board are provided to physically independent people. Regulations for this type of facility vary from state to state and from community to community within states.

A *rehabilitation center* is a specialty hospital accredited by the Commission on Accreditation of Rehabilitation Centers and Facilities. Its purpose is to restore a handicapped person to the highest possible physical, social, emotional, and vocational level. Its staff generally consists of physicians, nurses, social workers, and physical, occupational, and speech therapists. Representatives of many other professions are often found there as well.

A *hospice* is both a concept and a discrete entity. It focuses on the patient and his or her family rather than on the disease. Its purpose is to allow terminally ill patients to live out the last days of their lives as comfortably as possible. An organized hospice program provides health care personnel to deliver necessary services to patients and their families (15,16). The local cancer society or hospital would be able to answer questions about the existence of these resources within a particular community.

In addition to helping the physician and patient with the tangible aspects of planning for aftercare, the social worker is also able to help the patient and family with feelings and concerns that they may have about the illness and hospitalization. Patients and their families do not easily accept an altered state of health and frequently need help with these changed roles. This kind of help can be provided by the social worker in collaboration with the patient's physician and with other health care professionals who interact with the patient.

Hospital-based social workers serve their patients either by working directly with the patient and family as individuals or within groups led by the social worker. Social workers also work with community groups to develop additional services for patients. Along with other health care professionals, they assume responsibility for calling attention to gaps in services and the need for providing other services. They can provide a link between the community, the hospital, the staff of the hospital, and its patients.

CRITERIA FOR CHOOSING A SOCIAL WORKER

The NASW, the largest professional social work membership organization, publishes standards for the professional practices of social workers (17) and standards for social work personnel (18). The NASW defines six levels of social work personnel that represent different levels of education and experience. These six levels are:

1. *Social service aide.* Qualifications include high school diploma or practical experience.
2. *Social service technician.* Qualifications include completion of an organized social welfare program leading to an associate of arts degree or a bachelor of arts degree in another field.
3. *Social worker.* Qualifications include completion of a bachelor of social work program in an institution approved by the Council on Social Work Education.
4. *Graduate social worker.* Qualifications include completion of a master of social work program in an institution accredited by the Council of Social Work Education.
5. *Certified social worker.* Qualifications include completion of a master's degree program in social work plus accreditation by the Academy of Certified Social Workers (ACSW).
6. *Social work fellow.* Qualifications include completion of a doctoral program at an accredited school of social work or in a related discipline, with two years of specialization in an area of social work or certification by the ACSW and two years of social work experience in the field of specialization (18).

Included in the last two classifications are persons who are considered by the NASW to be capable of independent practice. Another group of persons considered capable of independent practice are those who are licensed in states with licensing laws as independent practitioners. As of January 1979, 25 states and Puerto Rico had licensing or certification laws. All other states are in the process of preparing licensing or certification laws.

Physicians who choose to employ a social worker can discuss their needs and the availability of qualified social workers with the director of a local hospital social work department or social work agency. In addition, the NASW and the Society for Hospital Social Work Directors have lists of persons who are qualified consultants to assist in the selection of social workers, including both the selection of persons for the job and in developing the job description and role for the social worker. If the inquiring physician is not sure how to reach a local group, he or she may write or call the national organizations of these two groups. It is important if one wishes to choose a social worker for practice in a primary health care setting that the social worker either have experience or training in the health care field or have access to consultants regarding the kinds of problems that occur in health care.

Westerman et al. state that,

> Together with cost-justification requirements will come increased public pressure for decentralization of professional responsibilities. Development of workable research and evaluation systems will undoubtedly produce results which reinforce the evolving belief that many health care tasks can safely be delegated to individuals with less technical training than is presently required. In the 1980s health professionals will not only be compelled to surrender veto power in the assignment of duties, but will likely need to demonstrate that any division of responsibilities represents an optimum distribution of resources and is consistent with the rationale of the delivery system (6).

Perhaps a primary care physician and a social worker working together represent such a "distribution of resources," which is not only cost effective but improves the quality of care to patients. Certainly, the addition of a social worker to a primary care practice represents a cost, but maybe a smaller and more productive cost than the addition of another physician to see patients who are not responding to traditional medical treatment.

REFERENCES

1. Klein P: *From Philanthropy to Social Welfare*. San Francisco, Jossey-Bass, Publishers, 1968.
2. Pray KLM: *Social Work in a Revolutionary Age*. Philadelphia, University of Pennsylvania Press, 1949.
3. American Hospital Association: *Essentials of a Social Service Department in Hospitals and Related Institutions*. Chicago, 1961.
4. Axinn J, Levin H: Money, politics, and education: The case of social work. *Hist Educ Q* Summer, 1978, p 145.
5. Professional Association: Council on Social Work Education: *Social Work Encyclopedia*. Washington, DC, National Association of Social Workers, 1977, vol II, p 1081.
6. Westerman JH, Spano RM, Keyes MA: Public accountability, quality assurance and social work. *Soc Work Health Care* 2:36, 1976.
7. Weiss E, English OS: *Psychosomatic Medicine*. Philadelphia, WB Saunders, 1949.
8. Twersky RK, Cole WM: Social work fees in medical care: A review of the literature and report of a survey. *Soc Work Health Care* 2:78, 1976.
9. Lum D: The social service health specialist in an HMO. *Health Soc Work* 9:43, 1976.
10. Bell C, Gorman LM: The HMOs: New models for practice. *Soc Work Health Care* 1:325, 1976.

11. Bergman AS: Emergency room: A role for social workers. *Health Soc Work* 1:32, 1976.

12. Joint Commission on Accreditation of Hospitals: *Accreditation Manual for Hospitals.* Chicago, Illinois, 1979.

13. Conway JB: The role of the social worker in discharge planning. Unpublished paper presented at the Middle Atlantic Health Congress, Atlantic City, New Jersey, May 18, 1977, Joint Session with Home Care Nursing and Social Work.

14. Department of Public Welfare, Commonwealth of Pennsylvania: *Medical Assistance Memorandum No. 61 Supplement No. 1.* Harrisburg, 1975.

15. Foster Z: Standards for hospice care: Assumptions and principles. *Health Soc Work* 4:117, 1979.

16. Millet N: Hospice: Challenging society's approach to death. *Health Soc Work* 4:130 1979.

17. National Association of Social Workers: *NASW Standards for Social Work Personnel Practices—NASW Policy Statements 2.* Washington, DC, 1975.

18. National Association of Social Workers: *NASW Standards for Social Work Manpower—NASW Policy Statements 4.* Washington, DC, 1973.

14
Principles of Management: Planning and Directing

Ross Arkell Webber

The crisis in health care in the United States is less of a medical crisis than a managerial crisis. Physicians are capable of doing more than economics or administrative effectiveness allow. The blame for this situation, however, does not fall solely on legislators or administrators. Physicians also deserve their fair share because frequently they have shirked administrative responsibility and demonstrated managerial ignorance.

In all realms of American life, we are coming to recognize that simply desiring more effective leadership is insufficient. Our wishes must be framed within the limits of administrative competence. In medicine, this framework will demand better relations and understanding between creators and implementors and between providers of specialist services and general administrators—in short, between physicians and managers. Even more important, it will require more physicians as managers.

Unfortunately, the motivation and thought processes of managers and physicians tend to be quite different and at times conflicting. Physicians tend to be driven more by achievement and distrustful of hierarchic power; managers tend to be influenced more by the motives of power and politics. As a result, many physicians put distance between themselves and administrators. Or they think that a professional administrator or office manager can take care of administrative detail without bothering physicians, who will be free to concentrate on what they know best. Such a point of view is sadly misguided because expertise and power are separated only at peril.

Even when a physician is in an administrative position (including that of running a private practice), he or she may denigrate the managerial component. Some see it as less intellectually challenging or less inherently valuable. The invidious distinction between professional and managerial effort is unnecessary and unfortunate. Organization and management are complex. Effective management does not reflect merely intuition or common sense. And efficient delivery of a prized service is a worthy objective. The physician as manager should not abdicate his or her responsibility to exercise leadership through planning and direction.

In this chapter, I shall address the dual objective of assisting physicians to understand management theory and to improve personal administrative effectiveness by discussing two administrative functions fundamental to management: direction or leadership based on understanding motivation, and planning organizational objectives and controlling performance. In Chapter 15, Hrebiniak will discuss two other functions essential to management: designing organizational stucture and managing organizational change.

MOTIVATING AND DIRECTING

Mankind has been described from more vantage points than has the proverbial elephant by blind men. Many, many conceptions of human nature exist. The conscious, or cognitive, approach will be emphasized here because it seems most applicable to what managers do. We assume that human behavior has purposes, that it is not random or unconscious. Most of the time, people more or less know what they are doing and why (1). We shall examine how motivation depends on expectations of need satisfaction, what needs exist, and how needs may be structured.

Motivation, Needs, and Expectations

Behavior is directed to obtain wants that will satisfy needs (2). Wants can usually be described easily; they are numerous and range from material specifics like bread and chrome-plated baubles to abstract states like security, love, prestige, and power. Whereas wants are apparently limitless, needs are not. Needs are relatively few, but they represent basic drives that motivate behavior in quest of a much larger number of wants.

People generally behave in various ways because they expect to satisfy certain basic needs (3,4). Their expectation is seldom certain but, rather a matter of probabilities. Whether a person performs a certain act (such as striving for an A in a course) depends on whether he or she believes that the behavior has a good chance of satisfying some underlying need and whether the need is important.

The strength of a person's motivation to behave is based on three characteristics of the situation. First of all, the person must satisfy his or her own questions about the probability of success. These questions are ones of "confidence." Will my behavior lead to obtaining the wanted goods, pleasures, or states of being? How likely is this goal? If I think that the probability is small that I can obtain the want, I am less likely to try. I am more likely to try if the odds seem in my favor. I am also unwilling to try if I don't feel that I have the necessary ability and am more likely to try if I am confident.

Second, there are questions of "instrumentality." Will the wanted goods or state of being bring pleasure (or avoid pain) by satisfying one or more of my needs? My motivation to behave to obtain the wants will be stronger if I believe that the probability is high that the obtained want will be instrumental to satisfaction of my need.

Finally, there are questions of "valence." Is my need worth the effort? How important is the need that will be satisfied in comparison with my other needs and my limited energy?

Research indicates that future physicians focus on medicine as their career much earlier than do young people who eventually enter other occupations (5). By about age 14, most future physicians seem to recognize that a medical degree is the desired want because it will be instrumental to satisfying many high-priority personal needs, especially security, esteem, autonomy, and achievement.

The Structure of Needs

Since needs are inferences and not physical facts, we cannot "prove" their existence. Some like hunger, are obvious, but others like competence are more subtle. Keeping this uncertainty in mind, I shall discuss what seem to be the basic needs motivating human behavior.

There has been much controversy about the number of needs that exist. Suggestions range from as few as three to more than 20. Alderfer maintains that most people are able to distinguish among only three kinds of needs (6):

1. Existence needs that relate to the biological necessities of life
2. Relatedness needs that deal with relations with other people
3. Growth needs that express personal development

Maslow's slightly more complex model postulates five needs arranged in a hierarchic fashion (7):

5. Self-actualization
4. Esteem
3. Love
2. Safety
1. Physiologic needs

For a need to be lower on the hierarchy implies that it is predominant. Physiologic needs are placed at the bottom because satisfaction of those drives is essential for the maintenance of life; they are predominant for motivating behavior.

The hierarchic model suggests that as physical needs are satisfied (at least to a minimal degree), new needs emerge to motivate behavior. This model implies that lower-level needs must be satisfied before upper-level needs begin to become motivating forces. Before we can become concerned about social esteem, we must have sufficient food and shelter. Before most of us become concerned about achievement, we must have some affiliation, and so on. Still, only relative satisfaction is necessary. We do not know what the proportions are, but we can assume some value below 100% satisfaction of a lower need before the next higher need becomes motivating.

In the years since this hierarchic model was advanced, there has been substantial research on the nature and impact of these needs on human behavior (8). Of special concern have been the upper levels of the hierarchy because "self-actualization" is difficult to define and too abstract a concept for many to understand. Originally, it conveyed a biologic image: that one had an ultimate need to fully actualize one's potential, to become everything one is capable of becoming. It now appears that self-actualization is a more complex phenomenon that includes elements of autonomy, power, achievement, and creativity.

Power can be a means that satisfies various needs. It can bring one safety through a private army; prestige if other people admire power; perhaps even a form of affiliation if slaves can be ordered to provide it. The need for power is different, however. It is satisfied by the intrinsic process of influencing others by exercising power. The need for power is measured by the person's concern about control of the means for influencing other people (9). Such concern may be inferred from emotional reaction to a dominance situation; for example, pleasure in winning or anger in losing an argument. It is what drives the political leader to pursue the feeling of being involved in decisions that affect others' lives (10).

The inverse of personal power is freedom from the power of others, or autonomy. Freedom from arbitrary and unilateral authority, even from the benevolent despot, is a persistent theme in history. Indeed, the drive for power has its roots in the helplessness of childhood when the child is dependent on and controlled by adults. The drive for autonomy reflects both fear of dependence on others for satisfaction of physiologic needs and desire to fulfill higher needs.

What may be the apex of human needs are the person's drives for achievement, creativity, and self-actualization, located at the top of the needs hierarchy. We are perhaps combining distinct motives, but they all point in the same direction: what a person can be, he or she must be. One should create and achieve everything of which one is capable. Overcoming challenging, difficult, and novel problems, creating new institutions and objects, developing one's attributes and capabilities are all sources of satisfaction (11).

Achievement is a confusing term for this need because achievement means so many things and brings so many rewards. Like power, achievement can be a want that satisfies several needs. The need for achievement, however, is satisfied by the process of expending effort and experiencing successful completion. In stories, the need takes the form of how the hero, through persistent efforts, overcomes great obstacles and obtains his or her distant goal (12). The emphasis is less on the goods or honors than on successful achievement and satisfaction with the process itself. Great achievements, of course, may bring social prestige, power, security, perhaps even love. As satisfying as such things are, however, they do not reflect the need for achievement. People with high achievement needs may like status and money as much as others do, but they are also concerned with the process of performing a task well, meeting high standards, overcoming difficult obstacles, and trying novel or creative methods (13).

The difference between people is the relative frequency and intensity of various drives. The self-actualizing person is more frequently motivated by competence and achievement needs; the other-directed person is more frequently motivated by social and prestige needs; and the fearful person is more apt to be motivated by safety and security. Each person has his or her own particular cycle of these needs, that is, how frequently and how strongly each need is felt. But almost all people possess all needs to some degree. The chemistry researcher with the Ph.D. may be mainly driven by desires for autonomy, competence, and achievement, but there are also needs for security and affiliation. The assembly line worker may be concerned mostly about money and security, but he or she does have needs for esteem and competence. The drives are not all equal in frequency, duration, or intensity, but all people possess all needs to some extent.

Influence Through Coercive and Reward Power

To lead or direct someone, it is necessary to influence them (14,15). And to influence, one must appeal to one or more of the needs discussed. The influence process depends on the follower as much as or more than it depends on the leader. It is a decision by the follower whether to respond that determines if the process will succeed.

Coercive power is based on a follower's perception that the influencer has the ability to punish, and that the punishment will be unpleasant or frustrating of some need. Reward power is based on a follower's perception that the influencer has the capacity to reward and that the reward will be pleasant or satisfying of some need. The influence process, exerted through fear or hope drawing on coercive or reward power, can work if logically and consistently applied. Nonetheless, it is not certain that it will work in a particular situation with specific people. Whether an influence process will motivate a person to behave in the desired way depends on the person's perception and judgment as to whether effort will lead to the reward offered (or lack of punishment promised) and whether this reward will satisfy a fundamental need. Thus, the motivation model discussed can be modified to include the influence process (Fig. 1).

As indicated in Figure 1, the potential follower's motivation and effort depend on:

a. His or her estimate of the probability that effort will meet the influencer's objective
b. His or her estimate of the probability that on meeting the objective, the influencer will dispense rewards or withhold punishment
c. His or her estimate of the probability that the rewards will satisfy some needs
d. How much he or she values satisfaction of these needs

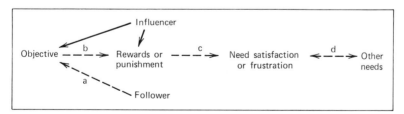

Figure 1. Influence model based on coercive and reward power. Solid lines indicate control by the influencer. Broken lines indicate decision made by the follower. The potential follower's motivation and effort depend on confidence, credibility, instrumentality, and valence. (Adapted with permission from Ross A. Webber, *Management: Basic Elements of Managing Organizations*. Homewood, Illinois, Richard D. Irwin, revised edition 1979. With permission. © 1979 by Richard D. Irwin, Inc.)

The follower's motivation and effort will be great if satisfaction of need is highly valued, if he or she thinks that the influencer's rewards will be instrumental in satisfying these needs, and if he or she thinks that his or her efforts will meet the influencer's objectives so that a reward will be given. Breaking the system at any point undermines the influencer's influence.

Credibility is important to the influencer; his or her threats and promises must be believed. When organized crime entered the loan sharking business, its credibility was one of its biggest assets. The borrower was influenced to pay back the loan on time because the borrower believed the lender's threats that he or she absolutely would be punished—no escape was possible. Indeed, the certainty of punishment is probably a stronger deterrent to undesired behavior than is the severity of punishment (16).

Emphasizing the positive reward for desired behavior is at the base of modern behavioral psychology and much ancient leadership practice (17). This reward may take varied forms in addition to money. The major arguments in favor of rewards over punishment are:

- The leader can clearly define the desired behavior, not just the undesired behavior. The fear approach implies that the follower has only two courses of action—what the leader desires and what he abhors. In fact, other alternatives may exist that the leader does not anticipate. The follower may choose one of these alternatives in hope of retaining some autonomy and still escaping punishment (18).
- Research suggests that fear of punishment often stimulates more effort, but the hope of a reward leads to greater follower understanding and satisfaction with what is expected (19). So under fear, a subordinate may work hard but at the wrong task. With hope of a reward, the subordinate is more likely to do what is desired and is happier doing it. The key is that the leader must know precisely what the follower is to do—and when it is to be done.

The primary motivation technique of management has been, and probably still is, to offer extrinsic rewards for desired subordinate behavior and performance. Money is the most common extrinsic reward, but managers have long dispensed other extrinsic rewards, including promotions, titles, public and private praise, fringe benefits, and status symbols like office size and furnishings. In recent years, interest in the use of nonfinancial rewards has grown, fueled by efforts to apply behavioral theory.

Recognizing good performance seems obvious to many managers, but it may well be that many organizations have become so bureaucratic and impersonal that no one pays attention to performance or takes time to express personal praise and gratitude. To an appreciable extent, in many organizations most extrinsic rewards are not given for performance but for loyalty and time; that is, employees are rewarded for seniority with promotions, larger offices, and better insurance plans. Rewards based on the calendar do motivate behavior, of course, but not especially performance. They primarily motivate employees to remain with the organization, which may be valuable to management but not necessarily relevant to performance.

The key in influencing behavior through hope of rewards is to link a pleasant outcome with desired behavior (20). Thus, management may dispense a reward that the employee perceives as valuable. There are three critical aspects of this process (21):

1. The reward, such as praise, must be contingent on good performance; it should not be given out all the time to everyone regardless of results.
2. The reward must be dispensed quickly.
3. The receiver must believe that the reward is instrumental to satisfaction of some need and subsequently experience this satisfaction.

For employees to respond affirmatively to a pay-incentive plan, they must trust management (and believe that management will not cut the rewards if they do well), understand the plan, and see a close relation between their performance and their pay. Management must stand by its word, keep its promises, and not offer more than it can deliver. It should ensure that the highest performers are the most satisfied. This approach will make it clear to others on what basis rewards are distributed. Employees should be able to observe that those who do better actually receive more than do average or unsatisfactory workers.

No one knows for sure how much this "more" should be. Existing incentive plans have been criticized as paying too little; it is maintained that a 10% bonus for a week, month, or even a year does not have sufficient impact (22). Something much larger, at least 30%, is probably necessary to substantially affect the recipient's life-style. Without such impact, the employee would not be too concerned about maintaining the increment through subsequent good performance. To pay such incentive earnings, however, requires management to make tough decisions differentiating between outstanding and average performers, because it would just be too expensive to pay large bonuses to everyone. Rather than upset nonrecipients, therefore, many organizations simply award 5–10% increases to everyone except the most incompetent. Such a policy does not motivate better performance; it simply encourages the average employee to remain with the organization (23).

The key is that increased pay should follow improved performance, not just be awarded beforehand in the hope that people will automatically try harder if they are paid more. To really increase one's effort for money would require these beliefs:

· Increased effort would lead to better performance.
· The employer can determine that performance has improved.
· Increased money will follow from this improved performance.
· The additional money will be valued because it would satisfy needs.
· Other needs for security, affiliation, and so on would not have to be unduly sacrificed.

This general influence model clearly defines the central leadership problem: to formulate, communicate, and ensure that the followers understand the path-goal relationships (24). The followers must understand the goals, the criteria for evaluating performance, the sanctions promised, and their meaning. The leader must design the system so that goal achievement leads to the follower's personal reward and satisfaction of need. A leader who does not do so will not be a leader, no influence will result, and there will be no followers.

Influence Through Other Forms of Power

When someone successfully influences another, we infer that the influencer possesses power (25). Thus, influence implies power, and power is necessary for influence. However, there are forms of power other than the coercive and reward powers discussed in the preceding section (26):

· Legitimate power is based on the follower's internalized values that convince him or her that the influencer has a legitimate right to influence that he or she is bound to accept. This relation is at the core of a traditional influence system, in which leaders are endowed with legitimate power called "authority" (27).

· Referent power is based on the follower's desire to identify with a charismatic leader whom he or she follows out of blind faith. The identification can be maintained if the follower behaves as the leader tells him or her to behave.

· Expert power is based on the follower's perception that the leader has special knowledge or expertise that can be useful in satisfying some of the follower's needs.

· Representative power is delegated upward to a leader by a group with an implied agreement to follow as long as the leader consults the followers and generally leads in the direction that they want to go.

Leadership is the use of these various power bases to influence or motivate people. Figure 2 illustrates the various forms of power and influence processes that will be discussed.

Tradition probably has been the most common influence mechanism in

Follower's Need Hierarchy	Influence Process	Leadership Style	Leader's Power Basis
Competence, achievement	Self-determination	Abdicative	
	Joint determination	Participative	Representative
Power, autonomy			
	Rational agreement		Expert
Esteem, prestige		Persuasive	
	Rational faith		
			Referent
Social, affiliation	Blind faith		
			Legitimate
	Tradition	Authoritarian	
Safety, security			Reward
	Fear-hope		
		Autocratic	Coercive
Physiologic			

Figure 2. Influence and leader's power basis. (Adapted with permission from Ross A. Webber, *Management: Basic Elements of Managing Organizations.* Homewood, Illinois, Richard D. Irwin, revised edition 1979. © 1979 by Richard D. Irwin, Inc.)

human history. The king is obeyed because he is the king, or because he is a representative of God, or as in ancient Egypt, because he is God, or at least because the people think so. As St. Paul remarked, "Let everyone submit himself to the ruling authorities, for there exists no authority not ordained by God." Response is quasi-automatic and almost unconscious, the kind of habitual obedience that is the intent of close-order drill learned during the first weeks in military training. Tradition may start out mainly as fear, but the response becomes institutionalized and internalized into the class structure and the ideology of the society. One responds out of respect for one's betters or because there is some natural social order that is customary and believed "right."

Tradition as the basis for obedience was commonly assumed in 19th-century management literature, when management structure was closely allied with the class structure of the society (28). It was assumed that "inferiors" should and would respond to "betters." Under this influence system, as with fear, it makes no difference whether the follower understands the reason for the directive or agrees with it, and he or she certainly has not participated in formulating the directive.

Although we Americans like to think of ourselves as egalitarian, we do have many superior-subordinate relationships that attempt to program obedience: parent-child, teacher-student, employer-employee. All have in common some traditional feeling that within certain limits, the subordinate will respond to the superior's suggestions (29). In 1938, the president of a large American corporation observed that the average worker in this country expected to do what he or she was told, within certain limits—what was termed a "zone of indifference" (30). The limits of that zone have probably narrowed in the past 40 years, however. We are less willing to respond automatically to authority and do what we are told than we once were.

The medical professions have been characterized by mixed feelings about legitimate authority. Physicians tend to distrust such institutionalized power, but nursing traditionally has shown enormous respect for the chain of command. Graduates of hospital schools of nursing have been especially socialized into respect for legitimate authority and the physician's power. Such automatic respect has generally been desired by physicians but is currently under question in university nursing programs, which are endeavoring to turn out more independent and questioning professionals.

Influence on the basis of blind faith reflects a kind of Alexander the Great or Napoleon syndrome. We respond to the great leader who has "charisma" (31). To the ancients, charisma was a gift of God, a gift of grace, or magical powers that were given to a few favored humans. Only fools would not respond to the charismatic leader. But what is the charismatic leader to us today? Haven't we outgrown the ignorance and superstition of earlier blind followers? Or has the source of authority shifted from magic to psychology?

People tend to respond to the leader who has characteristics that they admire, to the person who is a model of what they would like to be. Perhaps most fundamentally, they respond out of strong emotional attachment, even love for the leader, in whom they have blind faith. The relationship is personal rather than general, for charisma is not simply an attribute of the leader but the fit between his or her characteristics and the follower's needs (32,33).

Whenever the attempt to influence is based on fear, tradition, or blind faith and draws on coercive, reward, legitimate, or referent power, the influence process is essentially authoritarian. The leader tells the follower to do something; the follower responds because he or she fears being punished, wants the reward, feels a responsibility to obey, or loves the leader and believes in his or her abilities. In all four instances, the process is essentially a one-way authoritarian communication to which followers respond without questioning whether specific directives are appropriate to the task. They neither understand the reasons for the order nor necessarily agree with it.

Influence through faith is more limited than are the other authoritarian forms, however. The charismatic leader's power is partially dependent on performance. If the leader and his or her followers experience a series of failures, the leader's charisma and referent power will fade.

The charismatic leader influences people through his or her personality, not his or her position. Therefore, such a leader endeavors to interact directly with many people throughout the organization. The charismatic leader bypasses various levels of management because of a desire to bind people to himself or herself, not to his or her lieutenants. Franklin D. Roosevelt was often criticized as being a poor manager because his assignment of duties was sloppy and because he showed little respect for the structure of government. He would personally communicate with people throughout the system and give them projects, unknown to their peers or superiors. He cultivated individual, personalized relationships, not organizational, impersonal positions. General Robert Johnson, of the Johnson and Johnson Company, showed quite similar behavior. He would descend by helicopter on his plants unannounced, bypass the resident manager in charge, and move directly to employees at various levels. Such behavior can be upsetting to organizationally minded people, but it can create a sense of identification with the top and a willingness to sacrifice for the company that can be powerful.

Within medicine, the great surgeons have often exercised enormous influence by virtue of their referent power. Because their special skills were often dramatic (and their personalities likewise), and because they could publicly demonstrate their success, others tended to attribute power to them and to follow. The more quiet successes of the competent internist contribute less to charisma (34).

If we could count the number of incidents of influence in modern organizations, especially among managers and professionals, the most common influence process probably would be rational faith in expert power (35). The followers respond because they believe the leader, on the basis of some evidence that the leader has knowledge and ability. This influence process is similar to a patient's relationship with a physician. The patient can reach a somewhat rational judgment that the physician is qualified from the diplomas, license, and certificates on the office wall. Nonetheless, however rational the decision about the person, the response to specific suggestions is still based on faith.

Much of the time, a charismatic leader will draw on his or her expert power to persuade followers rather than ordering them. As a result, the followers will tend to feel that they share in the leader's power instead of feeling dominated by it. Success reinforces the power of the charismatic leader, and people respond out of rational and blind faith. Winston Churchill motivated his people because he persuasively articulated the challenge facing the nation and successfully built on their faith in and respect for him.

Not many possess Churchill's personality, but persuasive leadership may be the only option for a potential influencer who has no other power but expertise. Armed with knowledge, the leader attempts to convince others to follow this advice. Research suggests that persuasion will be more effective under the following conditions (36,37):

· If the influencer has high credibility based on perceived expertise and trustworthiness.
· If the influencer initially expresses some views that are also held by the audience or potential followers.
· If the information is perceived as privileged for a few, when large numbers want to hear it.
· If the influencer's personal appearance and characteristics please, or at least do not offend, the audience.

In addition, the following conditions can affect the possibility that persuasion will be an effective method of influencing others:

· If the followers have recently responded on a smaller but similar matter.
· If one side of the argument is presented when the audience is generally friendly or when the influencer's position is the only one that will be presented.
· If both sides of the argument are presented when the audience starts out disagreeing or when it is probable that they will hear the other side from someone else.
· Up to an indefinite limit, the more extreme the change the influencer asks for, the more actual change he or she is likely to get.
· When opposite views are presented one after another, the one presented last will probably be more effective.
· There will probably be more opinion change in the desired direction if the influencer explicitly states his conclusions than if he or she lets the audience draw their own (unless the audience is quite intelligent in which case allowing them to reach their own conclusions is desirable).
· Appeal to fear will frequently work if the influencer advances explicit, possible recommendations for action. However, if he or she makes no such recommendations, the appeal to fear may be rejected.
· Audience participation through group discussion and decision-making helps to overcome resistance. Having members of the audience state the espoused views is likely to increase adoption. The support of just one or two others can overcome the majority's initial resistance if the minority is consistent in expressing certainty.

Mutual Influence Between Leader and Follower

If a scientist places a pigeon in a cage with a feeding mechanism activated by a red button, the hungry bird will peck in various places in the cage. When the bird accidentally pecks a red button, the scientist reinforces the behavior by giving it a piece of corn. When the pigeon pecks the red button again, the bird again receives corn, and so on. Soon the pigeon will peck the button repeatedly. The scientist is training and controlling the pigeon, but the pigeon is also controlling

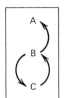

B's influence on C seems to be greater if C perceives B as having influence over A

Figure 3. Influence through representative power. B's influence on C seems to be greater if C perceives B as having influence over A. (Adapted with permission from Ross A. Webber, *Management: Basic Elements of Managing Organizations.* Homewood, Illinois, Richard D. Irwin, revised edition 1979. With permission. © 1979 by Richard D. Irwin, Inc.)

the researcher. All the pigeon has to do is peck a button, and the scientist gives the bird some food. In this operation, what is cause and what is effect (38)?

Thus, influence is reciprocal. To control, one must be controlled to some extent; that is, the influencer must be influenced (39,40). The fear-dispensing dictator must punish insubordination; otherwise, the dictator will lose his or her credibility (41). Similarly, a tradition-based system will collapse unless it provides its loyal, obedient supporters with warmth and security. The charismatic leader expecting blind faith must respond to certain demands of the followers. Basically, the charismatic leader must give of himself or herself; such a leader must allow his or her followers to see and touch him or her. Every influence mechanism and every leader thus implies two-way influence, some mutual control.

This mutuality has an important implication: influence is expandable. It is not a fixed pie that can only be divided; it is not a zero-sum game requiring a manager to lose influence when his or her subordinate gains. Both may gain increased influence as they mutually benefit from a relationship. As shown in Figure 3, influence downward may be enhanced rather than reduced by upward influence. Both managers and workers in more effective organizations perceive themselves as possessing greater influence. The greater the total influence everyone has in the system, the greater seems to be the total effectiveness of the system.

The vehicle for generating this greater influence is mainly through joint determination and participative leadership drawing on expert and representative power. When a follower has participated in determining what is to be done, he or she probably will understand the decision and agree that a certain course of action is necessary and proper. In this participation, the follower's higher-level needs are involved. The follower exercises some power, and he or she has an opportunity to express himself or herself and exercise his or her abilities. It is hoped that voluntary implementation will result from this participation and determination.

Participative leadership moves beyond the leader's power to recognize the follower's power. Their expertise is solicited and combined with the leader's, so that decisions are jointly reached. Their higher-level needs are energized through the joint-determination process.

Most practicing managers are not enthusiastic about participative leadership because they fear losing power. In addition, this influence style can be very time-consuming. Nonetheless, strong arguments have been advanced against older authoritarian styles (sometimes referred to as theory X) in favor of more participative approaches (theory Y) (42). To make comparison of the various points straightforward, they are arranged in parallel in Figure 4.

Arguments for Theory X—Authoritarian appeal to lower-level needs:

1. Authoritarian is the most predictable and effective style because everyone has physiologic, safety and security needs that most can satisfy only through money earned from a job.

2. Much work is unpleasant and many people are lazy. More or less, these conditions will always prevail, so authoritarian leadership is essential. Otherwise, most people will do as little as possible.

3. Authoritarian leadership is efficient because it is speedy; the superior simply tells the subordinate what to do, so no time is wasted in discussion. Too much concern for employees will only cripple managers, rendering them incapable of making tough decisions.

4. Authoritarian leadership is easier for most managers. They do not have to analyze the various needs of their subordinates because they assume a simple model of human nature—that people have low-level needs and must keep their jobs to satisfy them. This assumption of subordinate uniformity of physiologic and security needs makes this style especially effective for a large number of people. In addition, most manager's personalities are better suited to being "mature autocrats" than to being democratic leaders.

5. Authoritarian leadership is honest and straightforward: 'the superior (a) defines the desired behavior, (b) states

Arguments for Theory Y—Participative appeal to higher-level needs:

1. All people may possess lower-level needs, but they are not necessarily dependent on any one job to satisfy them. They may have skills that are in such demand that they have alternatives available, some of which may satisfy both lower-level and higher-level needs. Increasingly, mobile employees will move to these jobs.

2. Most people are not inherently lazy. The expenditure of physical and mental effort in work is as natural as play or rest. We are energetic and are excited by challenging and satisfying tasks. Frustrating work can be modified to release talent and drive; the job can be a vehicle for satisfying competence and achievement needs.

3. Nondirective leadership can lead to more creative and effective performance because people invest more of themselves in the task. They will exercise self-direction and self-control in the service to which they are committed. When people participate in defining organizational objectives and the system by which their performance is evaluated, they understand better and are more committed.

4. An increasing general educational level means that more people understand human complexities and desires for satisfaction of higher-level needs. The average manager or worker possesses more education than in the days when authoritarian leadership styles were developed; they are simply obsolete. As a result, many people are underutilized.

5. Participative leadership is more honest because the superior respects his or her subordinates, and because there

Figure 4. Comparing theory X and theory Y. (Adapted with permission from Ross A. Webber, *Management: Basic Elements of Managing Organizations*. Homewood, Illinois, Richard D. Irwin, revised edition 1979. © 1979 by Richard D. Irwin, Inc.)

the rewards and punishments, (c) judges the subordinate's performance and dispenses the sanctions, and (d) does not meddle with subordinates' personality, analyze their motives, or judge their lives. This frank approach is attractive to many who distrust the indirection of other styles of leadership.

is fuller communication about what each expects of the other.

6. Most subordinates expect superiors to be authoritarian; that is the way they have been raised and educated. A superior's departure from this expectation may be interpreted as weakness, and subordinates may walk all over the superior.

6. Subordinates increasingly want to influence the terms of this relationship. Children are not so automatically obedient because child-rearing and educational patterns have changed, to encourage increased participation, responsibility, independence, and self-control.

Figure 4. (continued)

Note that both sides in this debate accept the idea that the ultimate aim of the organization is effective and efficient performance. They differ on the means to achieve it (43). The authoritarians believe that strong management control and appeal to lower-level needs are more effective. The advocates of the nondirective, participative style believe that appeal to higher needs will draw more from people.

This philosophical debate is interesting but misleading because the distinction between ends of the needs-influence-leadership continuum is too simple. Effective leadership is not just being either hard or soft; it can require a manager to be both.

This perspective on leadership distinguishes between two facets of the process (44).

1. *Initiating structure and pressure for performance.* This facet is the degree to which the leader builds psychologic structure for followers by assigning particular tasks, specifying procedures, clarifying his or her expectations, and scheduling work to be done.

2. *Consideration and representativeness.* This facet is the degree to which the leader creates a supportive environment of psychologic support, warmth, and helpfulness by being friendly and approachable, looking out for subordinates' welfare, going to bat for them, and representing their interest upward.

Either one of these facets in the absence of the other tends to be associated with poorer performance, but in positive combination they are highly effective (45). In short, high management structure and pressure plus high representativeness is most likely to be associated with better subordinate performance, as shown in Figure 5.

Research findings that support two dimensions of leadership have led to a change of thinking among many theorists, who have suggested that managers can be both hard and soft, simultaneously task oriented and people concerned. A popular use of this concept has been to describe managers on a two dimensional

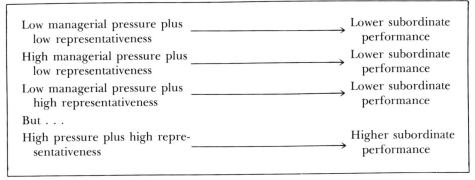

Figure 5. Performance and two dimensions of leadership. (Adapted with permission from Ross A. Webber, *Management: Basic Elements of Managing Organizations.* Homewood, Illinois, Richard D. Irwin, revised edition 1979. © 1979 by Richard D. Irwin, Inc.)

Managerial Grid ® of task and people orientations, rated on a scale of 1–9, as in Figure 6 (46).

PLANNING AND CONTROLLING

Planning can be visualized as a hierarchy related to the organizational hierarchy. As we go down this hierarchy, we move from top to bottom in the organization in terms of who performs the planning (47). We also increase specificity and detail and decrease the plan's time-span. This relation is illustrated in Figure 7. This hierarchy of planning from strategy to continuing objectives to specific goals originally was described for business organizations but is equally relevant for small medical organizations, such as a physician's office or a group practice.

Theoretically, such a hierarchy of plans means that if every unit understands its unit goals and reaches them successfully, the entire organization's specific goals and continuing objectives will be achieved. Whether this happy state is reached, however, depends on how well the objectives and goals have been defined and parceled out. The managerial task is enormously simplified if objectives are properly defined and allocated. Then, each lower manager will have a specific unit goal that he or she understands, that is within his or her ability, and for which he or she is responsible. Each lower manager knows how it is to be measured and when the deadline is.

The hierarchy of plans successively narrows the problems and alternatives confronting each layer of management. From the realm of all possible areas of actions in the world, the corporate strategy accepts some and rejects others. The continuing objectives eliminate more and the specific goals even more, so that the activities eventually become focused.

Even if the manager's goals and problems are narrower at the middle and lower levels, the ability to achieve them is helped by a knowledge of organizational strategy and an ability to link the unit's goals to the overall objectives. Indeed, subordinates' perceptions of the manager as an effective leader improve

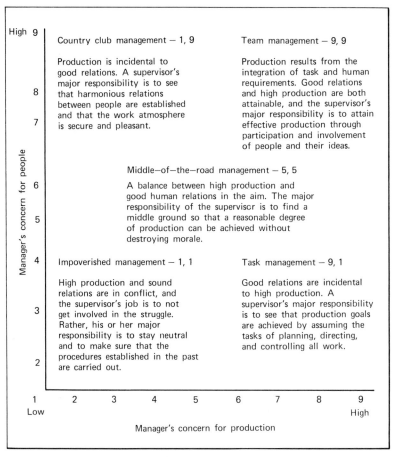

Figure 6. The Managerial Grid.® (Source: *The New Managerial Grid* by Robert R. Blake and Jane Srygley Mouton. Houston, Gulf Publishing, copyright © 1978, p. 11. Reproduced by permission.)

with their understanding of how the leader and they fit into the organization's planning and control process (48).

Defining the Organization's Mission and Strategy

The questions to be asked in defining the organization fall into four categories (49,50):

1. Services to be provided: What products or services will the organization provide and to whom?

2. Basic ways these services will be produced: What will the organization make, by what processes, and what will it buy from what sources?

3. Sequencing and timing of major steps: What moves will be made early, and what can be deferred?

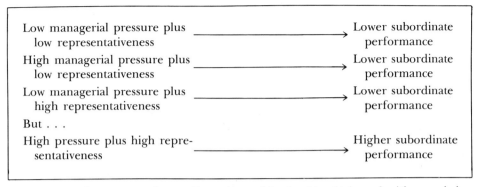

Figure 5. Performance and two dimensions of leadership. (Adapted with permission from Ross A. Webber, *Management: Basic Elements of Managing Organizations.* Homewood, Illinois, Richard D. Irwin, revised edition 1979. © 1979 by Richard D. Irwin, Inc.)

Managerial Grid ® of task and people orientations, rated on a scale of 1–9, as in Figure 6 (46).

PLANNING AND CONTROLLING

Planning can be visualized as a hierarchy related to the organizational hierarchy. As we go down this hierarchy, we move from top to bottom in the organization in terms of who performs the planning (47). We also increase specificity and detail and decrease the plan's time-span. This relation is illustrated in Figure 7. This hierarchy of planning from strategy to continuing objectives to specific goals originally was described for business organizations but is equally relevant for small medical organizations, such as a physician's office or a group practice.

Theoretically, such a hierarchy of plans means that if every unit understands its unit goals and reaches them successfully, the entire organization's specific goals and continuing objectives will be achieved. Whether this happy state is reached, however, depends on how well the objectives and goals have been defined and parceled out. The managerial task is enormously simplified if objectives are properly defined and allocated. Then, each lower manager will have a specific unit goal that he or she understands, that is within his or her ability, and for which he or she is responsible. Each lower manager knows how it is to be measured and when the deadline is.

The hierarchy of plans successively narrows the problems and alternatives confronting each layer of management. From the realm of all possible areas of actions in the world, the corporate strategy accepts some and rejects others. The continuing objectives eliminate more and the specific goals even more, so that the activities eventually become focused.

Even if the manager's goals and problems are narrower at the middle and lower levels, the ability to achieve them is helped by a knowledge of organizational strategy and an ability to link the unit's goals to the overall objectives. Indeed, subordinates' perceptions of the manager as an effective leader improve

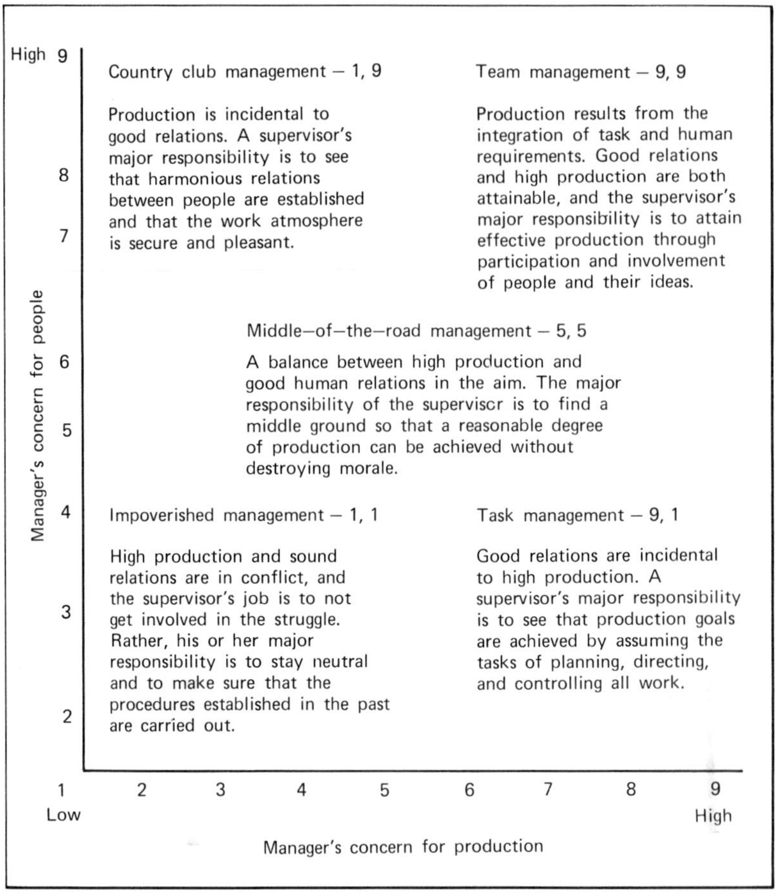
High 9
Country club management – 1, 9
Production is incidental to good relations. A supervisor's major responsibility is to see that harmonious relations between people are established and that the work atmosphere is secure and pleasant.
Team management – 9, 9
Production results from the integration of task and human requirements. Good relations and high production are both attainable, and the supervisor's major responsibility is to attain effective production through participation and involvement of people and their ideas.
8
7
6
5
4
3
2
Manager's concern for people
Middle–of–the–road management – 5, 5
A balance between high production and good human relations in the aim. The major responsibility of the supervisor is to find a middle ground so that a reasonable degree of production can be achieved without destroying morale.
Impoverished management – 1, 1
High production and sound relations are in conflict, and the supervisor's job is to not get involved in the struggle. Rather, his or her major responsibility is to stay neutral and to make sure that the procedures established in the past are carried out.
Task management – 9, 1
Good relations are incidental to high production. A supervisor's major responsibility is to see that production goals are achieved by assuming the tasks of planning, directing, and controlling all work.
1 Low
2
3
4
5
6
7
8
9 High
Manager's concern for production

Figure 6. The Managerial Grid.® (Source: *The New Managerial Grid* by Robert R. Blake and Jane Srygley Mouton. Houston, Gulf Publishing, copyright © 1978, p. 11. Reproduced by permission.)

with their understanding of how the leader and they fit into the organization's planning and control process (48).

Defining the Organization's Mission and Strategy

The questions to be asked in defining the organization fall into four categories (49,50):

1. Services to be provided: What products or services will the organization provide and to whom?
2. Basic ways these services will be produced: What will the organization make, by what processes, and what will it buy from what sources?
3. Sequencing and timing of major steps: What moves will be made early, and what can be deferred?

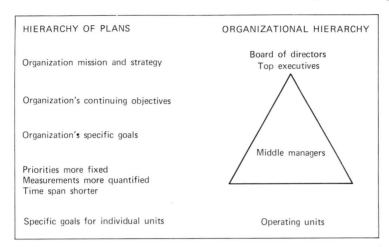

HIERARCHY OF PLANS   ORGANIZATIONAL HIERARCHY

Organization mission and strategy

Organization's continuing objectives

Organization's specific goals

Priorities more fixed
Measurements more quantified
Time span shorter

Specific goals for individual units

Board of directors
Top executives

Middle managers

Operating units

Figure 7. The hierarchy of plans. (Adapted with permission from Ross A. Webber, *Management: Basic Elements of Managing Organizations.* Homewood, Illinois, Richard D. Irwin, revised edition 1979. With permission. © 1979 by Richard D. Irwin, Inc.)

4. Targets to be met: What are the criteria for success, and what levels of achievement are desired?

Two different approaches for formulating strategy have been suggested: outside-in and inside-out (51).

The dream of the entrepreneur who starts a new organization is to discover an unfulfilled public need, a latent demand that people are just waiting to express for a not-yet-invented product or service. If the firm can develop such a product, it will be in the strongest market position. In this case, the firm's strategy will have been shaped by the outside environment. This method of formulating strategy is the outside-in approach.

In some cases, the demand is apparent, but the product or service is not. The oral contraceptive is an example: every pharmaceutical firm knew such a pill would sell, but they did not know how to make it. Management's response to such a clearly discernible potential need is technologic research and development.

Usually, however, the demand is latent: people have not really thought about what new product or service they want. They do not know what they are missing. In this situation, management's central strategy becomes "to create a customer." Ski-mobiles were not in great demand until companies began manufacturing, advertising, and selling them, but a substantial number of people readjusted their wants and expenditures to include ski-mobiles when they became available.

Making latent demands manifest is a more risky venture than is responding to a preexisting but unsupplied market. Identifying latent wants requires intuition and some faith. Most of all, it requires sensitivity to conditions and trends in the world outside the organization (52).

In essence, the outside-in approach to strategic planning requires the manager to monitor continuously the organization's environment to uncover latent demands for goods and services to which he or she can respond. The manager looks for unfulfilled needs that might be converted into wants that he or she can provide. The key seems to be for management to move with the environment rather than attempt to push the world into some shape that management envisions.

The inside-out approach is not a mutually exclusive alternative to the outside-in approach to planning strategy but is a complement to it. The inside-out approach is a necessity for the already successful firm. Management begins to apply this approach by asking itself what its particular skills and differential advantages are. What does the organization offer? What is unique about it?

For example, through the years, Minnesota Mining and Manufacturing Company has evolved into the 3M Company; its products went from sandpaper to roofing materials to reflective signs. These products are in widely different markets with different competitive conditions, but every product is based on a single technical skill—how to apply a closely controlled layer of material on a flexible base. It is a skill with wide application, and 3M is undoubtedly still looking for new ones.

The aim of the inside-out approach is to define the organization's mission in terms as broad as possible but to stay within the limits of its capabilities. As a senior IBM executive put it:

> We want to be in the problem-solving business—this is our mission. Our business is not to make computers. It is to help solve administrative, scientific and even human problems. If your mission is broad enough, you do not find one day that a competitor's new product has outmoded all your equipment (53).

In these examples, management examined what capabilities it possessed and how they might be expanded to new applications or generalized to serve others (54). In short, the organization determined what it had that others could be persuaded to use.

Continuing Objectives

Determining and communicating its continuing objectives makes the organization's strategic planning meaningful to its personnel. These objectives are the continuing concerns of the organization for at least the next five years, probably for the next 10 years, and perhaps forever. Years ago, Drucker pointed out what well-managed businesses have always known: managers should have multiple objectives in addition to profits (55). Here is his list:

· *Customer-client-market standing.* A firm should set objectives on where it wants to be relative to competitors. This objective might be market share, as indicated by the percentage of the total market compared with the competition, or a market niche where one enjoys a competitive advantage.

· *Productivity.* This objective is a ratio like efficiency rather than a measure of gross output. The ratio relates output of goods and services to input of resources, such as labor, hours, materials, and invested capital.

· *State of resources.* This objective relates to maintenance and reflects management's responsibility to protect its equipment, buildings, inventory, and capital funds.

- *Service.* To maintain market position and profitability, service objectives are essential to point out timely and appropriate responses to customers and clients.
- *Innovation.* This objective defines the need for development and delivery of new products or services to maintain market position.
- *Social contribution-public responsibility.* Although in the United States we believe in an inherent right of any person or group to form a business, no such organization has a right to continue unless society deems it valuable. Thus, this objective is concerned with the firm's impact on the environment and the quality of life.

The business objectives described above emphasize results, but we need to also recognize systemic or process objectives that apply to business, health care, and all other organizations (56). The distinction between these two categories is somewhat arbitrary, however, because one shades into the other. Nonetheless, time and attention must be allocated to the process objectives or results will not be maintained for long. The process objectives are:

- *Identification.* Clarity of purpose cannot be assumed. Attention must be devoted to achieving staff consensus and commitment to organizational objectives. This objective requires top management to act as internal salespersons selling the idea of the organization to its own people.
- *Integration.* No organization can exist unless personnel perceive some overlap between their personal objectives and management's objectives. This overlap may mean only exchanging their time for the organization's money, but it
- generally implies a feeling that needs like security, affiliation, and esteem are served by contributing to the organization. Thus, management should be concerned about integrating individual needs and organizational objectives.
- *Social influence.* To make problem-solving and goal achievement more simple, all organizations must distribute power and authority. We used to assume that power flowed from the top down in hierarchic fashion. However, this hierarchic power structure can no longer be assumed because of increased burdens on the top levels and changed expectations at lower levels. Therefore, the distribution of power should be as planned as are other aspects of management.
- *Collaboration.* No matter how well managed, all organizations composed of human beings will experience internal conflict. Rather than bemoaning this conflict as a sign of management's failure or personnel irrationality, management should see it as another area in which to set objectives. That is, management should institute means of managing conflict and measuring their performance in doing so.
- *Adaptation.* Again, no matter how well managed and well planned, all organizations confront changes in the environment. Competitors introduce new technology, market tastes change, and new laws are passed that threaten the institution's viability. Accordingly, management needs to set objectives for monitoring the external world and responding appropriately.
- *Revitalization.* This objective is the most ambiguous one, for it suggests the desirability of change for the sake of change, even though the organization is

not experiencing difficulty and nothing has dramatically altered in the outside world that demands adaptation. Management should be concerned with developing creativity to be ready for proactive rather than reactive responses.

Note that these continuing objectives have no priorities, numbers, or time limits. They simply define in qualitative terms the values that characterize the organization. Most organizations do not have a written statement embracing all their continuing objectives. Rather, these objectives exist in the combined minds of various executives and come into play only when specific goals are being formulated.

Setting Specific Goals

The list of continuing objectives for business and other organizations ignores the competition among them. Because we applied no priorities and set no deadlines for the various objectives, it was possible to discuss them without considering how they operate together. Simultaneously expanding profits and market share, for example, may be impossible, and improving productivity and curbing pollution may be mutually self-defeating (57). When the organization sets goals to be accomplished in a specific time period—next week, month, year, or decade—it encounters conflict among the continuing objectives.

The central difference between continuing objectives and specific goals is that the latter have time limits and measurements: profits should be up $100,000 in the next year; productivity up 10% in six months; market share increased by 5% in five years; capacity expanded by 300,000 tons in two years; occupancy rate increased to 90% from 75% in the next year; average patient length of stay reduced from 4.3 to 3.0 days; food costs per meal reduced from $3.15 to $2.60; and so on. For every specific goal, there should be a deadline for accomplishment and a criterion to measure performance.

Most desirably, each specific goal would be measurable on a bipolar scale (such as good-bad, accept-reject, go-no go) or in numbers (such as pounds, gallons, kilowatts, customers, percentages, or dollars). For each continuing objective, there should be a specific goal for the next relevant time period and a specific indicator by which achievement is to be measured (58).

If a continuing objective has no parallel specific goal for the next appropriate time period, managers are unlikely to devote much attention to it. Their energies will be focused on the specific goals by which their performance is being evaluated. Simply stating that "good patient care" or "high employee morale" are continuing objectives is unlikely to influence the behavior of managers concerned about the bed-occupancy rate, the net rate of return on investment, budget deficit, market share, or productivity. Even stating that the manager's goal is to improve morale by 15% in the next year will have little impact if no indicator is defined or no measurement is taken. To motivate the manager to attempt to improve morale would require more specificity.

The performance indicator will, in fact, measure the specific goal and hence its contribution to the relevant continuing objective. For the more easily quantifiable objectives, such as profitability and productivity, this relationship is clear.

For more subjective objectives, such as morale, however, the relationship between indicators and continuing objectives is more uncertain: turnover statistics
or a score on a test may not really measure morale.

Unfortunately, not all the continuing objectives can be converted into
quantifiable specific goals. How does one quantify public responsibility? Being a
good citizen? Achievement of identification, collaboration, or revitalization? Because such objectives are difficult to measure in quantitative terms, management
must often settle for qualitative statements that suggest what behavior most
probably indicates objective achievement. For example, contributing to the
United Fund and to private colleges may add to meeting social responsibility, not
breaking laws may mean good citizenship, conflict may be being managed well if
strikes are few, or hiring new managers may produce revitalization. These
conclusions are plausible, but proving them with numbers is difficult or impossible.

Control Through Performance Feedback

Whether expressed quantitatively or qualitatively, the specific goals are the basis
for instituting control (59). Feedback control picks up at the end of the planning
process when the specific goals of an employee, department, or organization
become the expected performance against which management will evaluate
actual results. The steps in control are as follows:

1. Communicating specific goals
2. Measuring actual performance
3. Reporting the actual performance to appropriate people
4. Comparing actual performance with specific goals
5. Deciding to do nothing, to correct behavior, or to modify goals

Feedback control is one of the most widespread phenomena of nature, as well
as of modern science and technology. It can be used effectively to improve
performance in the factory, the executive suite, or the physician's office.

Determining appropriate specific goals and performance indicators can be
difficult. The goals and indicators may influence behavior, but not necessarily in
a way that meets the organization's continuing objectives. Managers can develop
elaborate devices for adapting to controls by meeting the standards on paper,
but not always in ways that will promote effectiveness. Therefore, misdirected
control systems are one of the gravest threats to organizational initiative.

People will try to meet the numbers they are measured by. If they cannot
achieve these goals by accepted and desirable behavior, undesirable actions will
result. The Boy Scouts of America discovered that membership figures coming
from the field were false (61). The drive to increase membership had motivated
the field staff to increase the number of new members reported, but it had not
motivated them to increase the number of boys actually enrolled.

Controlling elements may suffer when objectives that can be quantified dominate nonquantifiable ones. If all continuing objectives could be converted into
specific numeric goals, the problem would not exist. But many objectives and

goals cannot be expressed numerically. In competition for a manager's time, numbers dominate. Thus, for some university football teams, measurable objectives like games won and tickets sold carry more weight than do nonquantitative objectives like developing young men's character or providing healthy recreation. Coaches are seldom fired for how the team played the game, but because it lost. It is the same in business. Objectives like profits, productivity, and growth receive more attention than do less quantifiable objectives like public responsibility, manpower development, or revitalization. Since the latter objectives are less easy to measure, evaluation is more subjective and more difficult to justify, and these objectives tend to be ignored. Unfortunately, such action may harm the organization in the long run because it means the deferment of important but more subjective objectives like public responsibility. Moreover, management has not been very clever in formulating performance indicators for such objectives.

It is not surprising that people do not like to be controlled. Even the word "control" has a negative connotation. Although it is natural for people to resent criticism, however, this reaction does not mean control can be eliminated. The common, stressful conditions that lead to anger about controls involve evaluations that are contradictory, uncontrolled, unpredictable, or unattainable (63).

Whether in industry or in health care, one of the most difficult positions is when one can look good on one performance criterion only by sacrificing one's evaluation on another criterion. It is unsettling to be told that one must do well simultaneously on contradictory or competing criteria. Ideally, management should prescribe unambiguous and mutually compatible performance goals that can be achieved simultaneously.

REFERENCES

1. Ryan TA: *Intentional Behavior: An Approach to Human Motivation.* New York, Ronald Press, 1970.
2. Currie L: Wants, needs, well-being, and economic growth. *J Econ Stud* 2:47, 1975.
3. Atkinson JW: *Introduction to Motivation.* Princeton, New Jersey, Van Nostrand, 1964.
4. Vroom V: *Work and Motivation.* New York, John Wiley & Sons, 1964.
5. Siegel E: Decision processes leading to career choices: A study of medicine and accounting. Wharton School, Philadelphia, 1978.
6. Alderfer CP: *Existence, Relatedness and Growth.* New York, Free Press, 1972.
7. Maslow A: A theory of human motivation. *Psychol Rev* 50:370, 1943.
8. Hall DT, Nougain KE: An examination of Maslow's need hierarchy in an organizational setting. *Organ Behav Hum Perform* 3:12, 1968.
9. Winter D: *The Power Motive.* New York, Free Press, 1973.
10. Quester GH: Priviness as the central goal of politics. *Publ Policy* 19:595, 1971.
11. Heckhausen H: *The Anatomy of Achievement Motivation.* New York, Academic Press, 1967.
12. McClelland D, et al: *The Achievement Motive.* New York, Appleton-Century-Crofts, 1953.
13. McClelland D: *The Achieving Society.* Princeton, New Jersey, Van Nostrand, 1961.
14. Tedeschi JT (ed): *Social Influence Processes.* Chicago, Aldine-Atherton, 1972.
15. Wheeler L: *Interpersonal Influence.* Boston, Allyn and Bacon, 1974.
16. Horai J, Tedeschi JT: Effects of credibility and magnitude and punishment or compliance to threats. *J Pers Soc Psychol* 12:164, 1969.

17. Wiard H: Why manage behavior? The case for positive reinforcement. *Hum Resource Manage* Summer, 1972, p 15.

18. Campbell BA, Church RM (eds): *Punishment and Aversive Behavior.* New York, Appleton-Century-Crofts, 1969.

19. Keller RT, Szilagyi AD: Employee reaction to leader reward behavior. *Acad Manage J* 19:619, 1976.

20. Lawler EE: *Pay and Organizational Effectiveness.* New York, McGraw-Hill, 1971.

21. Cammann C, Lawler EE: Employee reactions to a pay incentive plan. *J. App Psychol* 58:163, 1973.

22. Krefting LA, Mahoney TA: Determining the size of a meaningful pay increase. *Ind Relat* 16:83, 1977.

23. Merzberg F, Mausner B, Snyderman BB: *The Motivation to Work.* New York, John Wiley & Sons, 1959.

24. House RJ: A path goal theory of leader effectiveness. *Administ Sci Q* 16:321, 1971.

25. Etzioni A: *Comparative Analysis of Complex Organizations.* New York, Free Press, 1961.

26. French JRP, Raven BH: The bases of social power, in Cartwright D (ed): *Studies in Social Power.* Ann Arbor, University of Michigan Press, 1959, pp. 150–167.

27. Peabody RL: *Organizational Authority.* New York, Atherton Press, 1964.

28. Fayol H: *General and Industrial Management.* London, Pitman and Sons, 1949.

29. Bendix R: *Work and Authority in Modern Industry.* New York, John Wiley & Sons, 1956.

30. Barnard CI: *The Functions of the Executive.* Cambridge, Harvard University Press, 1938.

31. Weber M: *The Theory of Social and Economic Organization.* New York, Free Press, 1964.

32. Borgotta EF, et al: Some findings relevant to the great man theory of leadership. *Am Sociol Rev* 29:755, 1954.

33. Byrne D: *The Attraction Paradigm.* New York, Academic Press, 1971.

34. Coser RL: Authority and decision making in a hospital: A comparative analysis. *Am Sociol Rev* 23:56, 1958.

35. Albanese R: Criteria for evaluating authority patterns. *Acad Manage J* 16:102, 1973.

36. Zimbardo PG, Ebbesen EB: *Influencing Attitudes and Changing Behavior.* Reading, Massachusetts, Addison-Wesley, 1969.

37. Miller GR, Burgoon M: *New Techniques of Persuasion.* New York, Harper & Row, 1973.

38. Aldia O, Stachnik T, Mabry J: Of pigeons and men, in Ulrich R, et al (eds): *Control of Human Behavior.* Glenview, Illinois, Scott, Foresman, 1966.

39. Skinner BF: *Science and Human Behavior.* New York, Macmillan, 1953.

40. Skinner BF: *Beyond Freedom and Dignity.* New York, Knopf, 1971.

41. Mogy RB, Pruitt DG: Effects of a threatener's enforcement costs on threat credibility and compliance. *J Pers Soc Psychol* 29:173, 1974.

42. McGregor D: *The Human Side of Enterprise.* New York, McGraw-Hill, 1960.

43. Forrest CR, Cummings LL, Johnson AC: Organizational participation: A critique and model. *Acad Manage Rev* 2:586, October 1977.

44. Stogdill RM, Coons AE: *Leader Behavior: Its Description and Measurement.* Columbus, Ohio State University Press, 1957.

45. Patchen M: Supervisory methods and group performance norms. *Administ Sci Q* 7:275, 1962.

46. Blake RR, Mouton JS: *The New Managerial Grid.* Houston, Gulf Publishing, 1978.

47. Alderson W: Perspectives on the planning process. *Acad Manage J* 2:181, 1959.

48. Reimnitz CA: Testing a planning and control system in non-profit organizations. *Acad Manage J* 15:77, 1972.

49. Cohen KJ, Cyert RM: Strategy: Formulation, implementation, and monitoring. *J Business* 46:349, 1973.

50. Newman WH: Selecting company strategy. *J Business Policy* 2:60, 1972.

51. Kastens ML: Outside-in planning. *Manage Plan* 22:1, 1974.

52. Guth WD: Formulating organization objectives and strategies: A systematic approach. *J Business Policy* 2:24, 1971.

53. Maisonrouge J: quoted in *Harvard Business Rev* 50:45, January-February 1972.

54. Mintzberg H: Strategy formulation as an historical process. *Int Stud Manage Organ* 7:28, 1977.

55. Drucker P: *The Practice of Management*. New York, Harper & Brothers, 1954.

56. Bennis W: *Organizational Development*. Reading, Massachusetts, Addison-Wesley, 1969.

57. Hackman JT: Drawbacks of continuing corporate growth. *Harvard Business Rev* 52:6, January-February 1974.

58. Latham GP, Yukl GA: A review of research on the application of goal setting in organizations. *Acad Manage Rev* 18:824, 1975.

59. Ouchi W, Maguire MA: Organizational control: Two functions. *Administ Sci Q* 20:559, 1975.

60. Giglioni GB, Bedeian AG: Conspectus of management control theory: 1900–1972. *Acad Manage J* 17:292, 1974.

61. Camman C, Nadler DA: Fit control systems to your managerial style. *Harvard Business Rev* 54:65, 1976.

62. Warner WK, Haven AE: Goal displacement and the intangibility of organizational goals. *Administ Sci Q* 12:539, 1968.

63. Scott WR: Organizational evaluation and authority. *Administ Sci Q* 12:93, 1967.

15
Principles of Management: Organizational Design and Change

Lawrence G. Hrebiniak

Even a cursory examination of formal organizations—whether corporations, hospitals, or universities—reveals that they vary a great deal in many respects. Their products, services, and clients are quite dissimilar, and their organizational designs vary considerably. For example, the automotive firm is vertically integrated: it controls the flow of raw materials into the firm by owning the facilities that produce certain parts and raw materials, and it exercises control over the retail outlets that sell its products. By contrast, the hospital is not vertically integrated: it buys supplies from others, and it gives physicians almost unrestricted control over patient-care decisions. Moreover, control and coordination of tasks are organized differently in the hospital than are control and coordination in the profit-oriented automotive company. People working at the operative level in the two organizations are also quite dissimilar: they are assembly-line workers in one instance and physicians and nurses in the other.

In chapter 14, Webber discussed the role of people and planning in an organization. The purpose of this chapter is to help physicians deal effectively with large organizations by explaining organizational design and organizational change.

Much of the discussion will focus on the hospital as a matrix organization, a special form of organization. Before considering the matrix organization, however, it is necessary to clarify what is meant by organizational design and structure.

ORGANIZATIONAL DESIGN

Definitions

The terms "organizational structure" and "organizational design" are often used interchangeably. The way these terms are used normally does not cause a problem as long as their interchangeable nature is recognized. To avoid confu-

Table 1. Organizational Design: Primary and Secondary Variables

Primary Variables	Secondary Variables
Functional, project, or matrix organization	Centralization or decentralization of authority
Geographic dispersion	Control: self-control, professional control, or top-down bureaucratic control
Size	Coordination or integration mechanisms
Number of hierarchic levels	Participation or involvement in decision-making
Number and type of divisions	

sion, it is helpful to separate design (or structural) variables into primary and secondary variables (1). Table 1 provides examples of each type of variable. Primary variables describe the organization in a concrete or physical sense, in terms of its configuration, size, or geographic dispersion. Secondary variables describe how the organization functions; they include internal structure or operational processes, such as control, degree of central authority, or coordination mechanisms.

The two sets of variables are related, but there is no perfect or necessary correspondence between the two. For example, assume that there are two different organizations with product groups called divisions (Ford Division, Psychiatric Division, or Consumer Products Division), a primary design variable according to Table 1. It may be that division managers in one organization have complete authority to make decisions about investments, hiring policies, admissions, and a host of related factors. By contrast, managers in the second organization must seek approval from headquarters for virtually all major decisions. The first organization is decentralized, and the second is centralized; they are distinguished on the basis of a secondary variable. Despite their similarity on the basis of the primary design variable (division structure), the two organizations are quite different according to a secondary design variable (centralization of authority).

In addition, every organization is influenced by its environment (2). It engages in exchange with external groups—suppliers, professional associations, governmental regulatory agencies, patients, and unions—to attain necessary inputs and dispose of output. It somehow transforms inputs into output. The automobile firm sells cars and receives money, which, in turn, is used to manufacture additional cars. The hospital performs a valuable health service for clients; payment received is used to purchase equipment and pay the salaries of the professional staff, thereby ensuring the provision of future medical care. Every organization interacts and bargains with external constituents as it defines its own future.

Organizations transform the inputs into output; this process constitutes the technology of the organization, which is itself an important factor in determining the structure or design of the organization. In the university medical school, the interaction between students and professors is part of the conversion process. The technology in the mental hospital involves the direct interaction of the psychiatrist or psychologist with the patient. The general hospital uses its technology to transform sick people into well people.

Technologies differ in many respects, and these differences produce their own effects on the organization. Differing technologies determine the tasks performed, the level of professionalism, the number and the type of external linkages, and the control structure used. It is easy to see why the automotive firm is different from the hospital. The technologies are different, as are the tasks performed, the level of staff professionalism, and the means of coordination and control.

Examining organizations as open systems explains some of their differences. A hospital that must deal with a strong union, for instance, will have an industrial relations unit, whereas a nonunionized hospital will not. A for-profit hospital facing a large number of competitors will be organized so as to maximize efficiency and income, and it likely will not treat all types of patients. A teaching or university hospital will be organized quite differently because it must serve different external groups.

Different organizations will be confronted with different external forces, different technologies, and different products, and they should be organized to meet these different demands. There is no one organizational structure that is appropriate for every organization, but different organizations may have similar structures because of similarities in environmental influences, technologies, and products. An organization has several different design options; these options include purpose, process, and matrix designs. Many hospitals have adopted the matrix design.

Design Options

Consider first a small manufacturing firm with one product and a two-part (A and B) production process (3). The organizational design is relatively simple and is called purpose departmentation (Fig. 1). To manufacture an output, processes A and B are coordinated by the manager. For example, in a small health clinic, the administrator or physician may coordinate the flow of patients through two different departments, such as the x-ray department and the clinical laboratory.

When a second product is introduced, the manager has two design alternatives. The first alternative is to retain the purpose departmentation (Fig. 2) and create separate manufacturing processes (A_1 and B_1, A_2 and B_2) for each product. Ease of management is the principal benefit. Each product has its own

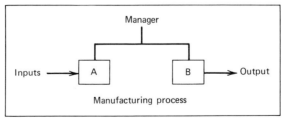

Figure 1. Purpose departmentation with a single product.

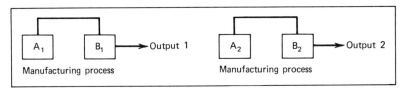

Figure 2. Purpose departmentation with two products.

organization, thereby eliminating the scheduling and coordination problems that would exist if both products relied on only one centralized process. As an example, Figure 2 suggests that the psychiatric department would have its own staff, as would the medical department.

There are potential costs, however, despite the simplicity of this design. The most important is that purpose departmentation can prevent the economies of large-scale production. The second alternative is to design the organization around common processes or functions (Fig. 3). The manager's task is to coordinate the flow of work for different products through a common facility enabling the component divisions of the organization to specialize according to the processes that they perform. As an example, Figure 3 suggests that both psychiatric and medical patients would use the same ancillary services; their flow would be coordinated by a general manager.

Process specialization, however, is not without its own problems. The benefits are those of specialization and economies of scale, but the problems result from the increased need for coordination. The problems become worse if the number of products (or types of patients) is increased. As the number increases, coordination costs increase.

There is a point at which the economic benefits of process specialization are outweighed by the costs of coordination. To avoid this problem, the manager can combine purpose specialization with process specialization in a division structure and reap the benefits of each (Fig. 4). When the costs resulting from coordination requirements approach the economic benefits derived from process specialization, the organization should be reorganized according to product, geographic area, or customer type. The organization should reincorporate purpose departmentation into the design by creating a division structure with process subunits. Each purpose grouping has its own process. For example, each school in the university would have its own faculty, research facilities, and fund-raising activities. In the industrial sphere, General Motors is composed of separate

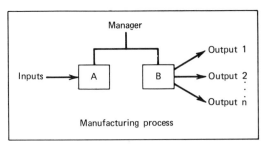

Figure 3. Process specialization.

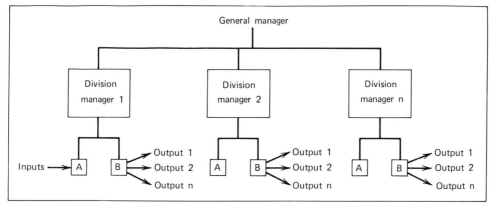

Figure 4. Division structure.

distinct divisions (e.g., Chevrolet and Buick), and each is able to develop its own manufacturing and sales process. The benefits are those of self-containment and independence; each dean or division manager need not be concerned with his or her counterpart in other divisions of the larger organization.

However, such a design is costly when there are interdependences, common communication requirements, and opportunities for cross fertilization across projects (4). To illustrate, consider an organization like the National Aeronautics and Space Administration (NASA). Many projects are the rule, but the organization is not separated into divisions. Manufacturing an advanced communications system for one satellite creates new technologies that can be adapted for use in other projects. An organizational design that allows functional areas to serve different projects for limited time periods, depending on the need, is well suited to organizations with many, but similar, projects.

The matrix design was created to provide the flexibility needed for these organizations (Fig. 5). In the matrix model of organizational design, employees from functional areas perform services for one project for a limited period of time. They become part of the project team for the duration of the project. They serve two supervisors. In Figure 5, Engineer B reports both to the chief of engineering and, while the project lasts, to the manager of Project 1. When the project is complete, the engineer leaves Project 1 to join a new project team. At some level, there is system-wide perspective to ensure that project deadlines are met and that needed personnel are allocated properly to meet deadlines and performance measures.

In brief, the matrix design stresses both horizontal and vertical communication; it is a project (or "purpose") organization superimposed on a functional (or "process") organization. Functional people can be moved to projects to solve problems as they arise. Emphasis is placed on getting the right people to deal with the problem and solve it without referring every problem up to the project manager, who, in turn, would be forced to make a decision and pass it back down the hierarchy.

There is bilateral dependence between project and function in the matrix. Project managers depend on the expertise of functional personnel; functional managers depend on project managers to use their employees' time and skills

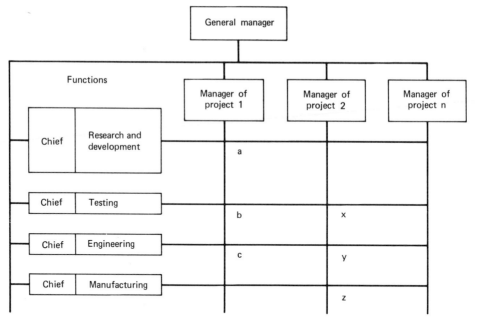

Figure 5. Matrix organization. The team working on Project 1 includes Employees a, b, and c. The team working on Project 2 includes Employees x, y, and z.

and justify their existence in the organization. The constraints of budget and time and the concern for a common, superordinate goal help ensure that functional employees are used properly and that deadlines, performance, and quality constraints are met.

The Hospital as a Matrix Organization

Because the hospital is an organization with many, but similar, tasks, it is well suited for the matrix form of management (Fig. 6).

Each patient is managed as a separate project supervised by the patient's physician. The physician arranges for the patient to receive services from a team of specialized employees, each of whom is drawn from a department in the hospital with its own director. As shown in Figure 5, there is bilateral dependence, and a superordinate goal (quality care) exists to integrate the system and guarantee efficient and effective performance.

A hospital employing the matrix design may have ambiguous lines of authority. There may be duality of control: nurses adhere to physicians' requests in certain matters, but in others, nursing supervisors have the final say.

Consider the methods for achieving coordination. The task is to coordinate (a secondary structural variable) within the matrix form of the organization (a primary variable). Table 2 shows some ways to achieve coordination. Hierarchic coordination, including reliance on rules, performance programs, and standardized procedures, is most feasible when tasks are relatively simple. As tasks become more complex, however, standard procedures or responses become insufficient, and it is necessary to provide for lateral coordination.

In a hospital or community health center, a common device for lateral coor-

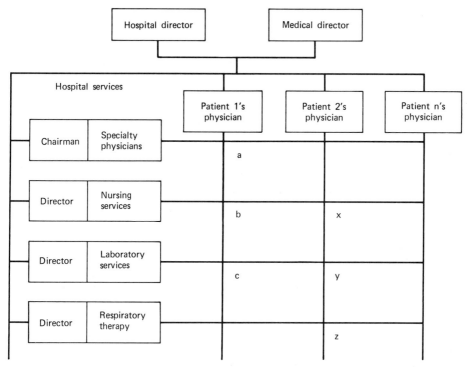

Figure 6. The hospital as a matrix organization. Patient 1 is cared for by Employees a, b, and c. Patient 2 is cared for by Employees x, y, and z.

Table 2. Means of Attaining Effective Coordination*

Means/Techniques	*Example*
Hierarchic coordination	
Traditional scalar hierarchy	This organization is the classic one, with hierarchically imposed rules, regulations, and standardized procedures
Staff personnel and departments	Staff are "assistants to" someone and back up the hierarchy
Automation	Information is processed and decisions are made by computers
Lateral coordination	
Management committees, task forces, or teams	These groups coordinate activities among independent or separate departments
Direct communication by persons from different departments	Personal contacts
Work teams made up of persons from different departments at the production level	The patient-care team uses the patient's medical record as a coordinating device
Integrators, integrating departments	Unit managers, scheduling departments, and expeditors

*Adapted from Neuhauser (5).

dination is the patient-care team (6,7). Team members bring their own expertise to the problem; they need not pass information on to superiors and wait for a decision. Thus, treatment is more timely. Team decision-making is also more suited to complex tasks for which no one person can collect sufficient information to make an effective diagnosis. Finally, the existence of the many perspectives of the team members (e.g., R.N.s, M.D.s, and social workers) helps to ensure that concerns are aired and political problems are avoided. Teams are not free of conflict, but they can coordinate the work of diverse kinds of employees for the benefit of the patient.

In summary, the matrix design of the hospital fosters flexibility and timely attention to patients' needs. To provide health-care services, emphasis is placed on lateral relations across different project areas.

Problems with Matrix Organizations

There are many conditions in the health industry that cause health care organizations to operate less smoothly than their private-industry counterparts. These problems stem largely from the power or influence structure in the health industry and the nature of the control, or incentive, system (2).

In health care, the physician enjoys influence over other professionals and administrators. The basis of this power is twofold. First of all, only the physician fully understands, interprets, and, most importantly, uses the technology of patient care. Because he or she has received formal medical training, the patient and hospital staff depend on the physician for expert health care; the physician is the sole "absorber of uncertainty" for others whose tasks rely on certainty and structure, for example, specific instructions for treatment and medication. Second, the physician brings in the paying customer, thereby providing the critical resource of income to the institution. The hospital administrator whose occupancy rate is low depends on physicians for increased admissions. To the administrator whose performance is being judged in terms of income, the physician is perceived as being responsible for the solution of the problem.

Under these conditions, the physician becomes increasingly influential, and the administrator or manager becomes increasingly dependent. A problem arises if this influence becomes more and more unilateral, with the physician wielding greater and greater control, for the matrix cannot operate easily under these conditions. Recall that for the matrix to function effectively, dependence cannot be unilateral. Thus, the hospital matrix requires that the physician and administrator keep lines of communication open. Each must confront issues openly, including conflicts, to maintain coordination.

The goals and the control system are related problems. The solution of conflicts in the matrix depends to a large degree on the existence of superordinate goals. That is, the control system must be unified around a common purpose. By contrast, the control system in a hospital is usually fragmented, not unitary (8,9). Physicians and other professionals often have a cosmopolitan outlook characterized by concern with external reference groups (colleagues), the desire to maintain professional standards and avoid organizational standards, and the desire to allow only professionals to monitor and evaluate the work of other professionals (10). These desires are often in direct conflict with administrative criteria that stress organizational control.

A fragmented control system with its inevitable conflict argues against the matrix design. Whereas the patient care team can focus on the superordinate goal of responding quickly and effectively to the needs of a single patient, a superordinate goal does not always exist for the hospital as an organization. A fragmented control structure with conflict between professionals and administrators does not maintain superordinate goals, nor does it allow open confrontation and solution of conflicts.

Therefore, an organization like a hospital, which has three "systems" (management, governance, and professional systems), may not be an extremely good candidate for the matrix design (11). Whereas concrete goals, clear formal authority, high task interdependence, and measurable performance criteria exist in most industries, the absence of these conditions complicates the matrix in hospitals and other health care organizations. The control system is fragmented by the professional identity system, which retains ultimate responsibility for standards of medical practice and which stresses the culture of medical science and downplays organizational identity and the governance system. The costs include poor communication between professionals and administrators and inadequate resolution of conflict.

There are steps that can eliminate many of these problems; they include the following (11):

· Clarifying the hospital's goals
· Budgeting both according to department and program (function and project) to encourage integrated activity
· Involving professionals in managerial tasks
· Planning resource management more deliberately
· Bringing physicians and other professionals into institutional budget discussions
· Using team approaches to decisions that affect both professionals and administrators
· Discussing problems, constraints, and opportunities in formal group sessions designed toward that end

The purpose is not to limit professional autonomy in health care organizations, for that would be disastrous. The purpose is to allow both professionals and administrators to work in a matrix organization and to unify their activity around the major tasks of the organization.

ORGANIZATIONAL CHANGE

Organizational design and the process of management are not static (2,12,13). The organization is an open system, dealing with external groups whose demands affect organizational structure and management. Both internal and external pressures continue to shape policies, design, and measures of performance as organizational change takes place.

The Environment and Change

The environment is important for organizational structure and management. Table 3 shows the effect of stability or uncertainty on structural variables, such as central decision-making and coordination. Organizations that face stable, predictable situations have fairly simple secondary structures; they use rules and standardized procedures for control and make most major decisions centrally. By contrast, where conditions are unpredictable and complex, one cannot rely on set procedures and rules for coordination. When the environment is uncertain, organizational design is more complex, and management becomes increasingly important. Changes in environmental certainty and complexity thus induce changes in organizational design and management.

Legal constraints place important pressures on hospitals, as evidenced by the effects exerted by the Office of Economic Opportunity, which enforces regulations about employment of minority groups. Other outside forces include the demands of patients, the actions of competitors, and technologic innovations.

Changes in the number of products or services provided, the types of patient treated, or the need for coordination of common services can affect organizational design. For example, a small general hospital can operate easily with a divisional structure (purpose specialization) by offering a limited number of services and having those services self-contained. Expansion of services, however, combined with an increased need to coordinate the flow of patients across the diverse service areas, can cause the hospital to change to a matrix structure. Similarly, technologic change can result in process specialization as many different departments or even hospitals must coordinate the movement of patients through a central facility or location where a piece of sophisticated equipment is located. The point is that organizational design is not immutable but, rather, is dependent on the forces and pressures placed on the organization.

Internally Generated Change

Change often results from the interplay of forces at the boundary of the organization with its environment, but change can also be generated internally.

Table 3. Nature of Organization Environments and Examples of Effects on the Organization

Environments	
Stable/Certain	*Shifting/Uncertain*
Simple in structure, e.g., its boundary-spanning components	Greater complexity of structure, e.g., greater number of boundary-spanning components
Centralization of decision-making, few functional divisions	Decentralization of decision-making
Adaptation by rules and performance programs	Adaptation by adjustment
Administration by rule enforcement	Less reliance on standard procedures and rules in administration

Internal change may occur without deliberate assessment of the external environment. Alterations in the flow of work, modifications in physical layout, changing spans of control, reassignment of personnel, and development of training programs seem, at first glance, to be examples of internal changes made without consideration of the outside environment. Yet, two points must be kept in mind. First, even these changes stem from the interplay of forces between the organization and its environment. For example, the development of new training programs is based on outside scientific developments and evidence concerning employees' social needs. Second, many changes within organizations can best be understood as the result of forces acting across the boundaries that separate subunits within the organization.

Resources and Change

A perceived need for change is a necessary, but not always sufficient, cause of change. Creating a better organization is one thing; having the resources to implement change is sometimes quite another. The resources needed to effect change include authority in matters pertaining to change. Physicians may be able to act autonomously in areas under their jurisdiction and to bring about a change because others recognize the change as necessary and legitimate.

The perceived need for change often varies directly with organizational professionalization; a high level of professionalization in an organization is an important resource for change. There is also a positive relation between professionalization and innovation; the greater the level of professionalization, the more likely people are to support innovative proposals.Therefore, in organizations like hospitals, the demand for excellence fostered by professional employees is an asset for change.

In cases where there exists an overriding concern with power and an avoidance of both risk and conflict, however, the climate is not conducive to change or the introduction of innovative procedures (14). Physicians and research scientists perform tasks filled with uncertainty. Control over one's project is a necessary condition of work, and attempts by the organization to impose administrative rules or bureaucratic procedures that limit self-control are strenuously opposed (10,15,16). The conclusions are fairly clear: organizational mechanisms geared toward control must be compatible with the needs of the professional staff for innovation. Administrative and professional staff must, therefore, confront these problems openly to ensure effective organizational performance.

Assessing Change

Assessing change is the important final step in the change process. Assessment is not always easy because the effects of change may not be clearly visible. Accurate assessment depends wholly on the type of change undertaken, the criteria against which change is evaluated, and the values of the persons involved in the assessment (2).

Consider the case of a manufacturing firm whose production process is obsolete, resulting in poor quality and loss of profit. The firm is likely to see the effects of new technology easily; any change in product quality is a direct result of technical change. Other situations, however, may be far less clear. For example, an attempt may be made to improve the nursing staff's response to patients' calls for assistance that involves a change in personal attitudes, but attitudes are not easily measured. Successful assessment depends equally on objective criteria and on the values and perceptions of the persons involved in the process. It is, therefore, not at all surprising that successful changes in technique are often reported by those responsible for developing and using them in the first place, especially in the absence of objective criteria.

OVERVIEW AND IMPLICATIONS

The organization is an open system constantly engaged in exchanges with its environment that generate pressures on the organization. Their strength depends on the organization's power over external elements and on its ability to reduce or eliminate dependence. Conversely, the pressures it feels depend on its vulnerability to the environment.

Organizational design and change are two outcomes of this exchange process. The matrix design is a response to increasing technologic complexity under conditions in which the organization can benefit most by sharing functional personnel across projects and decision-making is best decentralized.

It is important to remember that design affects people's tasks and can create "people problems." For instance, the demands for efficiency that created the assembly line also led to problems of boredom, alienation, and personnel turnover. The most obvious problem in the matrix organization is conflict. On the positive side, one important outcome of confronting conflict is problem-solving and maintaining task orientation. Another problem is frustration from unclear authority when, for example, a nurse has to deal with two supervisors—the physician in charge and the head nurse.

In brief, the manager and physician must be aware of the factors that affect organizational design and the problems created by organizational design and change. Understanding the problems of the hospital administrator can help the physician deal with the complexities of the hospital and large group practices. It can also provide a common ground for developing superordinate goals through proper task coordination and effective communication between administrative and medical staff.

REFERENCES

1. Melcher AJ: *Structure and Process of Organizations: A Systems Approach.* Englewood Cliffs, New Jersey, Prentice-Hall, 1976.
2. Hrebiniak LG: *Complex Organizations.* St. Paul, Minnesota, West Publishing, 1978.
3. March JG, Simon HA: *Organizations.* New York, John Wiley & Sons, 1958.
4. Galbraith J: *Designing Complex Organizations.* Reading, Massachusetts, Addison-Wesley, 1973.
5. Neuhauser D: The hospital as a matrix organization. *Hosp Administ* Fall, 1972, pp. 8–25.
6. Rubin I, Beckhard R: Factors influencing the effectiveness of health teams. *Milbank Mem Fund Q* 50:317, 1972.
7. Wise H, Rubin I, Beckhard R: Making health teams work. *Am J Dis Child* 127:537, 1974.

8. Hrebiniak LG: Job technology, supervision, and work-group structure. *Administ Sci Q* 19:395, 1974.

9. Woodward J: *Industrial Organization: Behavior and Control.* London, Oxford University Press, 1970.

10. Gouldner A: Cosmopolitans and locals: Toward an analysis of latent social roles. *Administ Sci Q* 2:282, 1957.

11. Weisbord M: Why organization development hasn't worked (so far) in medical centers. *Health Care Manage Rev* 17:28, 1976.

12. Thompson JD: *Organizations in Action.* New York, McGraw-Hill, 1967.

13. Lawrence P, Lorsch J: *Organizational and Environment.* Cambridge, Massachusetts, Harvard University Press, 1967.

14. Pelz DC, Andrews FM: *Scientists in Organizations: Productive Climates for Research and Development.* New York, John Wiley & Sons, 1966.

15. Blaw PM, Scott WR: *Formal Organizations.* San Francisco, Chandler, 1962.

16. Vollmer CR, Mills DL (eds): *Professionalization.* Englewood Cliffs, New Jersey, Prentice-Hall, 1966.

16
Reading the Medical Literature

Paul D. Stolley
Joan L. Davies

In the field of medicine, as in all scientific endeavor, the serious student must constantly read pertinent articles and keep abreast of new developments reported in the literature. The critical evaluation of scientific literature is a skill, which, like any other, requires practice and continual application for its successful acquisition. Furthermore, to critically evaluate research reports, one must understand the fundamentals of research strategies. A knowledge of statistical methods and reasoning is also necessary to be an informed consumer of research reports and scientific literature.

In chapter 17, Steinmann describes how the practicing clinician might undertake a clinical investigation; in this chapter, we shall describe the usual outline followed in medical and scientific articles and suggest questions the reader should ask in evaluating these reports; we shall also briefly describe the aims and applications of descriptive and inferential statistics as used in medical research. Our purpose is to leave the reader with a framework for the analysis of scientific articles that can be applied whenever it is helpful.

STRUCTURE OF SCIENTIFIC ARTICLES

Most articles start with a summary, or abstract, which should describe the methods used and the principal findings in concise form. One should read this summary carefully, since it will act as a guide for reading the rest of the article. The summary tells the important findings, and it is the reader's task to decide whether the conclusions are justified by the data presented.

The introduction to the article is designed to summarize the literature leading up to the present research or investigation. It should review the findings of previous investigators in an unbiased fashion and explain why the present research project was initiated and is important. In this section, the reader should try to identify the precise question or questions that the author or authors hoped to answer, in other words, the aims and objectives of their research.

247

The materials (or methods) section usually follows and should provide a detailed description of the research design, the research instrument or instruments, and the general content of the study.

The questions that one will want to ask when reading this section include the following:

1. Is the research design experimental or observational?
2. If it is experimental, was randomization carried out? How was randomization carried out?
3. Was "blinding" used so that neither the investigator nor the subject was aware of which group was receiving the tested intervention?
4. For both experimental and observational studies, was the number of subjects sufficient to show important differences?
5. If the study is observational, is it a cohort (prospective) or case-control (retrospective) design?
6. Is the study controlled? In other words, is there a comparison group? How was it chosen? Is is truly comparable?

Freedman et al., in their excellent book *Statistics* (1), advise:

When looking at a study, ask the following questions [Fig. 1]. Was there any control group at all? If so, how were subjects assigned to treatment or control: through a process under the control of the investigator (a controlled experiment), or through a process outside the control of the investigator (an observational study)? If it was a controlled experiment, was the assignment made using a chance mechanism (randomized controlled) or did it depend on the judgment of the investigator? With observational studies, and even with nonrandomized controlled experiments, try to find out in detail how the subjects came to be in treatment or control [groups]. How are the treatment groups similar? different? What factors are confounded with treatment—that is, what could explain a difference in response between the two groups, apart from treatment? What adjustments were made to take care of confounding? Were they sensible?

The results section of the article presents the findings and usually contains tabulated data and graphs describing the data. It is likely that the author's conclusions will stand or fall depending on the information found in the tables

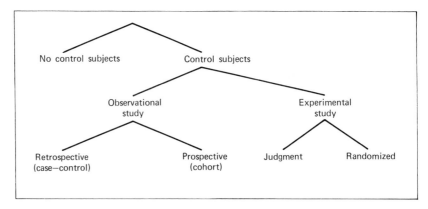

Figure 1. Classifying investigations.

presented and discussed in this section. Many find tables dull and tend to skip them in their reading of scientific articles. It would be a serious mistake to skip the tables: reading and interpreting tables is a necessary skill for the informed reader of medical literature.

When examining a table, the reader should note the following:

1. Is the table concise and yet still informative? Is the table comprehensive?
2. What is the source of the data? Are there any footnotes indicating the source?
3. Are the format, the strata, and the intervals in the body of the table all reasonable? Are there patterns and inconsistencies in the data?
4. What are the conclusions that can be derived from examining the tables (and graphs)?

The final part of the usual medical article is a discussion of the results. What do the results mean, and what are the implications of the findings? The value of many an otherwise excellent article has been diminished due to unwarranted speculations and overly broad conclusions that are based on limited data. The reader will want to ask whether the author's conclusions are justified by the data that they present. Is the explanation of their findings the only possible one? Is it the most likely? Does it best fit the facts?

ANALYSIS OF DATA

There is a universal trend in medical literature to apply statistical methods to the data. Statistics, when computed from data collected on a sample, may be either descriptive or inferential.

Descriptive statistics characterize the sample but do not lead to any conclusions about the population sampled. If the sample consists of patients with a specific disease, descriptive statistics might include the proportion of the patients identified through various medical centers, the proportion of the patients in the various stages of disease at diagnosis, and the mean age of the patients at diagnosis.

Inferential statistics are used to draw conclusions about the population sampled. The author may wish to generalize from a small case series seen in one clinic to a larger group of patients. Or the author may have samples from several populations; for example, one could look for a difference in the rate of lung cancer among workers exposed and not exposed to a suspected chemical carcinogen used in an industrial process. Inferences are usually in the form of a statement about the sampled population(s) accompanied by some measure of uncertainty. The two types of inferential statistics most commonly used in medical literature are tests of hypotheses (or tests of significance) and confidence intervals.

Hypothesis Testing

In hypothesis testing, the statement is either the acceptance or the rejection of a hypothesis concerning the distribution of a characteristic in the population or populations; the measure of uncertainty is the probability, decided in advance, that a correct hypothesis will be rejected. Hypothesis testing involves specifying the hypothesis to be tested (the null hypothesis), selecting a test statistic (a measure of the inconsistency of the data with the null hypothesis), and establishing a critical region (a set of values for the test statistic that are so inconsistent with the null hypothesis that this hypothesis will be rejected if one of these values is obtained from the sample). The critical region is often chosen to be the 5% of results that one is least likely to obtain if the null hypothesis is correct.

For example, consider patients with a specified condition randomly selected from all patients admitted to a hospital for this condition during a specified time period. All the specially selected patients are given a new drug, and the proportion showing improvement within one week is noted. It is known that one half of all patients given the standard treatment can be expected to show improvement within this time. One wishes to test whether the proportion of patients improving on the new drug is the same as the proportion improving on the standard treatment. Therefore, the null hypothesis is: "The proportion of patients improving on the new drug is no different than the proportion improving on the standard treatment or 0.50."

If 62% of 102 patients who received the new drug improve, it is not clear from simply inspecting the data that the difference between 0.62 and 0.50 reflects a real difference in the two treated populations or whether it occurred by chance. A test statistic can help the investigator make the decision. In this case, Z is an appropriate test statistic.

It is calculated as follows:

$$Z = \left| \frac{0.62 - 0.50}{\sqrt{(0.50)(0.50)/102}} \right|$$

As seen from the formula, the larger the difference between the proportion improving with the new drug and the proportion improving with the standard treatment, the larger is Z and the more inconsistent are the data with the null hypothesis. From tables, it can be determined that a 5% critical region for Z consists of those values greater than 1.96 (1–3). A calculated value for Z that falls in this critical region indicates that the results of the experiment would be unlikely to occur if the null hypothesis were correct. In our example, the calculated value for Z is 2.42, which is greater than 1.96 and thus falls in the critical region. We reject the null hypothesis and conclude that the level of improvement among patients receiving the new drug is not the same as the level of improvement among patients receiving the standard treatment. The difference in the improvement rates appears to be real and not due to sampling variation.

The Z test statistic is appropriate for only a small number of the investigations the physician will read about in the medical literature. Other common test statistics are the "chi-squared" test and "Student's t" test. Many others are used. The choice of a test statistic depends on how one selects a control group and measures the outcome, as well as on other factors.

Significance Testing

Although there are many different test statistics, it is not necessary to memorize the critical region for each one to determine if an investigator has correctly decided to reject the null hypothesis. In most cases and regardless of the test statistic used, the author will calculate a p value. A p value is the probability that the data (i.e., data that are at least as inconsistent with the null hypothesis as those observed) would arise by chance if the null hypothesis were correct. In the example used above, where Z equals 2.42, the p value would be reported as "$p = 0.008$."

P values must be interpreted with caution. A low p value indicates that one of the following is true: either the null hypothesis is correct and a very unlikely event has occurred, or the null hypothesis is not correct. If the p value is low, one must doubt the null hypothesis because of the tendency not to believe in rare events. However, a low p value says nothing about how the null hypothesis fails to describe the population or populations and nothing about the severity of the failure.

If the p value is lower than a chosen level, the results are said to be "statistically significant," and the null hypothesis is rejected. The chosen level is arbitrary, depending on the investigator's concept of a very unlikely event; a level of 5% is most commonly used in the medical literature. The lower the level chosen, the less likely one is to conclude that there is a difference when there is not (or, stated another way, to reject the null hypothesis when it is correct—a Type I error). By contrast, the lower the level chosen, the more likely one is to conclude that there is no difference when, in fact, there is (or, stated differently, to fail to reject a null hypothesis that is incorrect—a Type II error). In practice, the level chosen often depends on which error is more important to avoid.

Rejection of the null hypothesis (statistical significance) means that data at least as inconsistent with the null hypothesis as those observed would be unlikely to arise by chance. It is not proof of failure of the null hypothesis; if the hypothesis is correct and a level of 5% is used, 5% of such data are expected to be statistically significant.

Failure to reject the null hypothesis (lack of statistical significance) means that the data do not provide evidence against the null hypothesis since data this inconsistent or more so would frequently arise by chance. It is not proof that the null hypothesis is correct; the data may be consistent with several alternative hypotheses, including an incorrect null hypothesis.

Statistical significance must be distinguished from practical or clinical significance (importance). Since it is unusual that a hypothesis about a population is exactly correct, one can almost always show statistical significance if enough data are collected. Statistical significance does not necessarily mean that the failure of the hypothesis is of any practical or clinical importance.

In our example, the low p value allows us to reject the null hypothesis— patients who received the new drug did not have the same rate of improvement as did patients receiving the standard therapy. However, the low p value alone does not allow us to conclude that the better improvement was caused by the new drug, only that it was associated with the new drug. We must combine the low p value with other information to make a statement about the cause of the improvement. It may have been, for example, that only the patients most likely to improve were given the new drug or that the new drug was accompanied by more intensive nursing care or closer observation for complications—any one of these factors could explain the improvement. The overall design should have been constructed to prevent such factors from biasing the results. Unless the design is clearly described, it is impossible for the reader to evaluate causal inferences.

Confidence Intervals

Confidence intervals are closely related to hypothesis testing. The statement about the population or populations sampled is a set of estimates for one feature of the distribution of a characteristic in the population or populations. The measure of uncertainty is the proportion of such intervals that will actually contain the true population value. Thus, 5% of all 95% confidence intervals will fail to contain the population value. On the basis of the observed sample with 62% improvement, a 95% confidence interval for the proportion of patients improving with the new drug is (0.53, 0.71). A 95% confidence interval is usually the set of population values that would not be rejected by the sample results at the 5% level in hypothesis testing; it is a set of population values that are consistent with the data. As such, all the problems that arise in the interpretation of tests of hypotheses also arise in the interpretation of confidence intervals.

Cautions

Several cautions in the use of inferential statistics should be emphasized. The data should be of a quality worthy of statistical analysis and in a form amenable to statistical analysis. The methods chosen should be appropriate for the sampling scheme employed and the questions of interest. The population sampled should be clearly identified, and the assumptions involved in the use of inferential statistics should be justified for this population. Last, classic inferential statistics, such as hypothesis testing and confidence intervals, are based on the concept of controlled error rates in repeated sampling. They are, therefore, ideally suited for maintaining quality control in industrial processes, where the overall rate of error rather than an individual decision is important. In medical research, however, only one sample is usually available, and the motivation for testing is quite different. The correct interpretation of classic inferential statistics is limited, and caution must be taken that they are not interpreted in a way that is incorrect. There is no assurance that hypothesis testing will lead to a correct decision regarding the null hypothesis or that a confidence interval will encompass the true population value. Significance testing gives no indication of clinical importance, and p values alone contain no information about the magnitude of the discrepancy between the observed sample value and the hypothesized value. These statistical methods alone cannot be used to make causal inferences.

Statistical methods are an integral part of any research project involving samples. They enable the data to be summarized to characterize a sample in a meaningful way, and they allow inferences to be made about the population or populations from which a sample was drawn. Statistical methods enable one to measure the uncertainty in a statement made about the population or populations on the basis of a sample—the uncertainty introduced by the actual process of sampling.

SUMMARY

When reading an article in the medical literature, a tolerant yet critical attitude should be assumed by the reader. An understanding of the fundamental research strategies, the structure and format of medical articles, and the basic principles of statistics are prerequisites for judging the worth of a report. It is helpful to approach the article with an organized set of questions to aid in the analysis. An outline successfully used for many years is reprinted here (Table 1). Finally, the reader of medical articles should always keep in mind that it is

Table 1. Outline for Critique of a Medical Report*

Objectives of the research
   What are the objectives of the study or the questions to be answered?
   What is the population to which the investigators intend to refer their findings?
Design of the investigation
   Was the study an experiment, planned observations, or an analysis of records?
   How was the sample selected? Are there possible sources of selection that would make the sample atypical or nonrepresentative? If so, what provision was made to deal with this bias?
   What is the nature of the control group or standard of comparison?
Observations
   Are there clear definitions of the terms used, including diagnostic criteria, measurements made, and criteria of outcome?
   Was the method of classification or of measurement consistent for all the subjects and relevant to the objectives of the investigation? Are there possible biases in measurement, and, if so, what provisions were made to deal with them?
   Are the observations reliable and reproducible?
Presentation of findings
   Are the findings presented clearly, objectively, and in sufficient detail to enable the reader to judge them?
   Are the findings internally consistent? For example, do the numbers add up properly, and can the different tables be reconciled?
Analysis
   Are the data worthy of statistical analysis? If so, are the methods of statistical analysis appropriate to the source and nature of the data, and is the analysis correctly performed and interpreted?
   Is there sufficient analysis to determine whether "significant differences" may, in fact, be due to lack of comparability of the groups in sex or age distribution, in clinical characteristics, or in other relevant variables?
Conclusions
   Which conclusions are justified by the findings? Which conclusions are not? Are the conclusions relevant to the questions posed by the investigators?
Constructive suggestions
   Assume that you are planning an investigation to answer the questions put in this study. If they have not been clearly put by the authors, frame them in an appropriate manner. Suggest a practical design, criteria for observations, and type of analysis that would provide reliable and valid information relevant to the question under study.

Source: From Colton (3). By permission of Little, Brown and Company.

difficult to carry out research and easier to criticize it. The critic should be able to suggest constructive ways to improve the research and not merely complain of inadequacies. When searching for better ways to conduct the research, the reader may discover that there are none, and the investigators did the best they could given that particular research question and the population available to them.

REFERENCES

1. Freedman D, Pisani R, Purves R: *Statistics.* New York, WW Norton and Company, 1978.
2. Day RA: *How to Write and Publish a Scientific Paper.* Philadelphia, ISI Press, 1979.
3. Colton T: *Statistics in Medicine.* Boston, Little, Brown and Company, 1974.

17

How to Investigate a Clinical Problem

William C. Steinmann

The practicing clinican routinely investigates clinical subjects every day—the patients seen in the practice. In this chapter, I shall explain how the clinician can investigate patients in a formal way that makes the results valuable to other physicians. The clinical subjects in this case are diagnoses, therapies, and other questions of interest to the practitioner. The intent of this chapter is to provide an introduction to the rationale, background, and methodology for the investigation of clinical subjects.

We should begin by dispelling two myths and reviewing the logic for practicing clinicians taking part in clinical investigation or research. The first myth is that practitioners are too busy with clinical responsibilities to consider, much less conduct, an investigational study. A clinician in practice certainly does have heavy responsibilities related to daily patient care, but clinical investigation need not require much additional time. An example of such an investigation is the summary of a patient's adverse reaction to a new drug. The results may be important, will certainly be interesting, and will require a minimal commitment of time if a routine and effective system of data collection is built into the practice. Clinical investigation can be a major activity and can require a major commitment of time, but this factor is not an essential criterion for good research.

The second myth is that good research can be done only in "high-powered" medical centers. A good deal of expertise is available for scientific research in medical centers, and some research can realistically be conducted only in such centers. However, many original and important contributions can be made by clinicians in practice, independent of such institutions (1). Some examples include the early reports of major drug effects, such as those from thalidomide, and much of the evidence on the epidemiologic characteristics of communicable diseases.

The rationale for investigation of a subject in practice can be divided into two broad categories: the value or rewards to those who participate in clinical investigation and the value or contributions to patient care and medical knowledge in general. Investigation of a clinical subject invariably will contribute to the researcher's knowledge of the topic and complement the careful observations of daily practice. The literature review, critical observations, and data analysis involved in conducting a clinical investigation will enable the physician to learn more about the subject of the research and will stimulate the physician to think critically about other clinical issues. In addition to the rewards of better patient care and increased knowledge of diagnosis and therapy, clinical investigation can provide intellectual satisfaction and stimulation from clinical practice.

The practicing clinician is in a unique position to make useful contributions to medical knowledge. In medical and research centers, the referral patients may not be representative of the severity and distribution of disease in the general population. The clinician away from these centers often deals with a more representative cross section of the general population. Therefore, he or she can provide important data that may be unavailable to major centers and that may better reflect the characteristics of diagnosis and therapy in the general population. Furthermore, since the major medical or investigational centers often deal with unusual diseases or with patients with more serious forms of a disease, the clinical practitioner is in a better position to provide data from patients with common problems.

Another distinct contribution that can be made by the clinician in practice is the evaluation of long-term follow-up. Continuity of care is not often available in medical centers, and therefore studies requiring long-term follow-up in many cases can be better made by practitioners who follow their patients for long periods of time.

Finally, the physician in practice deals with a large and heterogeneous population with many different diagnoses and therapies. Therefore, he or she is often able to identify problems before they are recognized by major institutions. The best example is drug reactions. Practicing physicians often are the first to recognize unexpected side effects. The clinician can, and often does, first identify the problem for large-scale study by major centers.

THE ANALOGY OF CLINICAL PRACTICE AND CLINICAL INVESTIGATION

Clinical practice and clinical investigation have common components. Most of the skills required for investigation of a subject differ little from those used in the usual clinical evaluation of a patient. These skills include making observations, keeping records, asking questions, identifying problems, and choosing a plan of action. Except for choosing a plan of action, which includes knowledge of the appropriate study designs, most clinicians already possess the skills required to conduct clinical research and use these skills routinely in day-to-day practice. Indeed, the simplest clinical investigation requires no special design and is simply a description of experience, perhaps a case report of a single patient. Investigation can be more difficult, for example, reporting the experience from many patients or incorporating more complicated study designs, such as is required by controlled clinical trials. More difficult studies, which may require data-gathering techniques or experimental designs unfamiliar to most physicians, will be discussed later in this chapter. First of all, however, the components of clinical practice, which are already familiar, will be reviewed. Regardless of the type of study one may conduct, these skills are preparatory to any clinical investigation and are as important in carrying out clinical research as they are in providing good patient care.

Making observations of patients and recording them are routine and essential parts of clinical practice. Whether evaluating the causation of hypertension or following the response to a new antihypertensive drug, the physician's evaluation will depend on observing and recording the results. In investigating a clinical subject, physicians may want to review previous experience in a retrospective study to collect data. Only from recorded observations can this past experience be evaluated. If the research design is a prospective study in which patients are to be followed (e.g., the response of a group of patients to a new antihypertensive agent over time), observational and record-keeping skills will not only contribute to the patient's clinical care but will also provide the data for evaluating patients' collective experience. More complicated experimental designs require competent observational and record-keeping skills.

The ability to ask important questions is an integral part of daily clinical practice, whether interviewing patients or evaluating the appropriateness of diagnosis or treatment. Good clinical care should include questions about accepted diagnostic and therapeutic regimens. These questions will produce a critical evaluation of patient care and potential topics for evaluation. In the design of any clinical investigation, the ability to ask probing questions will be required to appraise the design and results of the investigation.

Every clinical disposition, whether diagnostic or therapeutic, requires some plan of action. Planning a clinical investigation is no different. Although investigations like case reports require little in the way of study design, most studies in clinical practice require a well-defined plan of action. Before discussing the various types of studies and the design of a research project, I shall review some necessary considerations for effectively making observations, keeping records, asking questions, and identifying problems that should be reviewed.

THE INVESTIGATION

Making Observations

Whether a study is planned before data are available or is based on patients' records, good data will be available only if the observations are reliable and valid. If the study is planned before data are collected, the necessary observations can be determined in advance. Being sure that observations are reliable and valid will allow physicians to collect useful data for future use, even when a study has not been planned at the time the observations are made.

The major criterion in generating reliable data is to make consistent and systematic observations. In clinical practice, measurements or observations may be repeated on the same patient or on different patients. Any comparison requires the observations to be made in a consistent manner. For example, suppose that a physician measures the blood pressure of a patient to monitor the effect of therapy. As happens with many patients, there may be a difference in pressure between the right and left arms. Suppose that the pressure is sometimes measured in the right arm and sometimes in the left. If the physician then decides to investigate the response of patients to a new drug therapy for hypertension, the results may be confounded by the failure to make and record uniform measurements (left versus right arm, sitting versus standing, large cuff versus regular cuff, and so forth). The major difficulty is that the physician will be unaware of the failure to perform a consistent and systematic measurement. He or she will not account for the effect and, unwittingly, will interpret the data to be reliable and a result of therapeutic intervention when they may reflect only unsystematic measurement and intraobserver bias. Inconsistent measurements by several observers will result in equally serious interobserver bias.

The major criterion in generating valid data is to make accurate observations. In practice, the accuracy of observations requires continual evaluation of all possible sources of bias and error. Observations, measurements, and clinical impressions should be made in an objective, unbiased manner as part of any daily clinical activity. The ability to suspend previous clinical beliefs usually will enhance objectivity and help ensure accurate observations.

Therefore, since physicians do not always know which data may be needed, it is important to routinely evaluate patients in a consistent, systematic, and accurate manner. So, if data are collected, they will be reliable, valid, and therefore useful. Equally critical observations will be required in the design and evaluation of the progress of any clinical investigation.

Keeping Records

Just as the medical record is essential in the continuous care of patients, the written record in clinical investigation serves as the central data base. Clinical investigation requires specific data, and it would be ideal if one could predict the topics of future investigation to ensure the needed data at the time that the investigation begins. Unfortunately, such predictions are not possible. In fact, it can be experience in clinical practice that provides the questions for investigation, often long after the records have been made. Therefore, it is necessary to keep good records that meet patient care needs but that are also useful for research purposes. Although designs will differ among various inpatient and outpatient settings, the records should meet some minimal criteria. They should include age, sex, race, diagnosis, medications, and accurate descriptions of diagnostic and therapeutic evaluations (2).

The problem oriented record popularized by Weed is a practical and effective way to meet the criteria for accurate recording of diagnostic and therapeutic evaluations (3,4). By use of the acronym SOAP, for recording Subjective information, or Symptoms, Objective information, Assessment of the results, and Plans for each problem, a systematic and consistent approach to record-keeping is provided. The system further contributes to clinical investigation by providing an easy method to find information on a specific problem in any record and by providing an excellent record for retrospective review of the chronology of a problem (5,6). The problem oriented record can also be used for discharge summaries and as a record of the history and physical examination (3).

A valuable aid for recording information over time is the flow sheet, or flow chart. In this format, history, physical examination, or laboratory results are recorded on a single page over time to provide a chronology of the results in a readily accessible and reproducible form (3).

Remember that any record must be legible. This prerequisite is particularly important if others help collect data from the records.

In addition to a well-designed and accurate record system, it is necessary to have access to records. For inpatient records, the ICDA (International Classification of Diseases, American version) provides a uniform and standardized classification for disease categories (7). The ICDA codes should be used for discharge diagnoses to enable easy recall of charts for patients with a specified disease. In addition to primary and secondary diagnoses, charts should include discharge summaries and any procedures that were performed. Discharge summaries should give a complete and accurate account of the hospitalization recorded in a consistent and systematic manner. For outpatients as well as inpatients, a diagnostic index should be maintained with patients' records filed under disease categories. Since the rubrics of the ICDA are oriented toward the types of morbidity and associated disease found in hospital settings, the ICHPPC (International Classification of Health Problems in Primary Care) has been devised to supplement the ICDA for classification of diagnoses in the ambulatory setting (8).

Fry has described a minimal system of basic information for the office-based physician that includes the diagnostic index, or registry, mentioned above, an encounter record, and an age and sex registry (2). The diagnostic index includes the patient's name and details that are entered under the disease category. Thus, access to a list of patients with a specified disease is readily available. A similar registry can be maintained for patients given a specific treatment. The encounter record or patient's chart provides an accurate account of the diagnosis and therapy. The age and sex registry contains these data under the patient's name and provides a valuable record of the patient population if calculation of prevalence or incidence rates is desired.

Computer technology has greatly simplified the record recall in inpatient settings and likely will be useful as a part of record-keeping and retrieval in outpatient settings as well (9).

Asking the Question and Identifying the Problem

A novice investigator may look at the research of colleagues and marvel at how simple their studies seem and at how obvious are the questions that they asked. Practicing clinicians are in a unique position to address these simple yet important questions. The problems are there; physicians must learn to look for them so that they can identify them.

In identifying a researchable question, the physician should choose an area in which he or she has experience. Choosing a familiar area not only enables the physician to use previous knowledge and experience in planning the study but also saves time and will minimize errors from unforeseen circumstances that may arise in the design of the study.

There are two ways to identify a subject for investigation. The first is to identify a problem in one's own practice. The second is to choose a problem already identified in the literature. They need not be mutually exclusive strategies. It helps to develop an ability to suspend previous clinical beliefs and adopt a reasonable amount of skepticism as one approaches the everyday routine of clinical practice. "Bland diets enhance the healing of duodenal ulcers." "Diabetics have an increased rate of glaucoma." Are these statements really true? A review of the literature may provide an answer, but often it will offer no more than anecdotal evidence, which can and should be tested in practice.

Defining the Problem

Once a problem or area of interest has been identified, the physician has started the investigation of a clinical subject, but more work is required before data can be collected.

The first step will be to gather the information that summarizes one's previous experience and personal knowledge in the area of interest. Past experience should be reviewed. Next, one must seek additional knowledge from other sources.

At the outset, it is often helpful to survey colleagues about their experience. This approach provides a stimulating exchange with colleagues and forces definition and redefinition of the pertinent issues. Remember, however, that their experience may be anecdotal. They may also know of local experts or resources, including published data on the subject. Although a medical library is helpful in researching literature, it is not essential.

The next step should be to look at textbooks that deal with the area of interest. Every specialty has numerous textbooks that give a description of the state of the art in the subject, but they often are quite general and surprisingly uncritical in their presentation. In addition, they vary widely in quality and may be several years out of date. Nevertheless, they will provide additional information and usually give several key references that can be reviewed. It is helpful to use 5-inch by 7-inch index cards to record notes from the references. In some cases, a monograph may be found by looking under the subject index in the library. These sources tend to be more informative and more critical and usually provide more references on the subject.

The third step is to review the journal literature for the most recent published research in the field. If the physician does not have access to a medical library, he or she can review the index of the journals that he or she receives, looking under the headings of the subject area and related areas. The pertinent articles can then be reviewed. Again, each cited reference of interest should be noted and recorded on an index card. Also, information on the article's content and methodology should be recorded.

The final step, if necessary, is to review the journal literature found in medical libraries. Here, instead of reviewing specific journals, one should review *Index Medicus*, which cites references from many journals under specific headings. *Index Medicus* lists references from many journals under both subject heading and author name and includes books as well as journals. One can identify headings in the subject area of interest and then look up these headings. Each volume contains the literature listings for a single year. During each year, an index is published each month, and all references are compiled at the end of the year into one annual reference. It is useful to begin by reviewing the first volume of each year, for it lists all the subjects and their associated headings for that year (listed as "medical subject headings"). This practice ensures that the headings being reviewed are included in that year. By reviewing the subject heading and then associated headings first, the physician may find other pertinent headings that may be more appropriate or that have not been considered.

One can then begin with the most recent volume and work back chronologically, but it is often helpful to review only the two or three most recent years' volumes and then skip back to volumes five and 10 years earlier since there may be little current work but a great deal of earlier work on the topic. This practice will also enable the researcher to note if any dramatic changes have occurred in the approach taken by previous authors.

It is a good idea to scan the headings and the available references in the volumes before selecting titles for review. In this way, the physician can estimate how many articles deal with the subject and select the best titles for review.

The Medical Literature Analysis and Retrieval System (MEDLARS) of the United States National Library of Medicine is a computer-based system for identifying references. Although it sounds attractive, the system has limited use. It is most helpful for researching a limited topic on which little is known. Without a well-defined, limited topic and the assistance of a librarian, MEDLARS may generate hundreds of titles, many of them useless. There is usually a fee for this service. All the titles should be reviewed before the original journals are sought. MEDLARS should not be considered a routine source of information, but it may be of value when the circumstances warrant its use. For medical literature since 1975, MEDLARS can also provide abstracts for some of the titles. However, abstracts are not available for all titles from 1975 since restrictions of some journals prohibit them.

The *Science Citation Index* may also be used if the name of a specific author who has written on the subject is sought. The listing for a particular paper, as well as a listing of all works that have cited it as a reference, will be found under the author's name. These titles can be used to see what others have said or done about the subject since the paper's publication. Additional bibliographies according to subject and author are available. The medical librarian can provide a list of them and their subject matter.

After review of four or five volumes of *Index Medicus* has been made, the investigator can collect the appropriate titles. The physician should make records of the article that seem appropriate. When a reference is found, a record of it may be made on an index card; the record should include the authors' names, title, journal volume, page numbers, and year. Fewer than 40 references should be collected for the first review. When they have been collected, the first articles can be reviewed.

Searching in the library for articles to review should be conducted in a systematic manner. First of all, it is helpful to put index cards in alphabetic order according to journal title since the journals are arranged this way in the library. One will not then have to double back to pull references. Five to 10 journals should be collected at a time and reviewed in groups. When a reference is reviewed, a record of it is made on the index card. A quick confirmation of accuracy ensures that the investigator can easily return to the reference or cite it correctly by using the reference card. In reviewing each article, it is best first to scan the article, including the abstract, methods, results, and conclusion. If the precursory review indicates that the article deserves further attention, the entire article or valuable segments can be read carefully. This method of review saves much time.

As these papers are reviewed, they should be critically evaluated (see Chap. 16). If they are good, they may give valuable leads to further work, and if they are not, their deficiencies may suggest new approaches.

A short summary of the article, which includes methods, results, conclusions, and other appropriate information, should be recorded for each article on the index card. If the paper is irrelevant, the physician should still record a brief summary, noting why the paper is not appropriate. Later on, the note may prevent needless repetition of effort. Also, the summary will be helpful if one decides to change or modify the topic.

Some time may be saved by looking up references in abstracting journals, such as *Excerpta Medica*. This resource gives a brief summary of the articles listed. However, these volumes are limited to certain subject areas and do not include all papers published in the area. One may therefore spend a great deal of time looking for an abstract summarizing an article only to find that it has not been included in the volume.

After the first review, a more complete review of titles may be necessary and can be performed by returning to *Index Medicus* to review other years or headings. In addition, major articles or review articles usually include bibliographies of pertinent references. These bibliographies may be consulted since they provide a useful resource to locate old articles. However, such bibliographies are usually not complete and should not be relied on as a complete review of the literature.

Specifying the Problem or Hypothesis

At this point, the researcher will know what previous work has been done in the area of interest, what additional work is needed, and the problems or questions that require investigation. Now the researcher is ready to state precisely the problem or hypothesis and plan the study design. However, one must be sure that the problem or hypothesis can realistically be investigated. It is not sufficient simply to restate the original problem. One must modify it so that it is feasible to investigate. These considerations are interdependent—the final statement of the hypothesis or problem depends on the type of study that can be done, and the type of study will depend on the hypothesis or problem.

Some practical matters must be considered to select the appropriate type of study and finalize the specifics of the study design, including the patients, the methods or resources, and time. These factors will now be reviewed. Further description of study design is available (10).

Considerations in Study Design

Patients

The availability of patients is obviously crucial. What kinds of patients and how many will the study need? These considerations involve not only practical decisions (e.g., the patients whom the physician actually sees in practice) but also technical decisions (e.g., how many patients are needed to attain statistical significance).

Methods and Resources

Second, one must consider the available data base and the materials and re-sources that the study may require. Any investigation will be limited by these considerations. We have already discussed one aspect of the data base, the patients. If a complete and accurate record is available, the data from patients should be retrievable. If not, access to reliable data may be a problem. Other methodologic or resource considerations include considerations of personnel, facilities, finances, ethics, and statistics.

Regarding personnel, the simplest study may require only the active partici-pation of the investigator. However, many clinical investigations require the help and services of additional personnel. Regardless of the number of participants, several issues must be considered: the kind of additional personnel and services required; an estimate of the anticipated time requirements for each worker during the entire investigation; the number of additional personnel that are required; evaluation of the availability of the personnel and assessment of their willingness to participate for the duration of the investigation; the anticipated cost of the personnel.

The same issues should be considered regarding facilities needed for the investigation.

Financial issues consist of two major considerations: the anticipated cost of the investigation and who will pay for it. The physician must consider the costs of personal time, personnel, and data generation, collection, and analysis. Many investigations will cost no money. However, all possible costs should be con-sidered and means arranged for funding before initiation of the investigation. If additional procedures are planned for patients, the payment for these costs must be considered.

Issues regarding the use or need for statistics in the study must be part of the consideration of methods and resources. If the design calls for the use of statistics, the investigator must consider the most appropriate statistical methods to meet the objectives of the study as well as to incorporate into the study design any requirements dictated by the statistical methodology.

There are two types of statistics: descriptive and inferential (see Chap. 16). Descriptive statistics usually require no additional skills beyond those that the investigator already possesses. Descriptive statistics require no manipulation of data other than total counts, such as the number of patients seen with a particu-lar diagnosis. Inferential statistics require manipulations and, except for the most simple tests, require either some experience or knowledge of statistics or expert consultation.

Studies that call for the use of inferential statistics include those comparing two groups, such as patients given different therapies. Differences between the two groups can be meaningful and significant, or they can be explained by chance. Inferential statistics are needed to determine the numbers required to provide convincing evidence of differences between the two groups and to define what is normal or expected in an observation or experiment.

If statistics are required in an investigation, several considerations are important: 1) Will the numbers be adequate, so that the planned statistical analyses can be performed? 2) Is the sample population representative, so that statistical analysis can be generalized to other populations? 3) Are the subjects to be compared actually comparable? 4) Has bias in the data collection been avoided? 5) Has the proper statistical unit been chosen? 6) Are the means available to analyze the data as the statistical method dictates (e.g., coding ability or computer capability)?

In general, if statistical analysis is planned or being considered, consultation with an expert should be obtained early so that appropriate considerations can be made in the design of the investigation. It is also helpful to imagine the results to be obtained from the study before the study is begun. If uncertainty exists regarding the need for statistical analysis, consultation should be obtained.

Statistical consultants can perhaps best be identified by colleagues who have performed research requiring statistical analysis. If this opportunity is not available, local universities can usually provide statistical support. If access is available to statistical support from a medical school, this resource is quite valuable since statisticians from these centers may have broad experience in clinical investigation. Several excellent reference texts are available and can provide a good understanding of the statistical skills most commonly used in the analysis of data from clinical subjects (11–13).

Although most studies do not require informed consent, ethical questions must always be considered in the conduct and design of an investigation (14). If the local hospital, medical school, or other institution has a committee on human experimentation, it should be consulted concerning the research plans, and its approval should be obtained. Some outside funding resources, such as the federal government, require approval by such a committee before funding can be granted.

Since there are no governing bodies that have jurisdiction over clinical studies unless outside funds are used, the investigator has the responsibility to protect the interests of the patients. There are several considerations that are helpful in ensuring an ethically sound clinical investigation.

1. What are the costs, effects, risks, or harms of the research to the patient or patient's family, as far as can be known?

2. In whose interest is the research? If not directly in the patient's interest, how can the patient's participation be justified?

3. Is the research project rational, logical, and of good design? Can participation be justified such that under similar circumstances, another patient might readily be expected to participate?

4. Can the patient or the patient's representative make a reasonably informed decision to participate?

5. Before a patient participates, do all parties have the facts straight?

The federal government has published a listing of registries that have guidelines for human research (15).

Time Requirements

The third consideration in the study design is the availability of time. When first beginning studies, one can easily underestimate the time required to perform a clinical investigation. Therefore, the physician will need to schedule time carefully and allow for time away from clinical practice. Time is also an important consideration in the study design. Some studies can be completed in a short time. Others will require a much longer time and more active involvement during the study. One should be sure when choosing a study that adequate time will be available to complete it.

Types of Studies

If the physician has never conducted research before, it would be easiest to start off with a simple study design. As skills develop, one may want to use more complicated investigative techniques that may require more complicated study designs.

The different types of studies used in clinical investigation can be divided into two groups, experimental and observational. Both are useful, and both have their limitations. Both can be used to evaluate diagnostic and therapeutic methods and other aspects of clinical practice.

The experimental approach is probably most familiar, since it provides the basic model for investigation in science. In an experiment, the investigator studies the effect of some factor that is under control. Control of some factor requires a carefully planned intervention, usually introduced by the investigator.

In the more usual approach, the investigator can only observe the occurrence of a variable in patients who are already segregated into groups on the basis of some experience or exposure. In this kind of study, allocation into groups is not under the control of the investigator. The study is observational since contrasts in outcome between study groups are observed, not created experimentally. The investigator takes a passive role, carefully observing according to a structured plan.

Although experimentation can establish the causal association of a factor with a disease more conclusively than observation can, observational studies have provided and continue to provide a major contribution to the understanding of many clinical problems. Observational studies are usually easier to carry out than are experimental studies, but they are still no less important. They are also usually less expensive and time-consuming than are experiments, but not always. Their major limitation is that some of the more rigorous analytic statistical tests cannot be applied to data obtained in this manner.

Experimental designs include the statement of hypothesis, identification of subjects, a planned and calculated intervention, and then follow-up evaluation of the effect of the intervention. An experiment may compare the relative effectiveness of two different therapies or the effectiveness of one therapy as compared with no therapy (control group). This design is usually more complicated and difficult to perform. It also may be more time-consuming and more expensive than an observational study. However, experimental design lends itself readily to statistical testing.

Investigations are sometimes classified as descriptive or analytic studies. These terms usually refer to the manner in which the results are stated and evaluated. If the effect of aspirin on 20 patients with arthritis is reported, the study is called a descriptive study. If the same effect is compared with the effect of no aspirin in 20 control patients and the results are tested for statistical significance, the study is called an analytic study.

STUDY DESIGN

Once the original problem has been defined, the practical considerations reviewed, the type of study chosen, and the hypothesis or problem statement delineated, one is ready to state the plan for study and specify the elements that are included. The plan for the entire study is called the study design, and a description of the design is called a protocol.

A protocol is absolutely necessary for every study regardless of how simple it might be. Protocols vary in organizational features, but basically they identify all parts of the study in a systematic manner. A protocol provides a check list to ensure that the investigator has considered the major aspects of study design. It also provides a ready means to describe the study to others. Sample tables and graphs can be used in the protocol to help illustrate the kind of data to be collected. Any request for funding should include a protocol. A review of the protocol will provide a review of the elements of a study design, as the following questions illustrate (16):

1. *What is the problem or hypothesis?* The answer to this question is a statement of the specific problem or hypothesis to be investigated. For example, the question: "What are the effects of the new antihypertensive drug?" may become: "What are the changes in diastolic blood pressure after three months of therapy with Drug X in patients who were uncontrolled on conventional antihypertensive drugs?"

2. *What is already known about the problem?* Here previous experience, personal discussion, and literature review provide the background and rationale for the investigation.

3. *What type of study will be used in the investigation?* The answer to this question is a statement of the specific type of study that will be used. One should demonstrate that the chosen investigation can meet the objectives of the project and how.

4. *Who are the subjects?* A study population should be identified. Include the manner in which the subjects will be chosen and the number to be studied. The physician must be sure that there are enough subjects to answer the question convincingly.

5. *What data are to be collected?* The answer to this question is a description of the data that are to be collected and the methods to be used to collect them.

6. *What intervention is planned, if any, and how are the variables to be defined and measured?* This description applies to an experimental design, such as the controlled clinical trial. If one plans an experimental design, the planned intervention is defined and stated carefully.

7. *How will the data be processed and analyzed?* The statistical methods that will be used to analyze the data are described. In addition, if the data are to be processed by use of a computer, describe plans for how the data will be coded and who will code them.

8. *What problems of ethics does this project raise?* This section includes a description of ethical considerations required for the investigation. Is permission needed from subjects, hospitals, or committees on experimentation?

9. *What is the expected timetable?* The answer to this question is a description of the time schedule for the completion of the investigation. This schedule provides guidelines for expected progress of the study. Also, it helps to ensure that adequate time has been allowed to complete all aspects included in the study design. Moreover, the time table provides a schedule that allows other participants involved to plan their time commitment for logistical and budgetary reasons.

10. *What is the cost of the investigation?* This section lists all the anticipated costs of the investigation. The physician should consider such costs as his or her own time, salaries for a research assistant, statistician, and other consultant, computer time and key-punching expenses, supplies, telephones, photocopying, equipment (e.g., calculators, typewriters, and new clinical equipment), space, administrative expenses, reprint reproduction or articles emanating from the study, and postage.

SUMMARY

The investigation of a clinical subject is part of any clinical practice. Investigation enhances patient care and is an important segment of medical knowledge and research.

Most of the skills required to study a clinical subject are routinely used by those in clinical practice to evaluate their patients. Critical use of these skills not only provides good patient care but is preparatory and part of any clinical investigation.

There are various types of studies that can be used for investigation of a clinical subject. The choice of study type depends not only on the definition of the problem but also on the practical considerations of patients, methods, resources, and time.

In any investigation, the study design incorporates all proposed or expected aspects of a study. The elements of the study design are well defined and clearly stated in the protocol.

REFERENCES

1. Pickles WN: *Epidemiology in County Practice.* London, Bristol, John Wright and Sons, 1939.
2. Fry J: Information for patient care in office-based practice. *Med Care* 9(Suppl): March-April 1973, pp. 35–40.
3. Weed LL: *Medical Records, Medical Education, and Patient Care.* Cleveland, The Press of Case Western Reserve, 1971.

4. Hurst JW, Walker HK: *The Problem Oriented System.* New York, Medcom Press, 1972.

5. Hurst JW: How to implement the Weed system (in order to improve patient care, education and research by improving medical records). *Arch Intern Med* 128:456, 1971.

6. Hurst JW: The art and science of presenting a patient's problems (as an extension of the Weed system). *Arch Intern Med* 128:463, 1971.

7. American Hospital Association: *International Classification of Diseases, 8.* American version. New York, 1975.

8. American Hospital Association: *International Classification of Health Problems in Primary Care.* Chicago, 1975.

9. National Center for Health Services Research: Automation of the Problem Oriented Medical Record. Rockville, Maryland, DHEW Publ. No. (HRA) 77-3177, 1977.

10. Hamilton M: *Lectures on the Methodology of Clinical Research.* London, Churchill Livingstone, 1976.

11. Swinscow TDV: *Statistics at Square One.* London, British Medical Association, 1976.

12. Hill B: *Principles of Medical Statistics.* New York, Oxford University Press, 1971.

13. Colton T: *Statistics in Medicine.* Boston, Little, Brown and Company, 1974.

14. Ramsey P: *The Patient as Person.* New Haven, Connecticut, Yale University Press, 1977.

15. National Institutes of Health: *New Regulations for the Protection of Human Subjects.* Booklet 45CFR. Bethesda, Maryland, 1978.

16. Warren MD: Aide-memoire for preparing a protocol. *Br Med J* 1:1195, 1978.

Index